Praise for Previous Editions

"Here's inspiration to turn off the television and head for the hills."
—*Napa Valley Register*

"If you like to hike, make the most of your outdoor adventures by toting this handy reference guide in your backpack. With author Matt Heid's insights, you're sure to wander through some of this scenic region's most stunning backcountry."
—*Spirit* magazine, Southwest Airlines

"A wonderful selection of trails, good writing, and helpful graphics makes this a choice guidebook for ambles in the special places of Northern California."
—Honorable Mention, 2001 National Outdoor Book Awards

"Before heading into the backcountry, a generation or two of hikers have packed an essential piece of equipment: a trusty Wilderness Press hiking guide."
—*Sacramento Bee*

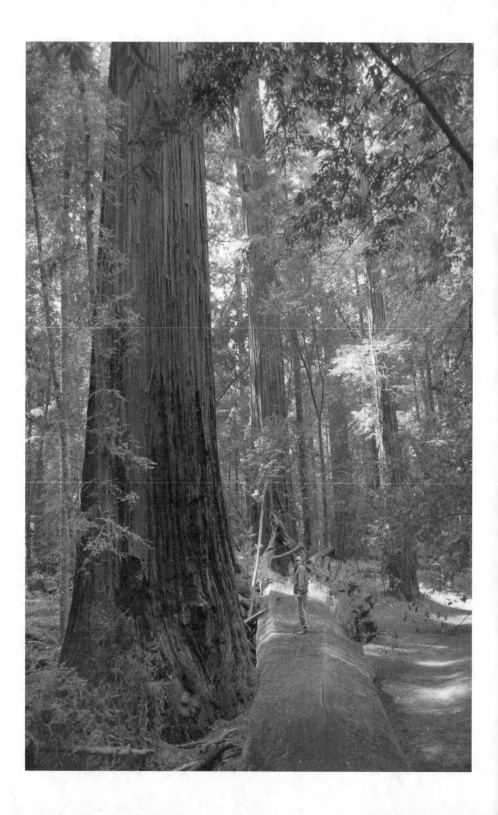

101 HIKES in Northern California

Exploring Mountains, Valleys, and Seashore

Matt Heid
Third Edition

WILDERNESS PRESS . . . *on the trail since 1967*

Dedicated to my mom and dad, for everything

101 Hikes in Northern California

Third edition, first printing

Copyright © 2000, 2008, and 2015 by Matt Heid

Editor: Kerry Smith
Project editor: Ritchey Halphen
Cover and interior photos: copyright © 2015 Matt Heid, except where noted
Topographic maps: © 2015 National Geographic Maps, with trails added by the author
Overview map and cover design: Scott McGrew
Text design: Larry P. Van Dyke
Proofreaders: Rebecca Henderson, Kate Johnson
Indexer: Ann Cassar / Cassar Technical Services

Library of Congress Cataloging-in-Publication Data

Heid, Matt, 1975–
  101 hikes in Northern California : exploring mountains, valleys, and seashore / Matt Heid.
  pages cm.

  Summary: "*101 Hikes in Northern California* by Matt Heid benefits readers by narrowing down the multitude of options for hiking in Northern California to the very best of the best adventures. It is distinct from other similar guidebooks in that it covers the northern two-thirds of the state, including nearly the entirety of the Sierra Nevadas south to Kings Canyon National Park and the entire Big Sur region along the coast south to Silver Peak Wilderness. It also provides significant geographic diversity: Hikes are spread out across the entire region. No matter where you are in northern California, you can find a hike in the book within a short drive. The guide is unique in the amount of natural history information it provides, especially the geologic stories of the featured destinations. It provides not just the essential directions for completing a hike, it enhances the experience by telling the story of how the landscape came to be the way it is." — Provided by publisher.

  ISBN 978-0-89997-781-2 (paperback) — ISBN 0-89997-781-2 — eISBN 978-0-89997-782-9

  1. Hiking—California—Guidebooks. 2. Trails—California—Guidebooks. 3. California—Guidebooks. I. Title. II. Title: One hundred one hikes in Northern California. III. Title: One hundred and one hikes in Northern California.
  GV199.42.C2H45 2015
  796.5109794—dc23
                                        2015008843

Manufactured in the United States of America

Distributed by Publishers Group West

Published by: 🝋 **WILDERNESS PRESS**
          An imprint of Keen Communications, LLC
          2204 First Ave. S., Suite 102
          Birmingham, AL 35233
          800-443-7227, fax 205-326-1012

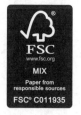 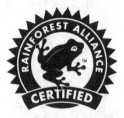

Visit **wildernesspress.com** for a complete listing of our books and for ordering information. Contact us at **info@wilderness press.com**, **facebook.com/wildernesspress1967**, or **twitter.com/wilderness1967** with questions or comments.

Cover photos: Front: Mounts Ritter and Banner rise above Ediza Lake in Ansel Adams Wilderness (see Hike 91). *Back:* (top) the rugged coastline south of Sonoma's Lost Coast (see Hike 40), (inset) old-growth redwood forest (see Hike 49).

Frontispiece: A hiker marvels at old-growth redwood forest along California's northern coast.

SAFETY NOTICE Although Wilderness Press and the author have made every attempt to ensure that the information in this book is accurate at press time, they are not responsible for any loss, damage, injury, or inconvenience that may occur to anyone while using this book. You are responsible for your own safety and health while in the wilderness. The fact that a trail is described in this book does not mean that it will be safe for you. Be aware that trail conditions can change from day to day. Always check local conditions, and know your own limitations.

Acknowledgments

Thanks go first to the countless rangers, public-land managers, and stewards of Northern California's natural treasures. They patiently answered my long lists of questions and were an invaluable resource in ensuring the accuracy of this updated guide.

Many wonderful people joined and supported me on this latest book-updating adventure, including my brother, John, and his family, Analise, Ansel, and Siena; my mom and dad; Joann Volinski; Chuck and Benjamin Kapelke; Tom Hruschka; Grant and Becky Wayman; and Bob and Marsha Lewis.

Thank you to Molly Merkle and Ritchey Halphen for your remarkable patience and exceptional work in bringing this latest edition to completion. And thank you to Colleen MacDonald, Suzanne Shaw, and everybody at UCS for providing me with the time and support needed for this update.

Lastly, I want to especially thank my beloved wife, Gretchen, for supporting my lifelong passion for the Northern California wilderness and perpetual dedication to this book. Thank you, Gretchen—I love you. And to my two young boys, Kieran and Rohan—someday soon we'll all hike the trails of Northern California together!

Hike on.

—*Matt Heid*
Bedford, Massachusetts
March 2015

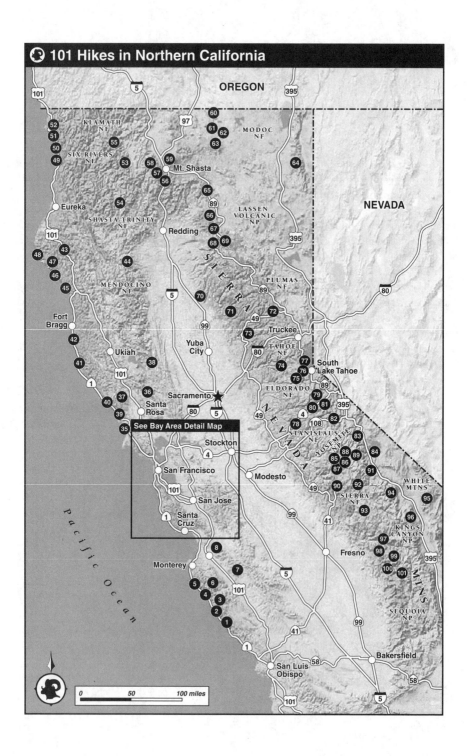

101 Hikes in Northern California

OREGON

NEVADA

Pacific Ocean

KLAMATH NF

SIX RIVERS NF

SHASTA-TRINITY NF

MENDOCINO NF

Eureka

Fort Bragg

Ukiah

Santa Rosa

Sacramento

Stockton

San Francisco

San Jose

Santa Cruz

Monterey

Mt. Shasta

Redding

Yuba City

Truckee

South Lake Tahoe

Modesto

Fresno

San Luis Obispo

Bakersfield

MODOC NF

LASSEN VOLCANIC NP

PLUMAS NF

TAHOE NF

ELDORADO NF

STANISLAUS NF

YOSEMITE

SIERRA NF

KINGS CANYON NP

SEQUOIA NP

WHITE MTNS

See Bay Area Detail Map

0   50   100 miles

Contents

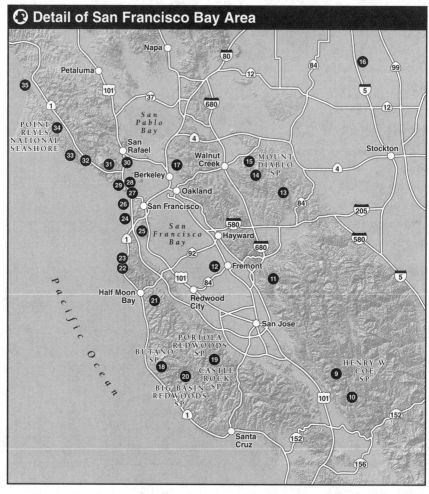

Preface

WELCOME TO THE total Northern California outdoor experience. Every aspect of the region's incredible natural diversity is found within these 101 hikes—the jagged granite of the High Sierra, the crashing surf of the Pacific Coast, the volcanic landscape of the Modoc Plateau, the rich diversity of the Klamath Mountains, the magnificent redwoods of the North Coast, the spectacular views of the Bay Area. Lakes, peaks, rivers, creeks, volcanoes, waterfalls, valleys, beaches, forests, meadows, wildlife, wildflowers, lighthouses . . . all can be found within these pages.

This book describes a greater area than most Northern California guidebooks. Stretching north from Sequoia National Park through the Modoc Plateau of northeast California, it includes virtually all of the Sierra Nevada. Sweeping north along the coast, from Big Sur to the Oregon border, it contains the Coast Ranges, the San Francisco Bay Area, and the Klamath Mountains. In total, this book covers the entire northern two-thirds of the state. And now this third edition opens up several new realms, with 18 entirely new trips and expanded coverage of the Sierra Nevada and North Coast regions.

The hikes were selected using three basic criteria, with each adventure including some combination of the following:

- **Isolation:** Wilderness is freedom, an escape from the trappings of society. The fewer people you encounter, the deeper your experience.

- **Scenic beauty:** Sweeping 360-degree vistas, exquisite works of nature, and the splendor of Northern California.

- **Unique destinations:** Redwood forests, giant sequoias, granite domes, marble mountains, thundering waterfalls—places unlike anywhere else on Earth.

While all of these hikes can be completed in a single day, more than half can also be done as overnight backpacking trips. Each hike includes summary information outlining the basics of the trip, detailed driving directions, an in-depth trail description, and the location of the nearest visitor center and campground. Backpacking information is provided for appropriate hikes. The hikes are broadly distributed across Northern California—no matter where you are, an adventure awaits nearby. Enjoy!

OVERVIEW OF HIKES

NO.	HIKE	DISTANCE (in miles)	ELEVATION GAIN (in feet)	TRAIL TYPE	DOGS ALLOWED	GOOD FOR KIDS	DIFFICULTY	BACKPACKING
1	Upper Salmon Creek Falls	5.2	1,000	↗	🐕		★★★	🥾
2	Vicente Flat	10.4	2,000	↗	🐕		★★★	🥾
3	Cone Peak	4	1,400	↗	🐕		★★★	
4	Ewoldsen Trail	4.5	1,500	↻			★★★	
5	Molera Beach	5	200	↻		👫	★	
6	Pine Valley	12	3,500	↗	🐕		★★★★	🥾
7	High Peaks Trail	5.3	1,650	↻			★★★	
8	Fremont Peak	1	350	↗		👫	★	
9	Coit Lake	12.4	3,800	↻			★★★★	🥾
10	Coyote Creek	12.1	2,500	↻			★★★	🥾
11	Sunol Backpack Area	5.9	1,100	↻	🐕		★★	🥾
12	Coyote Hills	2.5	400	↻	🐕	👫	★	
13	Bob Walker Ridge	5.8	850	↻	🐕		★★	
14	Mount Diablo	0.7	100	↻		👫	★	
15	Eagle Peak	4	1,800	↻			★★★	
16	Cosumnes River Preserve	3	10	↻		👫	★	
17	Wildcat Peak	7	1,000	↻	🐕		★★	
18	Little Butano Creek Canyon	8.8	2,100	↻			★★★	🥾
19	Castle Rock	5.2	1,200	↻			★★	🥾
20	Berry Creek Falls	9	3,200	↻			★★★★	🥾
21	Purisima Creek	7	1,200	↻			★★★	
22	Devil's Slide	2.6	3,70	↗		👫	★	
23	Montara Mountain	5.4	1,650	↗			★★★	
24	San Andreas Fault	3.5	50	↗		👫	★	
25	San Bruno Mountain	4.9	700	↗			★★	
26	San Francisco's Pacific Shore	5.5	500	↗		👫	★★	

OVERVIEW OF HIKES

NO.	HIKE	DISTANCE (in miles)	ELEVATION GAIN (in feet)	TRAIL TYPE	DOGS ALLOWED	GOOD FOR KIDS	DIFFICULTY	BACKPACKING
27	Golden Gate Bridge	2.4	60	↗		🧍	★	
28	Point Bonita	1	50	↗		🧍	★	
29	Gerbode Valley	6.1	1,500	⟳			★★	
30	Ring Mountain	3.2	600	⟳		🧍	★★	
31	Mount Tamalpais	6.8	1,900	⟳			★★★	
32	Martin Griffin Preserve	2.3	700	⟳		🧍	★★	
33	Alamere Falls	8.5	900	↗			★★	🎒
34	Sky and Coast Trails	10.8	1,800	⟳			★★★	🎒
35	Tomales Point	9	1,300	↗			★★★	
36	Table Rock	4.4	1,400	↗			★★★	
37	East Austin Creek	9.1	1,150	⟳			★★★	🎒
38	Cache Creek	10	1,100	↗	🐕		★★	🎒
39	Bodega Dunes	2.2	50	⟳		🧍	★	
40	Fort Ross	2.2	150	↗		🧍	★	
41	Manchester Beach	4	Negligible	⟳		🧍	★★	🎒
42	Fern Canyon	5	200	↗		🧍	★	🎒
43	Humboldt Redwoods	7	500	⟳			★★★	
44	Yolla Bolly Mountain	11.2	3,100	⟳	🐕		★★★★★	🎒
45	Lost Coast Trail	16.7	3,800	↗			★★★★★	🎒
46	Big Flat	17	50	↗	🐕		★★★	🎒
47	King Peak	5.1	1,950	⟳	🐕		★★★	🎒
48	Punta Gorda Lighthouse	6.4	100	↗	🐕		★★	🎒
49	Prairie Creek Redwoods	6.2	800	⟳			★★★	
50	Klamath River Mouth	1	Negligible	↗		🧍	★	
51	Damnation Creek	4.2	1,200	↗			★★	
52	Boy Scout Trail	5.6	750	↗			★★	

OVERVIEW OF HIKES

NO.	HIKE	DISTANCE (in miles)	ELEVATION GAIN (in feet)	TRAIL TYPE	DOGS ALLOWED	GOOD FOR KIDS	DIFFICULTY	BACKPACKING
53	Hogan Lake	7.6	2,700	↗	🐕		★★★	🚶
54	Canyon Creek Lakes	15	3,000	↗	🐕		★★★★	🚶
55	Marble Rim	17.4	2,800	↗	🐕		★★★★	🚶
56	Castle Dome	5.4	2,300	↗			★★★★	
57	Heart Lake	1.8	700	↗	🐕		★★	
58	Mount Eddy	10	2,100	↗	🐕		★★★★	🚶
59	Hidden Valley	6	2,300	↗			★★★★	🚶
60	Sheepy Ridge	0.6	180	↗	🐕	🧑	★	
61	Schonchin Butte	1.4	500	↗			★	
62	Valentine Cave	0.5	Negligible	↗		🧑	★	
63	Glass Mountain	1	50	↗			★	
64	Patterson Lake	10.2	2,900	↗	🐕		★★★★	🚶
65	Burney Falls	1.2	200	↻			★	
66	Magee Peak	12	3,200	↗	🐕		★★★★	🚶
67	Chaos Crags	4	1,050	↗			★★	
68	Brokeoff Mountain	7.4	2,600	↗			★★★★	
69	Devils Kitchen	5	700	↗			★★	
70	Big Chico Creek	3.5	600	↗	🐕		★★	
71	Feather Falls	7.4	1,650	↻			★★★	
72	Sierra Buttes	4.6–11	1,600–2,000	↗	🐕		★★★★	🚶
73	South Yuba River	8.8	1,800	↗	🐕		★★★	🚶
74	Rubicon River	6	500	↗	🐕		★★	
75	Island Lake	6.2	1,250	↗	🐕		★★★	🚶
76	Mount Tallac	9.2	3,400	↗	🐕		★★★★	🚶
77	Lake Tahoe	6.6	1,150	↗			★★	
78	Calaveras Big Trees	5.3	600	↻		🧑	★★	

OVERVIEW OF HIKES

NO.	HIKE	DISTANCE (in miles)	ELEVATION GAIN (in feet)	TRAIL TYPE	DOGS ALLOWED	GOOD FOR KIDS	DIFFICULTY	BACKPACKING
79	Grouse Lake	11	2,500	↗	🐕		★★★★	🥾
80	Mokelumne River	15.6	5,100	↗	🐕		★★★★★	🥾
81	Hiram Peak	2.4	1,250	↗	🐕		★★★	
82	Deadman Lake	4.5	1,700	↗	🐕		★★★	🥾
83	Green Creek	9	1,700	↗	🐕		★★★	🥾
84	Mono Lake	1.5	Negligible	↺		👫	★	
85	Nevada and Vernal Falls	5.9	1,900	↗			★★★	
86	Half Dome	16.4	4,800	↗			★★★★★	🥾
87	Sentinel Dome and Taft Point	5.2	1,150	↺			★★	
88	Clouds Rest	14	2,500	↗			★★★★	🥾
89	Ireland Lake	22.4	3,300	↺			★★★★	🥾
90	Mariposa Grove	5.8	1,100	↺			★★	
91	Ediza Lake	15	2,100	↗	🐕		★★★	🥾
92	Balloon Dome	9.9	2,300	↗	🐕		★★★★	🥾
93	Kaiser Peak	10	3,200	↗	🐕		★★★★	🥾
94	Little Lakes Valley	7	1,150	↗	🐕	👫	★★	🥾
95	Methuselah Grove	4.2	1,000	↺			★★★	
96	Palisade Glacier	17	5,200	↗	🐕		★★★★★	🥾
97	Yucca Point	3.4	1,150	↗			★★★	🥾
98	Redwood Canyon	10	1,900	↺			★★★	🥾
99	Pear Lake	12.4	2,750	↗			★★★★	🥾
100	Moro Rock	0.6	250	↗			★★	
101	Sawtooth Peak	13	4,500	↗			★★★★★	🥾

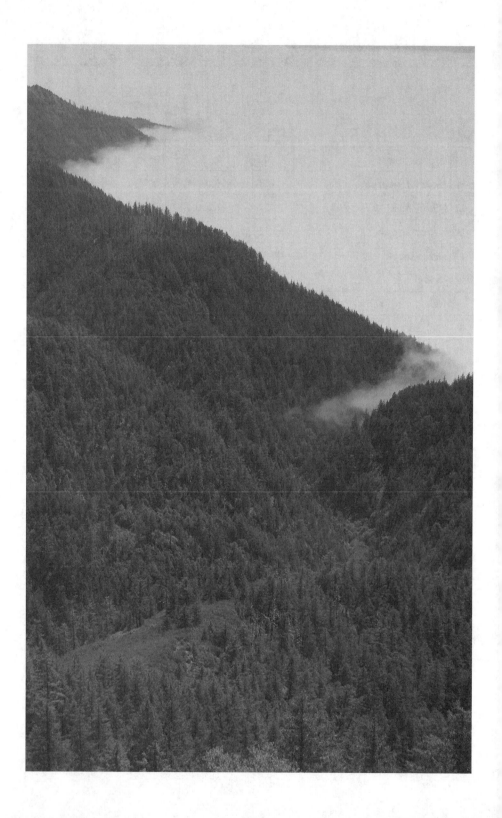

Using This Book

TO PREPARE FOR the total Northern California outdoors experience, first carefully read "Safety, Gear, and the Wilderness Ethic" (starting on page 5). Because selecting a hike can be an absorbing process, those unfamiliar with the state or unsure about where to visit should consult "Where Should I Go Hiking?" (starting on page 13). Those looking for a specific feature should consult the chart on page xii or "Hikes by Theme" on page 344. Otherwise, just flip through the pages to your desired area and evaluate each hike based on the information provided.

Beginning along the Pacific shore with the Big Sur region, the hikes are organized clockwise around the state: north through the Bay Area, Coast Ranges, and Pacific Coast to the Klamath Mountains; then inland east across the Modoc Plateau; and finally south through the Sierra Nevada to end in southern Sequoia National Park.

Each hike is organized into a standard, easily understood template and includes at-a-glance summary information, detailed driving directions, a detailed hike description, and some additional information about nearby facilities:

Summary Information

Title The specific destination or location visited by the hike.

Highlights The most exciting features of a particular hike.

Distance The total mileage of the hike as described. For point-to-point hikes, the one-way distance is listed.

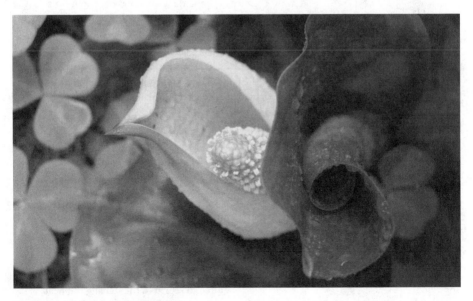

The distinctive flower of skunk cabbage

Total Elevation Gain/Loss The total amount of climbing and descending on the hike. This can be significantly greater than the difference between the hike's lowest and highest points.

Hiking Time The total amount of time required for the hike, including time for brief rest stops and a meal break on longer trips. Because this varies markedly depending on your physical fitness and pace, a range of times is usually given. The lower number indicates the amount of time in which a fit hiker can complete the hike, pausing only briefly for short breaks. The higher number is for hikers moving at a more leisurely pace and for anybody who likes to take extended breaks over the course of a journey. Remember that these times are only rough estimates and that hikes can potentially take longer for slower hikers and those with heavy backpacks.

It's important to be aware of your physical capabilities and limitations when selecting a hike. As a general rule of thumb, a reasonably fit hiker can expect to cover 2–3 miles per hour over level ground and on gradual descents, 1–2 miles per hour on gradual climbs, and only about 1 mile per hour—or 750–1,000 feet of elevation—on the steepest ascents.

Recommended Map(s) The best, most useful trail map for the destination, as well as the appropriate US Geological Survey (USGS) 7.5-minute topographic map. Many of the hikes can be completed using only the maps in the book or those available near the trailhead, but maps that are more detailed and comprehensive generally provide an extra measure of safety and comfort, especially on the more difficult and remote hikes. Most US Forest Service maps are available for purchase online at **nationalforest mapstore.com**. All USGS maps can be ordered online at **store.usgs.gov**.

Best Times The best times of year to do the hike. Note that many of the hikes can be done outside of the times listed, but weather or crowds will probably make them much less appealing.

Agency This line identifies the governing agency. Contact information is listed in "Nearest Visitor Center" at the end of each description. If the hike visits a designated wilderness area, it is listed here, followed by the governing agency for the location.

Difficulty This book uses a difficulty rating system of one to five stars. While all factors contributing to the overall challenge of the hike are taken into account, some general criteria for each level are as follows:

★ **EASY:** Typically short and level, these hikes can be done by anybody and have less than 500 feet of total elevation gain.

★★ **MODERATE:** Hikes on good trails with roughly 500–1,000 feet of total elevation gain. Suitable for any reasonably fit hiker.

★★★ **STRENUOUS:** Longer hikes with approximately 1,000–2,000 feet of elevation gain on trails that are often rocky and steep. Good fitness required.

★★★★ **CHALLENGING:** A very strenuous hike with roughly 2,000–3,000 feet of elevation gain in often remote regions on challenging trails. Experienced wilderness users only. Many are good overnight trips.

★★★★★ **EPIC:** An adventure with an elevation gain in excess of 3,000 feet on rough and difficult trails. Cross-country navigation skills are often required. Only the fittest individuals can complete these hikes in a single day. Excellent for overnight trips.

Trip Type Symbols

Out-and-back A hike that returns to the starting trailhead by retracing its route.

Loop or semiloop A hike that retraces little or none of its route to return to the starting trailhead.

Point-to-point A hike that ends at a different trailhead. A second car or a shuttle is required to return to the starting trailhead.

Other Symbols

🚶 **Backpacking** All hikes that can be done as **overnight backpacking trips** include this symbol. Specific backpacking information is listed at the end of each hike.

🐕 **Dogs** This symbol tells you which locations allow **dogs** in the backcountry.

👫 **Kids** Indicates hikes **well suited for young children.** Such hikes are short and easy, and they often have educational interpretive signs.

Hike Description

The body of the hike is broken down into three main sections:

The Hike Following the introductory material and background information is a brief overview of the hike, discussing seasonal differences, crowds, recommended equipment, special regulations, fishing possibilities, and the availability of water both at the trailhead and along the hike.

To Reach the Trailhead Concise driving directions to the start of the hike. This book assumes that you have a basic highway map of California. Mention is made if access requires a four-wheel-drive or high-clearance vehicle. Entrance fees are also included in this section.

Every vehicle's odometer is slightly different. Your mileages may vary from those listed here; any discrepancy should be consistent throughout the book.

Description The hike itself. Parenthetical notations such as (10,320') indicate elevation in feet. Parenthetical notations such as (2.7/8,750') are included at important junctions or landmarks. The first number represents the total distance from the trailhead in miles; the second identifies the elevation of the location in feet.

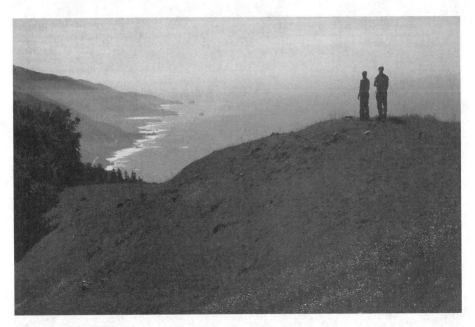

Oh, the seas of possibilities!

Nearby Facilities

Information about nearby facilities is displayed in a shaded box at the end of each hike:

Nearest Visitor Center The closest source of information to the trailhead and the best place to call for general information. Opening hours are included, but be aware that schedules are subject to regular change; these times should only be considered approximate. Unless otherwise mentioned, assume the hours are year-round.

Backpacking Information If the hike can be done as an overnight backpacking trip, this section discusses required permits, fees, quotas, and crowds. Campsite locations may be briefly mentioned, but they are not described in detail or discussed in the main description.

Nearest Campground The closest organized campground to the trailhead. *Organized* means that there are at least picnic tables, fire rings, and toilets. Water is available unless specifically mentioned otherwise. The total number of sites and camping fees is included as well. Be aware that prices always increase and that those listed should be considered approximate.

Additional Information Recommended websites for obtaining more information.

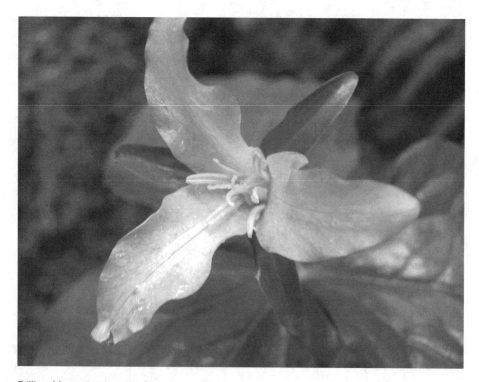

Trillium blooms in tripartite glory

Safety, Gear, and the Wilderness Ethic

Safety

Always tell somebody where you're hiking and when you expect to return. Friends, family, rangers, and visitor centers are all valuable resources that can save you from a backcountry disaster when you fail to reappear on time.

Know your limits. Don't undertake a hike that exceeds your physical fitness or wilderness abilities.

Try not to hike alone. A hiking partner can provide the margin between life and death in the event of a serious backcountry mishap.

Be prepared. Plan appropriately for the expected terrain and weather, and always carry essential survival gear.

Drink lots of water. Prevent dehydration and its accompanying dangers by consuming as much water as possible. Always purify water taken from rivers, lakes, and streams in the backcountry.

Animal Hazards

Bears

The grizzly bear is extinct in California, and only its smaller cousin the black bear still roams the mountains. Seldom dangerous, black bears will usually run away as soon as they spot you. In popular areas—Yosemite being the prime example—resident bears have learned that people mean food and exhibit no fear of humans. If a bear approaches, be loud and obnoxious, bang pots, throw small rocks, and try to frighten the animal away. Always avoid females with cubs, as the maternal instinct can make her attack if she feels her young are threatened.

When you are camping in bear country, it is imperative that you safely secure food and any scented items (toothpaste, deodorant, and so on) away from the campsite. Plastic bear canisters are now required in many locations, including Yosemite and Sequoia–Kings Canyon National Parks and most of Inyo National Forest. They are available for inexpensive rental from the primary visitor centers and ranger stations.

Hanging your food from a nearby tree is an option in less-traveled areas. To hang your food, divide it evenly between two stuff sacks and find a tree with a long, thin branch extending at least 10 feet from the trunk and at least 20 feet from the ground. Throw a rope over the branch using a weighted object of some kind, tie one of the stuff sacks to the end, hoist it to the branch, attach the second stuff sack as far above the ground as possible on the other end of the rope, and use a stick to push the second sack upward until it is level with the first.

Rattlesnakes

Common throughout Northern California below approximately 6,000 feet, these venomous snakes like to bask on hot rocks in the sun. They usually flee at the first sight of people and will attack only if threatened. Be wary when cruising

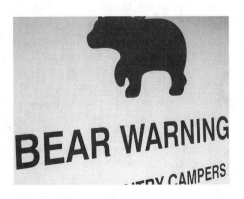

BEAR WARNING
...RY CAMPERS

off-trail, and don't put your hands where you can't see them when scrambling on rocky slopes.

If you do get bitten, the goal is to reduce the rate at which the poison circulates through your body—try to remain calm, keep the bite site below the level of your heart, remove any constricting items (rings, watches, and so on) from the soon-to-be-swollen extremity, and do not apply ice or chemical cold to the bite; this can cause further damage to the surrounding tissue. Seek medical attention as quickly as possible.

Ticks

These parasites love brushy areas at low elevations and are common throughout the state, especially during the rainy season. Always perform regular body checks when hiking through tick country. If you find a tick attached to you, don't try to pull it out with your fingers or pinch the body; removing it this way is difficult and can increase the risk of infection. Using an appropriate tool instead, gently pull the tick out by lifting upward from the base of the body where it is attached to the skin. Pull straight out until the tick releases, and do not twist or jerk as this may break off the mouth parts under your skin. A stiff pair of tweezers works well for this operation.

Lyme Disease

While this disease is present in Northern California, only one of the 48 tick species found in the state is capable of transmitting it: the diminutive western black-legged tick. Chances for exposure are low, though the risk is steadily growing. Again, always perform regular body checks when hiking through tick country.

Caused by a spirochete, Lyme disease is potentially life threatening and can be hard to diagnose in its early phases. Common early symptoms include fatigue, chills and fever, headache, muscle and joint pain, swollen lymph nodes, and a blotchy skin rash that clears centrally to produce a characteristic ring shape 3–30 days after exposure. If you fear that you have been exposed to Lyme disease, consult a doctor immediately. Note that the majority of infected people never see the tick that bit them.

Giardia

Giardia lamblia is a microscopic organism occasionally found in backcountry water sources. Existing in a dormant cyst form while in the water, the critter develops in the gastrointestinal tract upon being consumed and can cause diarrhea, excessive flatulence, foul-smelling excrement, nausea, fatigue, and abdominal cramps. While the risk of contraction is very slight, the potential consequences are worth preventing. All water taken from the backcountry should be purified with a filter, with a chemical treatment, or by boiling for a minimum of 60 seconds. Be especially vigilant about water sources near heavily used camping areas.

Deer Mice

There is no known cure for hantavirus, a rare but usually fatal pulmonary syndrome acquired by ingesting the urine, droppings, or saliva of infected rodents, or by touching your nose, mouth, or eyes after handling infected rodents, their nests, or droppings. Deer mice are 4–7 inches long, are gray to brown in color with white fur on the belly, and have large ears. They are common around the state. Never handle rodent nests, avoid buildings they inhabit, and never leave food sitting out.

Mountain Lions

Common throughout the state, mountain lions are rarely seen. If you do encounter a mountain lion acting aggressively, make yourself look as large as possible and do not run away.

Plants to Avoid

Poison Oak

If you learn to identify only one plant in California, it had better be this one. Poison oak grows throughout California below approximately 4,000 feet. A low-lying shrub or bush, it has glossy, oaklike leaves that always grow in clusters of three and turn bright red in the fall before dropping off in the winter. Both the

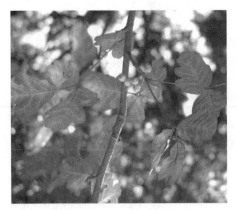

Poison oak leaves (photo: Jane Huber)

leaves and stems contain an oil that causes a strong allergic reaction in most people, creating a maddening and long-lived itchy rash that can spread across the body. Wash thoroughly after any exposure. Poison oak is mentioned in the hike description if it occurs along a given trail.

Stinging Nettle

Common along the coast, this spiny plant causes an unpleasant stinging sensation when any part of it comes in contact with your skin. It is also mentioned in the hike description when it appears along a given trail.

Physical Dangers

Lightning

Thunderstorms are common during the summer months and often bring lightning, especially at higher elevations. If you see a thunderstorm approaching, avoid exposed ridges and peaks, take shelter in low places, and sit on some sort of insulating material if you feel in real danger; your backpack or sleeping pad are good options.

Hypothermia

This life-threatening condition occurs when the body is unable to stay adequately warm and its core temperature begins to drop. Initial symptoms include weakness, mental confusion, and

uncontrollable shivering. Cold, wet weather poses the greatest hazard because wet clothes conduct heat away from the body roughly 20 times as fast as dry layers. Fatigue reduces your body's ability to produce its own heat; wind poses an increased risk as it can quickly strip away warmth. Immediate treatment is critical and entails raising the body's core temperature: Get out of the wind, take off wet clothes, drink warm beverages, eat simple energy foods, and take shelter in a warm tent or sleeping bag. Do not drink alcohol—this dilates the blood vessels and increases heat loss.

Heat Stroke

The opposite of hypothermia, this condition occurs when the body is unable to control its internal temperature and overheats. Usually brought on by excessive exposure to the sun and accompanying dehydration, symptoms include cramping, headache, and mental confusion. Treatment involves rapid, aggressive cooling of the body through whatever means are available—cooling the head and torso is most important—and drinking lots of fluids. Stay hydrated and be sure to carry some type of sun protection for your head if you expect to travel a hot, exposed section of trail.

Sunburn

The Northern California sun can fry you quickly—especially at higher elevations, where the air filters less of the damaging UV radiation. Always wear a broad-spectrum sunscreen that provides protection from both UVA and UVB rays (the SPF rating refers only to UVB protection). Wear pants and long sleeves when appropriate, plus a hat with a broad brim to protect your face and neck.

The Pacific Ocean

The dangerous waters of the Pacific are frigid, swirling with strong currents and undertows that can instantly suck the unwary out to sea. Rogue waves can always occur, sweeping the unsuspecting from seemingly safe rocks and beaches—especially during times of large swell. Unless you're confident in your abilities and knowledge of the ocean, don't tempt fate by going into the water.

Gear

Survival Essentials

You should always have the following:

Water Carry at least 1 liter of water (preferably 2), drink frequently, and have some means of purifying backcountry sources (chemical treatment or filter).

Fire and Light Bring waterproof matches and Vaseline-coated cotton balls (or other easy-to-ignite kindling) for starting an emergency fire, along with a headlamp or flashlight in case you're still hiking at night.

Survival Gear Pack heavy-duty garbage bags to use as emergency rain protection, shelter, and warmth, plus a whistle to signal for help.

First-Aid Kit At a minimum this should include an over-the-counter painkiller/swelling reducer such as ibuprofen; a 2-to 4-inch-wide elastic (ACE) bandage for wrapping sprained

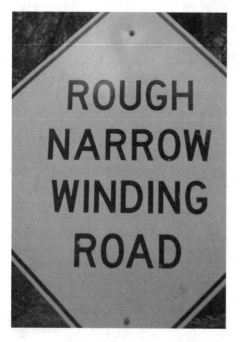

joints or other injuries; and the basics for treating a bleeding wound: antibiotic ointment, sterile gauze, small bandages, medical tape, and large Band-Aids. Prepackaged kits are readily available at any outdoor-equipment store.

Map and Compass To know where you are and to find your way home. Even the simplest compass is useful.

Knife A good knife or all-in-one tool can be invaluable in the event of a disaster.

Extra Clothes and Food Warm clothing can be critical in the event of an unexpected night out or a developing fog. A few extra energy bars can make a huge difference in morale and energy level if you stay out longer than expected.

Sun Protection Carry and use a broad-spectrum sunscreen that blocks both UVA and UVB, and protect your eyes with a pair of shades.

For Your Feet

Your feet are your most important piece of gear. Keep them happy, and you will be even more so. Appreciate them. Care for them.

Footwear Appropriate hiking shoes stabilize and support your feet and ankles while protecting them from the abuses of the environment. For most hikes in this book, a solid pair of mid-weight hiking boots is recommended, though a pair of lightweight boots or trail-running shoes can be adequate for hikers with strong ankles traveling over moderate terrain.

When selecting footwear, keep in mind that the most important feature is a good fit—your toes should not hit the front while going downhill, your heel should be locked in place inside the boot to prevent blister-causing friction, and there should be minimal extra space around your foot (although you should be able to wiggle your toes freely). When lacing, leave the laces over the top of your foot (instep) loose, but tie them tightly across the ankle to lock the heel down. Stability over uneven ground is enhanced by a stiffer sole and a higher ankle collar.

All-leather boots last longer, have a good deal of natural water resistance, and will mold to your feet over time. Footwear made from synthetic materials or a combination of fabric and leather is lighter and cheaper, but less durable. Many boots include Gore-Tex, a waterproof/breathable layer, a nice feature. Be sure to break in new boots before taking them on an extended hike.

Socks After armpits, feet are the sweatiest part of the human body. Unfortunately, wet feet are much more prone to blisters. Good hiking socks wick moisture away from your skin and provide padding for your feet. Avoid cotton socks, which become quickly saturated, stay wet inside your shoes, and take a long time to dry.

Most outdoor socks are a confusing mix of natural and synthetic fibers. Wool provides warmth and padding and, although it does absorb roughly 30% of its weight in water, is effective at keeping your feet dry. If regular wool makes your feet itch, try softer merino wool. Nylon, polyester, acrylic, and polypropylene (also called olefin) are synthetic fibers that absorb very little water, dry quickly, and add durability. Liner socks are a thin pair of socks worn underneath the principal sock and are designed to wick moisture away more effectively than thicker socks—good for really sweaty feet.

Blister Kit Blisters are almost always caused by friction from foot movement (slippage) inside the shoe. Prevent them by buying properly fitting footwear, taking a minimum of one to two weeks to break them in, and wearing appropriate socks. If the heel is slipping and blistering is occurring, try tightening the laces across the ankle to keep the heel in place. If you notice a blister or hot spot developing, stop immediately and apply adhesive padding (such as moleskin) over the problem spot. Bring a lightweight pair of scissors to cut the moleskin.

Outdoor Clothing

Fabrics Cotton should be generally avoided for outdoor activities. It absorbs water quickly and takes a long time to dry, leaving a cold, wet

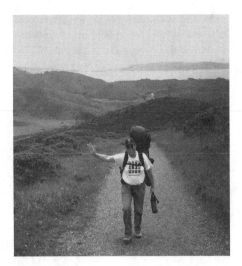

layer next to your skin and increasing the risk of hypothermia. Jeans are the worst.

Polyester and nylon are two commonly used, and recommended, fibers in outdoor clothing. They dry almost instantly, wick moisture effectively, and are of lighter weight than natural fibers. Fleece clothing (made from polyester) provides good insulation and will keep you warm, even when wet. Synthetic materials melt quickly, however, if placed in contact with a heat source (campstove, fire, sparks, and so on). Wool is a good natural fiber for hiking. Even though it retains up to 30% of its weight in water, it still insulates when wet.

Raingear/Windgear Three types are available: water-resistant, waterproof/breathable, and waterproof/nonbreathable. Water-resistant shells are typically (very) lightweight nylon windbreakers with a water repellent coating that wears away with use. The seams will not be taped. They will often keep you dry for a short period, but they'll quickly soak through in a heavy rain.

Waterproof/breathable shells contain Gore-Tex or an equivalent layer or coating and effectively keep liquid water out while allowing water vapor (that is, your sweat) to pass through. They breathe reasonably well until the outer fabric becomes saturated, at which point the breathability is lost and you will still get sticky and wet on the inside.

Waterproof/nonbreathable shells are typically coated nylon or rubber and keep water out but hold all your sweat in. Seams must be taped for them to be completely waterproof. Although wearing these on a strenuous hike causes a hot and sticky experience, they can be cheap and very lightweight. All three options effectively block the wind.

Keeping Your Head and Neck Warm Your body will strive to keep your torso, neck, and head a constant temperature at all times. Without any insulation, the heat coursing through your neck to your brain radiates into the air and is lost. Warmth that might have been directed to your extremities instead replaces the heat lost from your head. A thin balaclava or warm hat and neck gaiter are small items, weigh little, and are more effective at keeping you warm than an extra fleece.

Keeping Your Hands Warm Hiking in cold and damp conditions will often chill your hands unpleasantly. A lightweight pair of synthetic liner gloves will do wonders.

Backpacking Equipment

Backpack For overnight trips, a pack with a capacity of between 40 and 50 liters (roughly 2,500–3,000 cubic inches) is generally necessary, though dedicated ultralight hikers with the most compact and lightweight gear can get away with less. For longer trips, a pack with 60 liters (approximately 3,700 cubic inches) or more is recommended.

Just like footwear, the most important feature of a pack is a good fit. A properly fitting backpack allows you to carry most of the weight on your hips and lower body, sparing the easily fatigued muscles of the shoulders and back. When trying on packs, loosen the shoulder straps, position the waist belt so that the top of your hips (the bony iliac crest) is in the middle of the belt, attach and cinch the waist belt, and then tighten the shoulder straps. The waist belt should fit snugly around your hips, with no gaps. The shoulder straps should rise slightly off your body before dipping back down to attach to the pack about an inch below your shoulders—no weight should be resting on the top of your shoulders, and you should be able to shrug them freely. Most packs will have load stabilizer straps that attach to the pack behind your ears and lift the shoulder straps upward, off your shoulders. A sternum strap links the two shoulder straps together across your chest and prevents them from slipping away from your body.

Keep your pack's center of gravity as close to your middle and lower back as possible. Heavy items should go against the back, becoming progressively lighter as you pack outward and upward. Do not place heavy items at or below the level of the hip belt—this greatly diminishes your ability to carry that weight on the lower body.

Sleeping Bag Nights are surprisingly cool to cold in Northern California, especially at higher elevations. A sleeping bag rated to 20 degrees is recommended for all-purpose use, though a model rated to 0 degrees is often a better option in the spring and fall seasons or for people who prefer extra warmth.

Down sleeping bags offer the best warmth-to-weight ratio, are incredibly compressible, and will easily last 5–10 years without losing much of their warmth. However, untreated down loses all of its insulating ability when wet and takes forever to dry—a concern during long rainy spells. Some sleeping bags now offer water-resistant down, which reduces this risk.

Synthetic-fill sleeping bags retain their insulating abilities even when wet and are cheaper, but weigh more and are bulkier. Keep in mind that synthetic-fill bags lose some of their loft and warmth after a few seasons of use.

Sleeping Pad Sleeping pads offer vital comfort and insulation from the cold ground. Inflatable foam-filled pads are the most compact and comfortable to sleep on, but they're expensive and mildly time-consuming to inflate and deflate. Basic foam pads are lightweight, cheap, and practically indestructible. For three-season hiking, virtually all versions provide adequate insulation from the ground. Comfort makes the call.

Tent/Shelter Rains are infrequent during the Northern California summer—especially in the Sierra Nevada and Modoc Plateau—and there's often nothing to keep you from sleeping directly under the stars at night. Thunderstorms do occur but are usually short-lived, plus morning dew can be heavy at times, but in general a tent is optional during the summer season in many locations. (A small tarp for an emergency shelter is always worth carrying.)

Due to fog and wind, a tent is always advisable along the coast and in the wetter regions of northwest California. In winter and spring, a tent is essential across the state, while fall offers the greatest variability in weather, depending on your location.

If you prefer to carry a tent for shelter and privacy, a lightweight three-season tent is usually recommended. These days, a two-person backpacking tent typically weighs between 3.5 and 5 pounds. As a general rule, the lighter they are, the less spacious they are.

A rain fly that extends to the ground on all sides is critically important for staying dry. Leaks are typically caused by water seeping through unsealed seams or contact between a wet rain fly and the tent body. Seal any untaped seams that are directly exposed to the rain or to water running off the fly, paying close attention to the floor corners of the tent body. Pitch the tent as tautly as possible to prevent a wet and saggy rain fly from touching the tent body.

Stability in wind is enhanced by pole intersections—the more poles and the more times they cross, the stronger the tent will be in blustery conditions. Placing a tarp between the tent floor and the ground will not only protect the floor from ground moisture and wear and tear, but it also will increase the lifespan of your tent. Most tents these days have an optional footprint with dimensions that exactly match the floor—a nice accessory.

Ultralight floorless shelters are a weight-saving option and often use trekking poles for support. They can save a pound or more of weight, but come with some sacrifices, including decreased bug resistance and the need to pitch them in an appropriate site that will not allow rainwater to run underneath.

Cooking Equipment A stove is necessary if you want hot food on the trail. Three types are available. Canister stoves run on a pressurized butane–propane blend. Simply attach the stove burner to the fuel canister, turn the knob, and light. Such stoves are simple, safe, cheap, and have an adjustable flame. Their safety and simmerability make them a good choice for summer backpacking. However, the canisters can be hard to find outside of outdoor-equipment stores, are expensive and hard to recycle, do not work below freezing, and heat very slowly when less than a quarter full.

Alcohol stoves are compact, extremely lightweight, and a popular choice for long-distance hikers. The fuel is readily available but burns much less hot than butane–propane blends or white gas and takes notably longer to boil water.

Liquid fuel stoves run on white gas contained in a self-pressurized tank or bottle. White gas is inexpensive, burns hot, is widely available around the world, and works in extremely cold conditions. However, you must work directly with liquid fuel to prime the stove, adding an element of danger. Liquid fuel stoves are also expensive, produce flames that are prone to flaring up, and may not be adjustable for simmering. Liquid fuel stoves are a good choice for those interested in winter camping or international travel.

A simple 2- to 3-quart pot is all that you usually need for backcountry cooking. A black, or blackened, pot will absorb heat more quickly and increase fuel efficiency. A windscreen for the stove is invaluable in breezy conditions. The only dish needed is a plate with upturned edges, which can double as a broad bowl—a Frisbee works particularly well. Don't forget the silverware (or plastic). Lastly, bring an insulated mug to enjoy hot drinks.

Other Good Stuff A nylon cord is useful for hanging food, stringing clotheslines, and guying out tents. A simple repair kit should include needle, thread, and duct tape. A plastic trowel is nice for digging cat holes. Insect repellent keeps bugs away. Sandals or running shoes are a great relief from hiking boots after reaching camp. A pen and waterproof notebook allow you to record outdoor epiphanies on the spot. Extra sealable plastic bags or garbage bags always come in handy. Compression stuff sacks will reduce the bulk of your sleeping bag and clothes by about a third.

The Wilderness Ethic

In order to preserve the wilderness for future generations, follow some simple guidelines to leave no trace of your passage:

Respecting the Land Do not cut switchbacks. Stay on the trail as much as possible.

Camping Camp at established sites. Select a location that has adequate water runoff, and don't dig ditches around your tent. Keep your camp clean and never leave food out.

Fires Campfires should always be made in a fire ring. Use preexisting rings if available;

otherwise, scatter the stones and ashes before you leave. Keep fires small and use only material that is already dead and down. Avoid making campfires in heavy-use areas and at high elevations where firewood is scarce. Make sure the fire is completely out before leaving.

Sanitation Choose a spot at least 200 feet away from trails, water sources, and campsites. Dig a cat hole 6 inches deep, make your deposit, and cover it with the soil you removed. Do not bury toilet paper.

Garbage Carry out all garbage and burn only paper.

Group Size Keep groups small to minimize impact. Maximum group size allowed varies by location but is usually 10 persons or fewer.

Animals Do not feed wild animals.

Noise Be respectful of other wilderness users. Listen to the sounds of nature.

Meeting Stock on the Trail Move off the trail on the downhill side, and stand still until the animals pass by.

Where Should I Go Hiking?

THE HIKES IN this book range from supremely easy to incredibly difficult, and you should be able to find a hike that fulfills your personal sense of adventure in the region you wish to visit. For an overview of the difficulty-rating system, please see "Difficulty" on page 2. For those looking for a specific trail feature, the hikes are summarized in chart form on page xii and organized by theme beginning on page 344. Read on for a summary of the regions covered in this book, their weather, the best times of year to hike, and the agencies that govern the lands encompassed by these hikes.

California Dreaming

For the purposes of this book, Northern California can be divided into four regions:

The Central Coast, Bay Area, and Coast Ranges (Hikes 1–42)

The North Coast and Klamath Mountains (Hikes 43–58)

Shasta and the Modoc Plateau (Hikes 59–70)

The Sierra Nevada (Hikes 71–101)

Each region is described briefly in the introduction to its respective section.

Northern California Weather

The overall weather in California is closely linked to the sun's relative position with the Earth. As the sun's rays strike more directly north of the equator in spring, the air it warms in the tropics rises into the upper atmosphere and moves north over the Pacific Ocean. Cooled as it travels, the air sinks back down to the surface to form an area of high pressure over the north Pacific known as the Pacific High.

As the summer progresses, the high becomes increasingly stable and prevents low-pressure storm fronts in the Gulf of Alaska from reaching Northern California.

As a consequence, summers are almost entirely devoid of rain. Localized thunderstorms do occur—especially in the high mountains—but generally the entire state basks in never-ending blue skies and sunshine. Summers on the coast are remarkably different, however: The same Pacific High that keeps storms away also creates northwest winds that almost continually buffet the shoreline. Warm, moisture-laden summer air condenses into fog over the cold Pacific waters, which is then pushed onshore by wind and the land–sea temperature differential. Summer on the coast can seem a lot like winter.

As the sun begins to strike north of the equator more obliquely in October, the entrenched Pacific High keeps storms away for most of the month while the decreasing temperatures

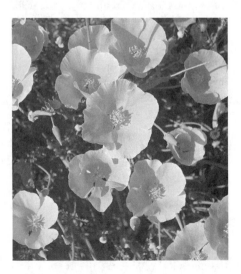

California poppies

greatly reduce the incidence of fog. It is California's choicest month of weather. Storms return by November, striking the North Coast first and then gradually reaching farther south as the Pacific High deteriorates. By January, storm after storm is hitting the state, inundating it with heavy rainfall and deep snow. Sunny breaks do occur between storms, but they are generally short-lived. February is the wettest month, and storms can continue well into April, although sunny spring days usually begin to occur in March. As a more direct angle of sunlight hits the north once again, the cycle repeats itself.

A Month-by-Month Playbook

The following is a brief description of the hiking opportunities available each month. Bear in mind that many hikes can be done year-round or at times not explicitly mentioned below.

January

Winter storms begin drenching the cold state, and only low-elevation regions near the coast are free from snow. Last year's brown slopes begin to explode with green grass, and powerful winter waves often break, making a coastal trip very worthwhile during sunny spells. The storms also cleanse the pollution from the air, making this the start of prime hiking season for views in the Bay Area—try Morgan Territory (Hike 13), Mount Diablo (Hike 14), San Bruno Mountain (Hike 25), or Mount Tamalpais (Hike 31). Redwood forests are always open for hiking on rainy days and big surf often booms below Devil's Slide (Hike 22). Crowds are all but nonexistent.

February

The wettest month of the year hammers at the state, making hiking a challenge. Stay coastal and in the Bay Area if the weather breaks. Pinnacles National Park (Hike 7) is a great place to visit on sunny days. The adventurous can go looking for bald eagles around Cache Creek (Hike 38), or for the abundant birdlife in Cosumnes River Preserve (Hike 16) or at Tule Lake (Hike 60). Crowds remain absent.

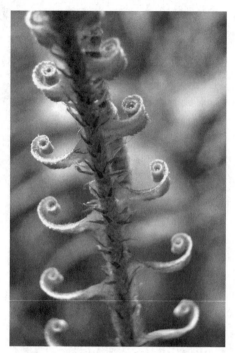

Ferns are a constant companion throughout Northern California's seasons.

March

A highly variable month, March can continue to bring wintry storms or break into long stretches of warm sunshine. Regardless of how frequently they come, the first spring days arrive this month and herald the start of wildflower season. Open slopes along the coast burst with color, views remain generally clear throughout the Bay Area, and oak woodlands flourish green. Big Sur (Hikes 1–6) can be downright hot during sunny spells.

April

Though much like March, April has increasing sunshine and warm weather. Fog can already begin to reappear on the coast, making this the last good month for fog-free coastal adventuring. Oak woodlands explode with wildflowers and Henry W. Coe State Park (Hikes 9 and 10) is a choice destination. This is also a great time for a coastal adventure north of the Bay Area, especially the North Coast region (Hikes 45–52).

Pummeled by rain and/or fog much of the year, the area experiences some of its nicest weather this month, when tourist crowds are absent.

May

The winter snowpack begins to melt at higher elevations, and hikes below 5,000 feet open for the season. In the northern Coast Range, Yolla Bolly Wilderness (Hike 44) often provides one of the season's earliest higher-elevation destinations. Mountain rivers rage with snowmelt, the waterfalls of Feather Falls (Hike 71) and Yosemite Valley (Hike 85) are spectacular, and deep river canyons offer summer heat and wildflowers, including the South Yuba River (Hike 73). Warm, sunny days on the coast are intermittent as the fog begins to increase, hills in the Coast Ranges begin to brown, and summer haze begins to collect, ending the prime Bay Area hiking season. Crowds remain surprisingly light until Memorial Day, when the summer hordes instantaneously appear.

June

The winter snowpack continues to melt, but hikes above 8,000 feet usually remain snow covered and inaccessible all month. The cable route on Half Dome (Hike 86) is usually put up early in the month, and Sequoia and Kings Canyon National Parks (Hikes 97–101) offer great early-summer adventures. Coastal fog continues to increase, and the heat in the Coast Ranges and Sierra foothills starts to become oppressive. The summer crowds come out in force at popular destinations.

July

Unless it has been an unusually heavy winter, virtually all hikes are open by July and the three-month high-elevation season has begun. While the Sierra Nevada is the destination of choice, with its wide variety of alpine hikes, also consider a trip north to Mount Shasta and the Klamath Mountains (Hikes 53–59). Wildflower season begins to taper off as the month progresses. Fog and crowds are heavy along the coast. Avoid the Fourth of July weekend if at all possible.

August

Though much like July, the very highest elevation hikes to Palisade Glacier (Hike 96) and Sawtooth Peak (Hike 101) sometimes don't become snow free until this time. Coastal fog is as thick as it gets, statewide temperatures max out, and crowds remain heavy all month long.

September

This is a great month to be anywhere in the mountains. Summer vacation ends for a lot of people on Labor Day and crowds suddenly vanish, yet the weather typically remains ideal across the state. It's a good time to visit the Trinity Alps (Hike 54), Lake Tahoe (Hikes 76–77), and trips in the eastern Sierra. Coastal fog begins to diminish, and high elevations become increasingly cold at night.

October

This is a great month to be anywhere in California. It is the month of Indian summer, when the sun shines day in and day out, coastal fog finally disappears for the season, and fall colors fluoresce in the mountains. Hot summer weather lingers on a tour of the Modoc Plateau (Hikes 60–69) as the aspens of empty South Warner Wilderness (Hike 64) rustle gold in the breeze. Higher-elevation hikes usually remain open, but nighttime temperatures often drop below freezing. Be aware that hunting season opens early in the month on national forest lands; wearing bright colors is a good idea. Near the end of the month, temperatures begin to swing markedly and the first winter storm often strikes the state.

November

Much of California closes to hiking as snow begins falling in the mountains and a chill sets in at higher elevations. Intermittent winter storms occur and air quality and visibility start to improve in the Bay Area. Fall lingers in the low-elevation foothills of the Sierra Nevada for the first half of the month—Rubicon River (Hike 74) is a pleasant destination. Stay coastal or in the Bay Area otherwise.

December

Daylight dwindles to a minimum as California slips into the depths of winter and hiking days get shorter. Weather is variable; long stretches of rain, cold snaps, and sunshine can all occur. Remain strictly coastal or enjoy views in the Bay Area.

The Different Governing Agencies

This book visits a wide variety of parks and forests managed by a number of different governing agencies. Regulations often vary by location but generally are the same within each group. The four most commonly visited areas in this book are national parks, state parks, national forests, and wilderness areas managed by national forests. A miscellany of other governing agencies are represented as well, including the Bureau of Land Management and various city and county parks.

National Parks

Run by the federal government (Department of the Interior), national parks are designated to preserve and protect unique natural features and wilderness. Generally very user friendly, they tend to draw substantial crowds and often have amenities like small stores, hot showers, and well-maintained campgrounds. Free park maps are handed out, and driving is easy. Regulations are generally strict—car camping is permitted only in designated sites, wilderness permits are always required for overnight trips into the backcountry, trail quotas are common, and dogs are never permitted on the trail. Entrance fees are charged for all national parks.

State Parks

Run by the state of California, state parks are generally small and protect a wide variety of natural features. They are common along the coast and tend to be the most costly places to visit—day-use fees are always charged, and

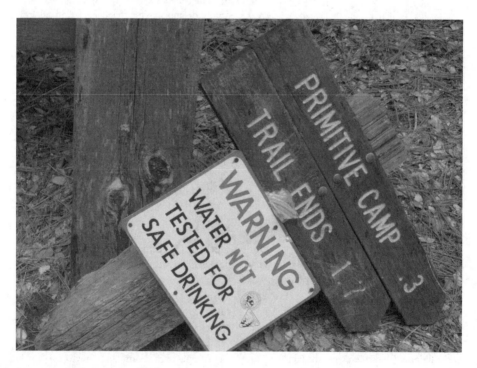

Be prepared. Adventure awaits.

state park campgrounds are among the most expensive in the state. Regulations are generally strict—car camping is permitted only in designated campgrounds, backcountry camping (when possible) is usually allowed only at designated trail camps, and dogs are never allowed in the backcountry. All state park campgrounds operate on the same reservation system; call 800-444-7275 or visit **reserve america.com** to reserve a site.

Note that the budget for the California state park system is often in flux and is almost always underfunded. Staffing and available amenities often vary from year to year as a result. In some cases, entire parks have closed during the off-season (typically November–April). Other parks have reduced the open seasons for their campgrounds and backcountry trail camps at times. The situation is fluid and will likely remain so in the months and years ahead. Call ahead to check current park status, especially if you're planning a visit during the off-season.

National Forests

As "the land of many uses," national forests are America's playgrounds. Run by the federal government (Department of Agriculture), the US Forest Service manages the land for a wide variety of purposes—logging, ranching, hunting, and hiking are all permitted—and regulations outside of wilderness areas are generally much fewer than on other public lands.

Dogs are allowed, camping is permitted virtually anywhere, wilderness permits are not required for backcountry camping, and no use fees are charged. A campfire permit is required for the use of stoves and campfires, obtainable free from any Forest Service ranger station and valid across the state for the entire year.

Roads are generally poor, commonly unpaved, and often challenging and confusing to navigate. National forest maps are usually remarkably accurate, indicate areas of private property, and are all but essential for road navigation. Organized national forest campgrounds are plentiful across the state and tend to be inexpensive, but they often lack amenities (pit toilets are common).

Wilderness Areas

Managed to protect the land's wilderness aspects, designated wilderness areas can be found in national forests throughout the state, as well as some state and national parks. No roads exist, all motorized vehicles are prohibited, and logging is not permitted. Wilderness permits are required in all but the most remote areas and can be obtained free at any nearby ranger station. Due to heavy use, the wilderness areas in the Sierra Nevada are more extensively managed—trail quotas are often in effect for backpackers. Dogs are usually allowed, and backcountry camping is permitted almost anywhere. Facilities and amenities are nonexistent—come prepared.

Other Agencies

City and county parks are common in the Bay Area and are almost all day-use only. Entrance fees are usually charged. Dogs are generally not permitted, but a few exceptions exist, most notably in the Bay Area's East Bay Regional Park District. The Bureau of Land Management manages a few regions covered by the book. Much like national forests, they have few regulations and almost no amenities or facilities. Dogs are permitted.

Other Considerations

Children

While this book is not designed for families with young children, several short hikes are perfectly suitable for the youngest hikers; look for the symbol in the trip header or the chart on page xii, or check the complete list in "Hikes by Theme" on page 344.

Campgrounds

Campgrounds vary markedly depending on location. State and national park campgrounds are generally the most luxurious, but they're often expensive and crowded. If you can cope with pit toilets, US Forest Service campgrounds are usually much more basic, smaller, and cheaper.

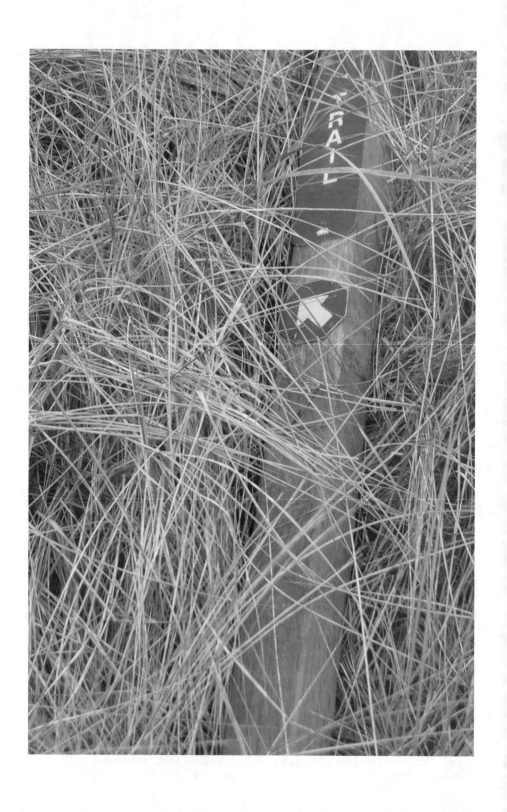

The Central Coast, Bay Area, and Coast Ranges

STRETCHING FROM Silver Peak Wilderness on the southern end of Big Sur to the northern end of Hwy. 1 in Mendocino County, this region encompasses the stretch of coastline accessible from Hwy. 1, all of the Bay Area, and the interior Coast Ranges. The overall topography is one of low mountain ranges divided by broad valleys—interrupted by the unique world of the San Francisco Bay Area. While the coastline is generally rocky and characterized by steep bluffs and headlands, beaches are also common.

Annual precipitation is high on the coast but diminishes rapidly as you go inland, creating habitat for lush redwood and mixed-evergreen forests near the Pacific, and extensive oak woodlands farther east. Going from south to north, precipitation generally increases while average temperatures decrease, leaving the southern regions hotter and drier for most of the year. Dense fog is common along the coast during the summer months, snow seldom falls anywhere in the region, and most of these hikes can be done year-round. Highlights of the region include rolling oak woodlands flushed green in spring, foaming surf on the dramatic Pacific Coast, lush redwood forests, and the endless variety of hikes and views available in the Bay Area.

HIKE 1 Upper Salmon Creek Falls 🥾 🚶 🐐

Highlights	Waterfalls, woodlands, and wildflowers
Distance	5.2 miles round-trip
Total Elevation Gain/Loss	1,000'/1,000'
Hiking Time	3–5 hours
Recommended Maps	*Big Sur and Ventana Wilderness* by Wilderness Press, USGS 7.5-min. *Villa Creek* and *Burro Mountain*
Best Times	Year-round
Agency	Silver Peak Wilderness, Los Padres National Forest
Difficulty	★★★

ON THE SOUTHERN EDGE of the Big Sur region, a little-traveled pocket of coastal mountain grandeur awaits within Silver Peak Wilderness. Far-reaching vistas look out across the ocean, perennial streams swirl beneath lush forest, and several quiet backcountry campsites entice you to spend the night.

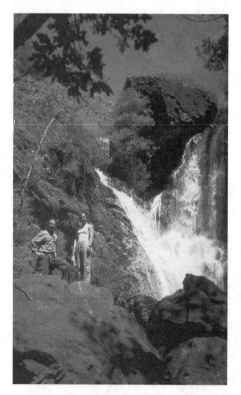

Salmon Creek Falls (photo: Analise Elliot Heid)

The Hike first ascends to nearby Salmon Creek Falls, a dramatic cascade within eyeshot of Hwy. 1, and then travels along the mossy corridor of Salmon Creek to reach Upper Salmon Creek Falls. An iridescent pool shimmers at the base of this misty gem, a refreshing swimming spot on hot summer days. Fog can be thick in the summer months and poison oak is ubiquitous year-round. No water is available at the trailhead, though Salmon Creek is regularly accessible.

To Reach the Trailhead Follow Hwy. 1 to the signed Salmon Creek Trailhead, at a tight bend in the highway 8 miles south of Gorda, 7 miles north of Ragged Point, and 1.5 miles north of the posted San Luis Obispo County line. Park in the wide turnouts on either side of the highway.

Description From the trailhead, follow Salmon Creek Trail as it climbs a moderate grade along the south bank of Salmon Creek. The falls are clearly audible and you quickly reach an unmarked junction leading downward to the base of the cascade (0.1/230'). A side trip not to be missed, the 200-foot spur drops past fragrant bays and mossy boulders to reach the mist-cloaked cascade.

After exploring the falls, don't be taken in by the heavily used, steep spur that continues up Salmon Creek to rocky promontories above the falls. Many hikers mistake this spur for the Salmon Creek Trail, following it until it disappears into oblivion a mile upstream. Instead, carefully retrace your steps to the earlier junction, bear left, and continue climbing a moderate grade up the south canyon wall. The trail soon switchbacks past a seasonal creek and reaches a rocky viewpoint (0.3/760') overlooking the lower Salmon Creek drainage.

Notice the diverse plant life and dramatic shift in vegetation in the surrounding canyon. A lush riparian forest of alders, maples, and bays lines the ravine's floor but quickly transitions to a drier coastal scrub zone of sagebrush, sticky monkeyflower, and coffeeberry bushes. Higher up, a rocky arid zone is populated by hardy succulents such as Our Lord's candle, a

yucca that dies soon after sprouting its large stalk of cream-colored blossoms.

Onward, the trail switchbacks past a conspicuous mound of light green, slippery serpentine (0.5/760'), California's state rock. Formed atop ancient seafloors that tectonic activity later smashed into Big Sur, serpentine produces nutrient-poor soils that are inhospitable to most plant life. A few "serpentine endemics" have adapted, however, including California poppies, yucca, and other tenacious succulents.

The trail passes several unobstructed ocean views as it climbs the north-facing slopes, winding through dense coastal shrub and

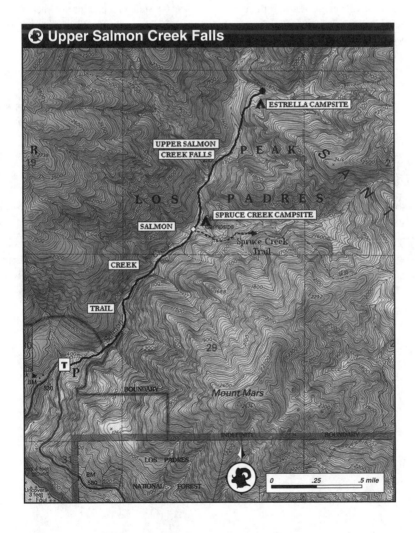

Upper Salmon Creek Falls

beneath shady live oaks and bays. Fragrant black sage and sagebrush thickets line the trail, as do mats of hedge nettles boasting deep lavender blossoms in spring. Just past a dry creek bed, you reach a crest (1.5/1,050') then gradually descend past groves of Douglas-fir, tan oak, and bay amid dense huckleberry bushes. The trail contours along the south canyon wall, hopping across two seasonal creeks. Fifty feet past the last creek, you reach the signed junction for Spruce Creek Trail (1.8/1,010').

Bear left to continue on Salmon Creek Trail as it heads steadily downslope past large old-growth Douglas-firs and vine-like poison oak. You soon reach Spruce Creek Camp (2.0/750'), where three idyllic campsites line the confluence of Salmon and Spruce Creeks.

Past the camp, the hike begins a moderate climb of the north-facing slopes in the shade of young Douglas-firs, bays, oaks, and ceanothus, which fills the spring air with a lilac aroma from profuse blue flowers. The trail skirts high above the creek past small rapids and swirling emerald pools; a few small washouts require careful footing.

To reach Upper Salmon Creek Falls, watch for a steep spur on your left, just before a bend in the trail (2.6/1,140'). More reminiscent of a deer trail, the steep and precarious path drops 150 feet over loose rock and past poison oak to reach the base of the falls, a refreshing grotto of mist and spray that is well worth the effort. After a refreshing dip, retrace your steps to the trailhead. Alternatively, you can continue another 0.6 mile along Salmon Creek Trail and ascend 300 feet to Estrella Camp, where two pleasant campsites perch along the banks of Estrella Creek.

Nearest Visitor Centers Big Sur Station, 831-667-2315, just south of Pfeiffer Big Sur State Park on Hwy. 1, is open daily 9 a.m.–4 p.m. Memorial Day–Labor Day; the rest of the year it's open intermittently depending on staffing availability. Also try King City Ranger Station, 831-385-5434, at 406 S. Mildred Ave. in King City; take the Canal off-ramp from Hwy. 101, go east on Canal, right on Division, and left on Mildred. It's open Monday–Friday 8 a.m.–4:30 p.m.

Backpacking Information Spruce Creek and Estrella Camp are both ideally situated for an overnight trip. Several sites feature picnic tables and fire rings. A valid campfire permit is required.

Nearest Campground Plaskett Creek Campground (43 sites, $22) is 4 miles north of Gorda along Hwy. 1. Eighty percent of the sites are reservable year-round; visit **recreation.gov** or call 877-444-6777.

Additional Information www.fs.usda.gov/lpnf

HIKE 2 Vicente Flat

Highlights	Golden coastal bluffs and ancient redwoods
Distance	10.4 miles round-trip
Total Elevation Gain/Loss	2,000'/2,000'
Hiking Time	6–10 hours
Recommended Maps	*A Guide to Ventana & Silver Peak Wilderness* by the US Forest Service, *Big Sur and Ventana Wilderness* by Wilderness Press, USGS 7.5-min. *Cone Peak* and *Lopez Pointi*
Best Times	Year-round
Agency	Ventana Wilderness, Los Padres National Forest
Difficulty	★★★

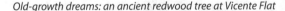

EXTREME TOPOGRAPHY defines the coastal flanks of Cone Peak, where soaring ridges and chasmic valleys crease the mountainside. The area is also known for its exceptional biodiversity, from wildflower-painted grasslands to yucca-studded chaparral, fluttering oak woodland to towering old-growth redwood forest. And don't forget the sweeping ocean views, which look out for miles across a glittering aquamarine sea.

The Hike ascends nearly 2,000 feet above the wave-swept coast and then traverses inland to reach Vicente Flat along redwood-lined Hare Creek. Open terrain allows dramatic coastal and canyon vistas as the trail initially climbs the grassy slopes, then heads inland through an increasingly lush forest to reach Vicente Flat, which offers campsites in a sun-drenched meadow or beneath old-growth trees. Spring welcomes a profusion of wildflowers to the

Old-growth dreams: an ancient redwood tree at Vicente Flat

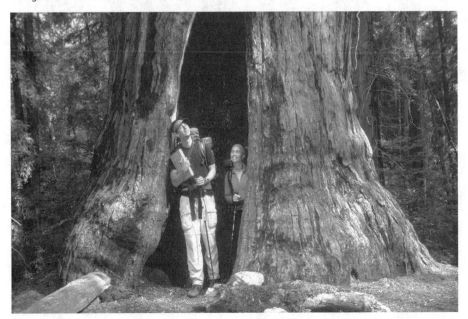

☉ Vicente Flat

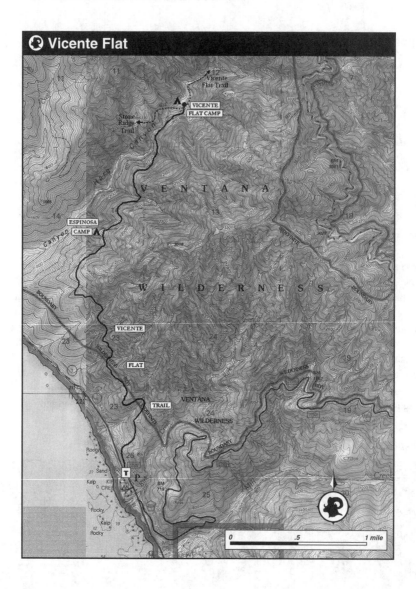

otherwise golden slopes. Summer brings view-shrouding fog and the majority of visiting hikers. At other times of the year, you may have the trail entirely to yourself. Water is available near the trailhead in adjacent Kirk Creek Campground.

To Reach the Trailhead Take Hwy. 1 to Kirk Creek Campground, 38 miles south of Pfeiffer Big Sur State Park and 36 miles north of Hearst Castle. The trailhead is on the east side of Hwy. 1, across the road from the campground.

Description From Hwy. 1 (0.0/190'), Vicente Flat Trail quickly climbs a series of switchbacks past coastal scrub. Flowering lupines, poppies, sticky monkeyflowers, and sagebrush highlight the hillside in spring. In 0.3 mile you cross a minor gully, head toward a minor saddle, then turn north across rolling grasslands and coastal chaparral. After crossing a gully choked with invasive blackberry and broom species, listen for water trickling from a nearby spring (0.9/700').

The grade steepens as the trail passes scattered yuccas, spiny testaments to the aridity of these exposed slopes. You next reach a ridge (1.4/1,000') offering spectacular views of the convergence of land and sea. Continuing, the trail quickly enters the Ventana Wilderness and reaches shade beneath a canopy of oaks, madrones, and bays. You follow the ridgeline through four gullies and past a dense band of redwoods, then climb steeply to a prominent ridge (2.9/1,610'), where exceptional views entice you to linger. To the east, 5,155-foot Cone Peak (Hike 3) and its neighbor, double-notched Twin Peak, loom over Hare and Limekiln creeks. Hare Canyon is one of the state's deepest gorges; Limekiln Canyon boasts the steepest coastal slope in the Lower 48.

The trail now descends off the ridge, veering northeast through varied microclimates that support a range of drought-tolerant and moisture-loving plants. The contrast is stark— yuccas dot the arid slopes, while moisture-reliant redwoods cluster nearby in damp gullies. You next reach a short spur to Espinosa Camp (3.4/1,660'), marked by a large fallen redwood 100 yards past a major gully.

The spur leads 100 feet to several small campsites atop a minor ridge in the shade of live oaks, bays, redwoods, and rare, endemic Santa Lucia firs. Rock outcrops offer unobstructed views toward the coast. This is an excellent picnic or overnight spot, though the nearby gully is usually dry. The continuing hike contours inland along the slopes, rounds a prominent ridge, and reaches the first reliable water source, a creeklet cascading past redwoods and ferns. Open grassy slopes return as the trail tops out at 1,860 feet and begins a gentle descent to Vicente Flat.

You cross three rubble-strewn gullies (4.1/ 1,800'), their adjacent marble faces misted in winter by a seasonal flow. After the next dry redwood gully, the trail contours north and enters dense woods a quarter mile before reaching Hare Creek and several large redwoods. A few feet farther, a spur cuts upstream to a pair of sites in the open meadow of Vicente Flat itself. The main trail continues a short distance to the Stone Ridge Trail junction (5.2/1,620'); beyond lie many beautiful campsites in the redwoods.

Nearest Visitor Center Big Sur Station, 831-667-2315, just south of Pfeiffer Big Sur State Park on Hwy. 1, is open daily 9 a.m.–4 p.m. Memorial Day–Labor Day; the rest of the year it's open intermittently depending on staffing availability.

Backpacking Information No wilderness permit is needed, but a valid campfire permit is required. The established tent sites of Espinosa and Vicente Flat Camps are exceptional places to spend the night.

Nearest Campground Kirk Creek Campground (33 sites, $22) is located at the junction of Hwy. 1 and Nacimiento Rd. Eighty percent of the sites are reservable year-round; visit **recreation.gov** or call 877-444-6777.

Additional Information www.fs.usda.gov/lpnf, ventanawild.org

HIKE 3 Cone Peak 🐾🐕

Highlight	Unobstructed views atop the highest coastal summit in California
Distance	4.0 miles round-trip
Total Elevation Gain/Loss	1,400'/1,400'
Hiking Time	2–3 hours
Recommended Maps	*A Guide to Ventana & Silver Peak Wilderness* by the US Forest Service, *Big Sur and Ventana Wilderness* by Wilderness Press, USGS 7.5-min. *Chews Ridge*
Best Times	April–November
Agency	Ventana Wilderness, Los Padres National Forest
Difficulty	★★★

THREE MILES FROM the ocean, Cone Peak rises a mile to the sky. In summer 1999, most of Ventana Wilderness burned. Cone Peak, the dominant mountain of the southern wilderness, burned with it. Life has since rebounded on these sheer slopes, yet does little to hide the seamless joining of ocean and sky, the towering coastal vistas, or the sweeping panorama of the Santa Lucia Mountains.

The Hike climbs to the fire lookout atop Cone Peak (5,155') on steep but short Cone Peak Trail. It's important to time your visit correctly. The 5-mile dirt access road closes after the first heavy winter rains (typically in December) and usually reopens in March, though this varies from year to year; call ahead to check if you're planning a trip in early spring or late fall. Crowds and coastal

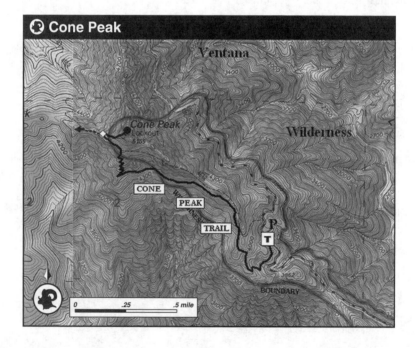

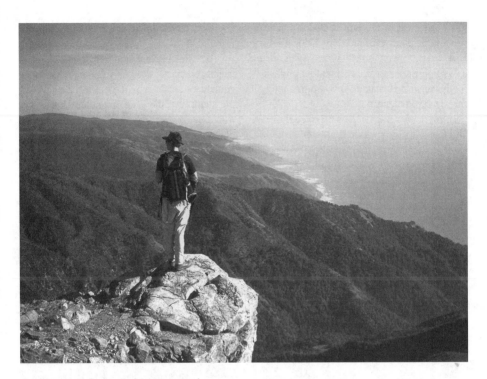

Looking south from mile-high Cone Peak

fog are heaviest in the summer. No water is available at the trailhead.

To Reach the Trailhead Take Nacimiento Rd. east from Hwy. 1—the turnoff is by Kirk Creek Campground 4 miles south of Lucia. Be aware that Hwy. 1 is subject to washouts and closures, especially in the winter. Follow sinuous Nacimiento Rd. as it climbs 2,800 feet in 8 miles to the divide, and turn north on rough and unpaved Cone Peak Rd. Low-clearance vehicles should have no problem making it to the trailhead, 5.2 miles down this road by a small turnout.

Approaching from the east, take Hwy. 101 to the Hwy. G14/Fort Hunter Liggett exit just north of King City. Follow G14 south for 19 miles and turn right (west) on Mission Rd., passing immediately through an always-open fort entrance gate. Bear left on Nacimiento Rd. 3.0 miles past the gate and left again 0.9 mile farther—be watchful as the intersection signs are not obvious. From here, it is 18 increasingly narrow miles to Cone Peak Rd., where you proceed as described above.

Description From the trailhead, the trail initially strikes west to quickly attain a nearby saddle. The cliffs of Cone Peak and the fire lookout are clearly visible to the northwest, and Hare Canyon can be seen slicing southwest down to the ocean. Far down the canyon is a dense patch of green, a stand of coastal redwoods very near the extreme southern limit of their range. Beneath them hides Vicente Flat (Hike 2). Briefly remaining on the ridge, the trail then drops inland and passes thickets of manzanita, wartleaf, and other regenerating shrubs before switchbacking up to a second saddle (0.5/4,030').

As the trail begins its long coastside traverse to approach the peak from the west, the devastation of recent fires is evident in the bare hillsides. Fires sweep through the dry chaparral about once every 20 years as part of a natural process of plant regeneration. Known as the Kirk Creek Fires, the 1999 blaze began during a dry lightning storm in September and eventually consumed 90,000 acres—more than half the area of Ventana Wilderness.

Only a few scraggly oaks survived the blaze and Coulter pine snags still protrude from the slopes like old burnt matchsticks. The exposed trail traverses below the summit cliffs before beginning a tightly switchbacking ascent along a steep and rocky spur ridgeline. A small patch of unburned forest grows below the trail as it climbs to a junction with the Gamboa Trail immediately below the summit (1.8/4,830').

The walkway surrounding the lookout is usually open to the public, though the views are equally tremendous on the summit itself. Looking southwest, the scale of land and sea is distorted by your elevation—notice the tiny bridge of Hwy. 1 at Limekiln State Park far below. Turning northeast, the tall rise of 5,862-foot Junipero Serra Peak is one of the few distinguishing peaks in this land of sheer, naked topography. Southeast, the broad valley of Fort Hunter Liggett can be distinguished beyond the low nearby ridges. Heading downhill, you return the way you came.

Nearest Visitor Centers Big Sur Station, 831-667-2315, 10 miles north of the entrance for Julia Pfeiffer Burns State Park and just south of Pfeiffer Big Sur State Park on Hwy. 1, is open daily 9 a.m.–4 p.m. Memorial Day–Labor Day; the rest of the year it's open intermittently depending on staffing availability. Also try King City Ranger Station, 831-385-5434, at 406 S. Mildred Ave. in King City; take the Canal off-ramp from Hwy. 101, go east on Canal, right on Division, and left on Mildred. It's open Monday–Friday 8 a.m.–4:30 p.m.

Backpacking Information Backpacking is permitted along this hike, though not recommended due to the lack of campsites and water. No wilderness permit is needed but a valid campfire permit is required.

Nearest Campgrounds Kirk Creek Campground (33 sites, $22) is located at the junction of Hwy. 1 and Nacimiento Rd. Eighty percent of the sites are reservable year-round; visit **recreation.gov** or call 877-444-6777. Inland, try Nacimiento Campground (8 sites, $15, no water), on Nacimiento Rd. 3.5 miles east of Cone Peak Rd.

Additional Information www.fs.usda.gov/lpnf, ventanawild.org

HIKE 4 Ewoldsen Trail Ⴑ

Highlights	Quiet redwood forest and aerial ocean views
Distance	4.5 miles
Total Elevation Gain/Loss	1,500'/1,500'
Hiking Time	3–4 hours
Recommended Map	USGS 7.5-min. *Partington Ridge*
Best Times	September–May
Agency	Julia Pfeiffer Burns State Park
Difficulty	★★★

BIG SUR IS exceptional country. Open redwood forest lines creeks gurgling clear as glass, mountains rise thousands of feet above the foaming surf, and bare golden hilltops offer sweeping vistas of it all.

The Hike A steady ascent along Ewoldsen Trail takes you through a creekside redwood forest on your way to a viewpoint atop an open bluff more than 1,600 feet above the sea. Crowds are constant on the Big Sur coast and— due to the limited amount of public land directly along the coast—all hiking trails receive heavy use. This is not a hike for solitude, and summer months are the worst for crowds. Water is available at the trailhead.

To Reach the Trailhead Take Hwy. 1 to the Julia Pfeiffer Burns State Park entrance, 11 miles south of Pfeiffer Big Sur State Park on the central Big Sur coast. There is a $10 day-use fee, valid for all Big Sur area state parks.

Description From the trailhead in the upper parking lot (0.0/280'), the path immediately enters the redwood forest and passes along a wooden fence before dropping down to a picnic area by McWay Creek. The open forest here is much different from the temperate rain forest more commonly associated with redwoods farther north. Here, at the southern limit of their range, the trees are only able to find adequate moisture for growth along the small creeks and

McWay Falls

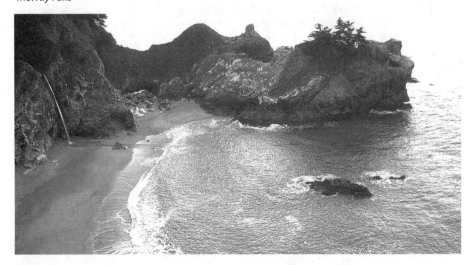

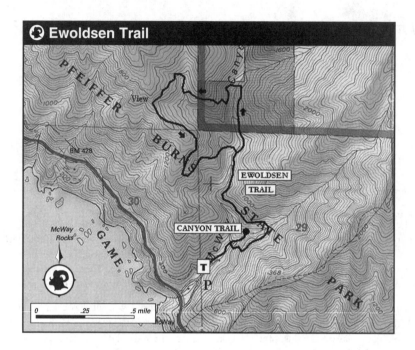

rivers that slice the Big Sur coast. The drier conditions prevent the redwoods from obtaining the colossal size of their northern counterparts and eliminate the dense understory and thick moss normally present. A few small patches of redwood sorrel, ferns, and seasonal wildflowers can be found among the litter of the forest floor, but generally the forest is remarkably open.

Crossing the clear creek by a run-down barn, the trail begins climbing through an area good for bird-watching. American dippers can often be observed ducking in and out of the water as they look for aquatic insects and other snacks on the creek bottom. Small brown creepers are easily identified overhead by their ability to ascend trees vertically, spiraling around the trunk as they go. The junction for Canyon Trail is soon encountered (0.2/400'); it's a quick and worthwhile 0.1-mile side trip leading to a delightful bench by a cascading ribbon of water.

Back on the main trail, you climb steeply above the canyon on a few switchbacks as

tanoak begins to appear trailside. After crossing the south fork of the creek, the trail traverses the slopes and passes through a dramatic vegetation change, where redwoods suddenly disappear into thick chaparral. Large redwoods reappear as you rejoin the creek and reach a junction by a small bridge (1.6/880'). This is the start of the loop. Go right, passing several substantial trees as the trail winds along the creek. You next turn west and ascend through coast live oak and California bay to the high point of the hike where spectacular views await (2.7/1,700').

Hwy. 1 winds along the edge of the continent below and the aquamarine clarity of the ocean often allows you to distinguish a sandy bottom. Looking south, several drainages are identifiable beyond that of McWay Creek, overshadowed by peaks of the high ridge rising abruptly and paralleling the coast a short distance inland. From this viewpoint, the ridgetop is still more than 2,000 feet above you, and the tallest summit visible south is nearly

4,000 feet high and less than 3 miles from the ocean—imposing topography indeed. This is also a good spot to look for red-tailed hawks and other raptors scanning the bare hillsides for lunch. From here, the trail drops behind the ridge, losing views as it makes a half-mile traverse before cutting back to quickly descend to McKay Creek and the junction at your loop's end. Head right to retrace your path to the trailhead.

Nearest Visitor Center Big Sur Station, 831-667-2315, 10 miles north of the entrance for Julia Pfeiffer Burns State Park and just south of Pfeiffer Big Sur State Park on Hwy. 1, is open daily 9 a.m.–4 p.m. Memorial Day–Labor Day; the rest of the year it's open intermittently depending on staffing availability.

Nearest Campground Pfeiffer Big Sur State Park has 218 sites ($20–$35, depending on site and time of year). Reservations are essential in the summer; visit **reserveamerica.com** or call 800-444-7275.

Additional Information **www.parks.ca.gov**

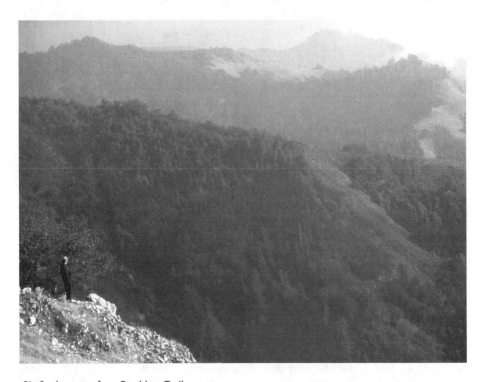

Big Sur bonanza from Ewoldsen Trail

HIKE 5 Molera Beach ⊘

Highlight	Peace and quiet on the beach
Distance	5.0 miles
Total Elevation Gain/Loss	200'/200'
Hiking Time	3–4 hours
Recommended Map	USGS 7.5-min. *Big Sur*
Best Times	September–May
Agency	Andrew Molera State Park
Difficulty	★

FOR CONSTANTLY BEING by the ocean, there is remarkably little coastal access from Hwy. 1 on the Big Sur coast. The jagged rocks and sheer cliffs that make the region so spectacular also make finding a beach, much less a secluded beach, a difficult proposition. Luckily there is Andrew Molera State Park and its 2-mile-long stretch of sand, whose farther end offers an opportunity to escape the crowds and commune peacefully with the sea.

The Hike explores the length of Molera Beach, traveling to its end before returning along the low bluffs. This is a tide-dependent hike, and the beach is treacherous and impassable in places during high tides, making it necessary to walk along the bluffs during these times. Tide tables are usually posted on the information sign in the parking lot, or you can check at Big Sur Station before heading out. Those arriving around high tide should hike first along the bluffs and return along the beach closer to low tide. Due to the treacherous nature of ocean currents here, swimming is deemed unsafe. Be aware that the seasonal starting footbridge across Big Sur River is removed after the first heavy winter rains, making it necessary to ford the swollen river during the winter months. Water is available at the trailhead. Dogs are prohibited.

To Reach the Trailhead Take Hwy. 1 south of Carmel for 22 miles to the park entrance and substantial parking lot. Approaching from the south, the turnoff is 4.2 miles north of the park entrance for Pfeiffer Big Sur State Park and is a hard, dogleg left turn. There is a day-use fee

of $10, valid for all Big Sur area state parks. It is possible to reach the trailhead by public transportation on Monterey-Salinas Transit Bus 22, which runs two to three times daily from downtown Monterey to Pfeiffer Big Sur State Park from Memorial Day to Labor Day, weekends only during the rest of the year. Call 888-678-2871 for current schedule and fare information, or visit **mst.org**.

Description From the trailhead, cross Big Sur River on the narrow footbridge and bear right on Beach Trail. Paralleling but beyond sight of the river, you pass the Creamery, a former pasture slowly being replanted with native vegetation. Twisted sycamores, arroyo willows, black cottonwood, red alders, and a few redwoods line the river, and chest-high bush lupines dot the open meadow. Looking behind you to the east, a prominent ridge of the Santa Lucia Range is visible. Composed primarily of granite transported from the south along the San Andreas Fault, the mountain range owes much of its sheer topography to the erosion-resistant nature of its granitic rock. The Creamery is also an excellent area for viewing birdlife—killdeer, black phoebes, and Cooper's hawks can often be spotted.

Continuing toward the beach, notice the incredibly grizzled redwood tree across the meadow on your left before you turn back toward the river. Then pass thick patches of poison oak and coffeeberry, which is easily identified by the dark black berries that ripen in the fall. Driftwood shelters and other interesting

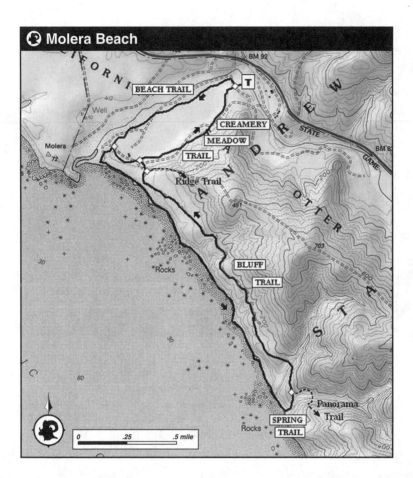

constructs fill this first sandy area where you turn south and begin the beach walk.

The low bluffs along the beach expose the variegated hues of intensely deformed rocks. While part of the Franciscan Complex, they have been more heavily metamorphosed than similar exposures found farther north in California, as a result of the numerous northwest-trending faults associated with the San Andreas Fault, which slice apart the Big Sur region and intensely shear the adjacent rock. The rare mineral almondite is exposed in places, coloring the white sand purple where it has eroded onto the beach. Rounded granite stones are also present, washed down from the Santa Lucia Mountains.

Sea lions, seals, and even sea otters can sometimes be spotted offshore as you go (barefoot) up the beach. Crowds diminish and rocky

points hem in secluded stretches of sand as you continue, eventually reaching the junction for Spring Trail, your access to the return route on the bluffs above.

Eighty feet of climbing up a narrow gully brings you to Bluff Trail—go left back the direction you came. Coyote brush, poison hemlock, California poppies, and more lupine cover the open blufftops along the trail back toward the Creamery. At the bluffs' end, the trail intersects Ridge Trail—go left again, immediately dropping down to a wide dirt road. Bearing left here returns you to the Beach Trail. Turning right down the road takes you winding along the opposite side of the Creamery close to several large coast live oaks, before the road rejoins the Beach Trail at the footbridge over Big Sur River.

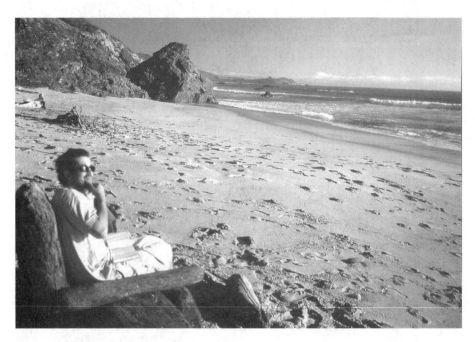

Relaxing on Molera Beach

Nearest Visitor Center Big Sur Station, 831-667-2315, 10 miles north of the entrance of Julia Pfeiffer Burns State Park and just south of Pfeiffer Big Sur State Park on Hwy. 1, is open daily 8 a.m.–6 p.m. Memorial Day–Labor Day; the rest of the year it's open daily 8 a.m.–4:30 p.m.

Nearest Campgrounds Andrew Molera State Park has 24 walk-in campsites available in a large meadow near the Big Sur River on a first-come, first-served basis ($25 per site, register at the entrance kiosk, with a maximum of 4 people per site and no dogs allowed). The closest developed campground is Pfeiffer Big Sur State Park (200 sites, $35–$50, depending on site and time of year). Reservations are essential in the summer; visit **reserveamerica .com** or call 800-444-7275.

Additional Information **www.parks.ca.gov**

HIKE 6 Pine Valley 🥾🧍🐕

Highlights	Sandstone cliffs, ponderosa pines, and an emerald swimming hole
Distance	12.0 miles round-trip
Total Elevation Gain/Loss	3,500'/3,500'
Hiking Time	6–8 hours
Recommended Maps	*A Guide to Ventana & Silver Peak Wilderness* by the US Forest Service, *Big Sur and Ventana Wilderness* by Wilderness Press, USGS 7.5-min. *Chews Ridge*
Best Times	September–May
Agency	Ventana Wilderness, Los Padres National Forest
Difficulty	★★★★

PONDEROSA PINES STAND sentinel above wildflower-strewn meadows in the heart of Ventana Wilderness. Cliffs and stones surround this broad valley, echoing stories of the Esselen people who once called this region home. A waterfall rushes out of sight nearby, pouring into a glittering pool. And on the way into peaceful Pine Valley, you'll enjoy far-reaching views of the ridge-rippled landscape that defines the Santa Lucia Mountains.

Note that in 2008, the massive Basin Complex wildfire scorched the majority of Ventana Wilderness, including the majority of this hike. Much of central and lower Pine Valley was spared, however, including the area around Pine Falls— now more of an oasis than ever. As the land and vegetation continue to regenerate, encroaching brush may pose some challenges on this hike— check with the Forest Service for the latest trail conditions before you head out.

The Hike approaches the Ventana Wilderness from the east via rough and unpaved Tassajara Road. The route first follows Pine Ridge Trail from China Camp, rising and falling along an overgrown ridgeline punctuated by several excellent views. It then turns northwest at Church Creek Divide and slowly descends Carmel River Trail into the open terrain of Pine Valley. The route is ideal in spring and fall, when temperatures are moderate and storms infrequent. The winter months can be quite pleasant as

well, though freezing temperatures and strong storms occur at times. The heat, flies, and mosquitoes of summer are best avoided. No water is available at the trailhead. Poison oak is plentiful—be watchful.

To Reach the Trailhead From points north, follow Hwy. 1 to Carmel and take Carmel Valley Rd. (County Rd. G16) east for 23 miles to

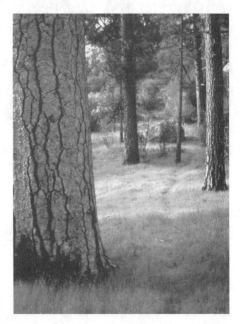

Ponderosa pines rise above the grasslands of Pine Valley.

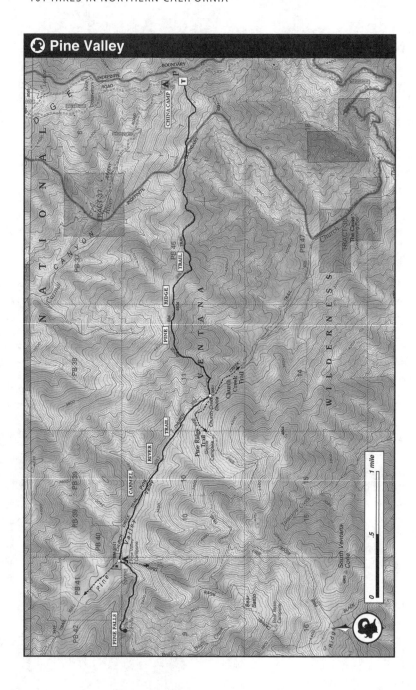

Pine Valley

Tassajara Rd. Turn right on Tassajara Rd., bear left in 1.3 miles at the fork with Cachagua Rd., and continue on Tassajara Rd. for another 10.7 miles to the China Camp entrance; the pavement ends 1.8 miles past the fork. Park at the large turnout across from the camp entrance. The trailhead is 100 feet farther south on the camp side of the road.

From points south, take Hwy. 101 to Greenfield and exit on Rte. 101 Business, the town's southernmost exit. Turn left on Elm Ave. (County Rd. G16) a half mile later and proceed 5.8 miles to Arroyo Seco Rd. (County Rd. G17). The two roads merge for 6.5 miles and then fork. Bear right and continue 17 miles on Carmel Valley Rd. to Tassajara Rd. Turn left and proceed as above.

Description From the marked trailhead (0.0/4,350'), Pine Ridge Trail gradually climbs 400 feet and then descends the same elevation through brush dominated by ceanothus and tan oak. After this scratchy welcome to the wilderness, you traverse steadily upward to emerge from the worst of the overgrown sections at the route's high point (0.6/4,750'). Views look south over the Church Creek and Tassajara Creek drainages, west toward the Coast Ridge, and southeast toward 5,862-foot Junipero Serra, which rises above the unseen Salinas Valley. Cone Peak (Hike 3) perches atop the farthest visible ridge to the south, 17 miles away.

The route cruises near the ridgeline through golden grasslands, charred forest, and thick new growth. Oak woodlands and stalks of Our Lord's candle, a large and easily distinguished yucca, punctuate the scenery as you next ascend and top a minor saddle before continuing upward to another, more prominent saddle. Views vanish briefly as the trail switchbacks southwest and then climbs north to the second highest point along the route (2.1/4,740'). From this point onward, it's all downhill to Pine Valley.

The trail turns southwest on a steep grade, dropping 850 feet through open woodlands carpeted with spring wildflowers. A final series of switchbacks deposits you at Church Creek Divide and a four-way trail junction (3.6/3,650'). The divide forms a deep saddle between two west-trending ridges and sits atop the 29-mile-long Church Creek Fault, a splinter fault of the greater San Andreas Fault system. The grinding faults of the area pulverize adjacent rock, which then erodes away to form distinctively straight valleys. Here the Church Creek Fault has created linear Church Creek canyon southeast of the divide, and the upper Carmel River valley (including Pine Valley) to the northwest.

The divide also separates the watersheds of the Carmel River, which has its headwaters in Pine Valley, and the Salinas River, which initially flows southwest before turning north, eventually entering the sea some 80 miles north of the Carmel River mouth.

From the divide, turn north and follow Carmel River Trail toward Pine Valley. The trail slowly descends, crossing over the usually dry headwaters of the Carmel River, and then eventually levels off. As the gradient eases, sandstone cliffs appear to your right, water trickles audibly off to your left, and ponderosa pines begin to rise from open meadows.

For thousands of years, Pine Valley was home to the Esselen people and provided them with fertile hunting, gathering, and living grounds. The Esselen may have used fire to clear underbrush and maintain the pine stands and broad meadow, where deer, rabbits, antelope, and even bears commonly grazed.

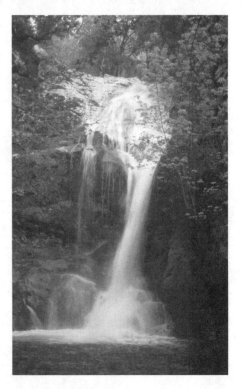

Hidden Pine Falls

In the adjacent forest, doves, quails, and other game birds flocked beneath the abundant canopy of oaks, bays, pines, and madrones. Wild roses grow in dense thickets on the east edge of the valley, perhaps cultivated by the Esselen for straight, strong arrow shafts. Beneath the sandstone cliffs, women took harvested acorns from the surrounding oak woodlands and ground the nutritious meat into flour. Their mortar holes still pepper sandstone outcrops just downstream from the Pine Valley–Pine Ridge Trail junction.

A large gate marks the official Pine Valley entrance (5.3/3,140') at a junction with the Pine Valley–Pine Ridge Trail and the route to Pine Falls. To make the trip to this waterfall oasis, be prepared for some hiking excitement—the 0.7-mile one-way journey follows a path that is narrow, overgrown, and washed out in a few precarious places. From the junction, turn left and cross the river. Head downstream a few yards and then recross the river past the first of three small unofficial campsites. The route now closely follows the river, crisscrossing it multiple times as it winds downstream through a lush riparian environment.

You eventually emerge at an overlook directly above 50-foot Pine Falls (6.0/2,700'). The descent to its base can be hazardous, as you must clamber across slick boulders. A conveniently placed rope may be available to help you negotiate the final 20 feet to the crystal clear pool. Enjoy a brisk plunge and then return the way you came.

Nearest Visitor Center King City Ranger Station, 831-385-5434, is located at 406 S. Mildred Ave. in King City. Take the Canal off-ramp from Hwy. 101, go east on Canal, right on Division, and left on Mildred. It's open Monday–Friday 8 a.m.–4:30 p.m.

Backpacking Information: Campsites and water are abundant in Pine Valley. A valid campfire permit is required.

Nearest Campground China Camp (9 sites, free) is adjacent to the trailhead. No water is available.

Additional Information www.fs.usda.gov/lpnf, ventanawild.org

HIKE 7 High Peaks Trail ○

Highlights	Monoliths of towering volcanic rock, prairie falcons, and California condors
Distance	5.3 miles
Total Elevation Gain/Loss	1,650'/1,650'
Hiking Time	3–4 hours
Recommended Map	USGS 7.5-min. *North Chalone Peak*
Best Times	October–May
Agency	Pinnacles National Park
Difficulty	★★★

THE STORY OF THE PINNACLES began some 28 million years ago when the Pacific tectonic plate first made contact with North America near present-day Los Angeles, and pushed an active underwater volcanic ridge beneath the continent. Widespread geologic havoc followed, and the first strands of the San Andreas Fault began forming. Shortly after this collision, 23.5 million years ago, rising magma escaped onto the surface through one of the many newly formed fractures and created a large, short-lived stratovolcano 24 miles long and roughly 8,000 feet high. Straddling the young San Andreas Fault, the volcano was quickly ripped in two as lands west of the fault were pushed northwest. The western half of the volcano was then tilted by associated splinter faults, protecting it from erosion until it was once again exposed at the surface. It slowly weathered to form the spectacularly unique peaks of the Pinnacles, 195 miles away from its eroded-rock counterpart in Southern California.

While numerous volcanic rocks compose the Pinnacles, the two most common (and easily identifiable) are volcanic breccia, a mess of angular fragments welded together into the reddish rocks of the High Peaks, and flow-banded rhyolite, a fine-grained lava that preserves its original flow patterns. Several excellent sources of information on the local geology are available at the visitor center, including a guide to the Pinnacles Geological Trail, the first half of which is along this hike.

The Hike climbs from Bear Gulch Nature Center along the Condor Gulch and High Peaks Trails, winding through wild volcanic formations before dropping steeply back down to Bear Gulch Picnic Area. The best time to come is February. You have to time your visit to avoid winter storms, but the reward is early wildflowers, crystalline air, flowing streams, green hillsides, and, most of all, solitude. The air, the water, and the green all remain from March through May—supplemented by a greater explosion of wildflowers—but the solitude vanishes, especially on weekends. An average of 400,000 people a year visit this small park, and most of them come during this time. In the summer months temperatures are sizzling and average almost 100°F during the day—don't bother. The fall is mild but brown and dry. Water is available at the trailhead.

To Reach the Trailhead Take Hwy. 25 South from Hollister for 35 miles to the posted turnoff for the Pinnacles on Hwy. 146. Approaching from the south, Hwy. 25 can be accessed from Hwy. 101 via Hwy. G13 at King City. Park in the nature center parking lot, 5 miles past the turnoff. The trailhead is across the road. While it is also possible to approach the Pinnacles (but not this hike) from the west through Soledad, there is no connection on Hwy. 146. There is an entrance fee of $10, which is valid for 7 days.

Description From the trailhead (0.0/1,650'), you begin climbing on the Condor Gulch Trail through large gray pines and deciduous blue oaks, quickly passing above a maintenance station. As you ascend, coast live oaks can be spotted in the riparian valley below. Toyon soon appears by the path, a shrub easily identified by its stiff, toothed, elliptical leaves and bright red berries, which first appear in December. At the first switchback, a rounded squat formation dubbed the Hippopotamus sits across the small gully. Looking like a stack of chips, Casino Rock is visible to the north. The trail then leads to an overlook where a small runnel of water gurgles down in season.

From the overlook, you leave the gulch behind and wrap around the ridge above you. Where the trail winds through open chaparral dominated by chamise, good views east of deeply furrowed San Benito Valley open up.

Views to the north appear as you intersect High Peaks Trail (1.7/2,290')—go left. This is a good place to start looking for California condors. Since 2003, the park has taken part in the California Condor Recovery Program. Several dozen juvenile condors have been released here in recent years and more than 60 currently live in the region. Look for these majestic—and enormous—endangered birds early in the morning and just after sunset. Also keep an eye out for prairie falcons. Every year from January through June, roughly a dozen pairs of these raptors nest in the cliffs of the Pinnacles and can often be seen swooping between the peaks. They are readily identified by their pointed wings, narrow tails, quick wingbeats, and distinctive cries.

Curving through massive boulders and outcrops, the trail then offers up views of the Balconies, a large, deeply sliced outcrop visible northwest. Reaching a junction with Tunnel Trail (2.3/2,480'), continue straight on High Peaks Trail to begin an exciting section where bolted iron railings provide handholds for steep

The volcanic jags of Pinnacles National Park

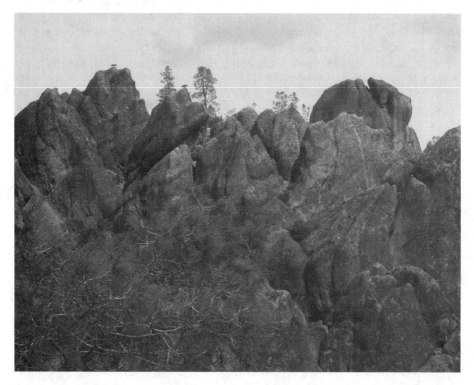

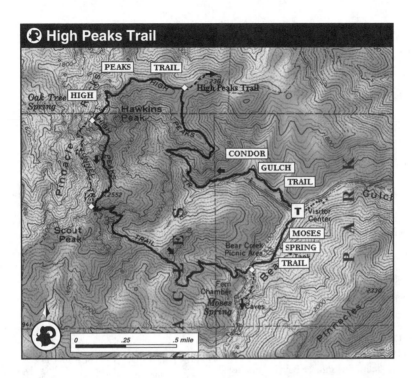

stairways whose steps are mere scoops in the rock. Passage is tight beneath Condor Crags, and descending those scoops is challenging; you soon reach a junction on the opposite side (3.0/2,470') where an outhouse is conveniently situated.

Keeping left on High Peaks Trail, you begin the steep switchbacking descent to Bear Gulch. You pass the aptly named Anvil along a brief level section before continuing down past large manzanitas to the junction with Rim Trail (4.5/1,600'). Descend left past Discovery Wall among handsome coast live oaks, and then go left again at the Moses Spring Trail junction (4.8/1,550') to quickly reach Bear Gulch Picnic area. Cross the road and follow the easy path back to the visitor center.

Nearest Visitor Center Pinnacles Visitor Center, in Pinnacles Campground, 831-389-4485, is open daily 9:30 a.m.–5 p.m.

Nearest Campground Pinnacles Campground (83 sites) is on Hwy. 146, near the park's eastern boundary; the fees are $23 per tent site for up to 6 people and $36 for RV sites with hook-ups. Reservations are recommended for weekends year-round; visit **recreation.gov** or call 877-444-6777.

Additional Information nps.gov/pinn

HIKE 8 Fremont Peak ⟋ 👥

Highlight	Superlative view of the entire Monterey Bay
Distance	1.0 mile
Total Elevation Gain/Loss	350'/350'
Hiking Time	1 hour
Recommended Map	USGS 7.5-min. *San Juan Bautista*
Best Times	After winter storms
Agency	Fremont Peak State Park
Difficulty	★

ATOP FREMONT PEAK on March 6, 1846, John C. Frémont defiantly raised the first American flag in California. Three days later, as he sat surrounded by Spanish forces threatening to attack, his flagpole blew down. Taking this as a bad omen, Frémont departed and left behind this unrivaled panorama of Monterey Bay.

The Hike is a quick and easy ascent of Fremont Peak (3,169'), a prominent summit due east from the center of Monterey Bay. Unparalleled views are the reason to come here, making it critical to correctly time your visit. The air is cleanest and the grass greenest immediately following winter storms, but air quality rapidly declines without rain and will usually begin to deteriorate within 24 hours. Prepare for chilly and windy conditions during the winter months. Fog can completely obliterate the view during the summer. Crowds are minimal, especially in the winter. Water is available in the nearby campground.

To Reach the Trailhead Take Hwy. 156 east of Hwy. 101 for 3 miles to San Juan Bautista and head south on the Alameda (Hwy. G1). Approaching from the east, the turnoff is 9 miles past the junction of Hwys. 156 and 25. Immediately bear left on San Juan Canyon Rd. (Hwy. G1) at the complex four-way intersection and proceed 11 miles to the upper parking lot at road's end. There is a nominal day-use fee.

Description From the trailhead, proceed up the paved road signed AUTHORIZED VEHICLES ONLY. A singletrack dirt trail quickly splits off across from a few, stout Coulter pines, passing through coyote brush punctuated by some valley oaks and small madrones. It wraps around the western slope where the antenna complex comes into view. A series of short switchbacks leads you to the rocky summit.

Savoring the view, ignore the antennas as you behold the curving expanse of Monterey Bay. Its southern arm is formed by the Monterey peninsula, visible beyond the city of Salinas. Its northern end contains south-facing Santa Cruz on its shores. Two main rivers drain into Monterey Bay: the longer Salinas River on the south, which flows 190 miles northwest through the broad Salinas Valley, and the Pajaro River on the north, which flows by Watsonville before entering the bay near its center. Between the two is Elkhorn Slough, a tidal embayment extending 7 miles inland whose mouth is marked by the enormous 500-foot-high boiler stacks of the Moss Landing Power Plant. The slough is a haven for birdlife—it once held the North American record for the most bird species seen from a single location in one day (116). The broad alluvial plain around Monterey Bay is rich agricultural land and annually produces the country's largest crop of artichokes.

Immediately offshore of Elkhorn Slough is the beginning of Monterey Canyon, California's deepest submarine canyon. Twisting slightly southwest, it reaches a depth of 6,000 feet less than 15 miles from the shore, almost twice the elevation of Fremont Peak, which is 16 miles from the shore. To create so deep a

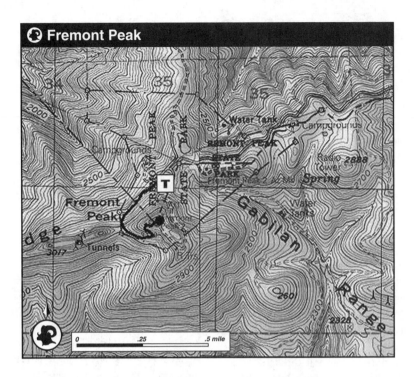

submarine canyon requires erosive power far greater than that provided by the current rivers that flow into Monterey Bay. To explain its origin, theory holds that in the recent geologic past (up to 5 million years ago) a large amount of California water drained through present-day Monterey Bay unhindered by any Coast Ranges, carving a deep offshore canyon over the course of millions of years. As the San Andreas Fault system moved Monterey Bay north, the rising Coast Ranges limited its drainage basin to its current watershed. Cold water upwelling from March through September funnels nutrient-rich waters up Monterey Canyon, providing sustenance for the incredible diversity of sea life that makes Monterey Bay world famous.

Nearest Visitor Center There is no staffed visitor center. Call 831-623-4255 for general information. An astronomical observatory near the summit offers public programs; call 831-623-2465 or visit **fpoa.net.**

Nearest Campground Fremont Peak State Park Campground (25 sites, $25) is below the summit and is lightly used except on the busiest weekends. For reservations visit **reserve america.com** or call 800-444-7275.

Additional Information www.parks.ca.gov

HIKE 9 Coit Lake ♻🚶

Highlights	Ridges, lakes, and remote adventure on the edge of the Bay Area
Distance	12.4 miles round-trip
Total Elevation Gain/Loss	3,800'/3,800'
Hiking Time	6–10 hours
Recommended Maps	*Henry W. Coe State Park Trail and Camping Map* by Pine Ridge Association, USGS 7.5-min. *Gilroy Hot Springs*
Best Times	December–May
Agency	Henry W. Coe State Park
Difficulty	★★★★

IN HENRY COE STATE PARK, the largest state park in Northern California, the towering bulwark of Wasno Ridge guards the approach to the southern backcountry, where a furrowed land of ridges, valleys, and solitude awaits the stalwart hiker. In 1775–76, a Spanish expedition led by Juan Bautista de Anza attempted (and failed) to find a route through this convoluted region. The Spaniards dubbed this area "Sierra del Chasco" ("Mountains of Deception"); they would be the last Europeans to visit the area for nearly a hundred years.

Today wide fire roads and clearly marked trails make navigation far easier—but the steep terrain is as taxing as ever. Wasno Ridge rises more than 1,500 feet above the trailhead, a heart-pumping obstacle that keeps hiking traffic to a minimum. Beyond it lie small Kelly Lake and larger Coit Lake, the second biggest in the park, as well as extensive views across the rumpled terrain.

In September 2007, a large wildfire scorched 40,000 acres within Henry Coe, including most of the park's eastern half. Known as the Lick Fire, the conflagration reached as far west as Coit Lake, where you can still find evidence of the blaze. The damage was not cataclysmic—most of the park's oak trees survived the blaze—but trails and large swaths of the landscape in the burned areas were significantly affected. Wildfires are a natural part of the park's ecosystem, and the backcountry is rapidly recovering, a process on full display around Coit Lake.

The Hike begins from the Coyote Creek Trailhead on Coe's southwestern edge, steeply ascends Wasno Ridge on singletrack trails, and then follows old ranch roads past Kelly Lake and over another ridge to Coit Lake. The return route follows a series of more gradual trails down the flanks of Wasno Ridge. The open terrain of oak woodland and chaparral provides excellent views throughout. Bass and crappie are abundant in both lakes for anglers. Water is usually available from Coyote Creek at the trailhead, and from several springs and ponds en route (a filter is strongly recommended). The hike can be completed year-round (Kelly and Coit lakes are reliable water sources), but the baking heat, shadeless slopes, and increasingly funky water make this a less attractive option in summer and fall.

To Reach the Trailhead Take the Leavesley Rd. exit from Hwy. 101 in Gilroy and follow it 1.8 miles east to New Ave. Turn left, follow New Ave. 0.6 mile to Roop Rd., and turn right. Follow Roop Rd., which becomes Gilroy Hot Springs Rd. and reaches Coyote Creek County Park on the left in 3 miles. You pass Hunting Hollow Trailhead 3 miles later on the right and reach the Coyote Creek Trailhead 1.7 miles farther at a bridge. There is an $8 day-use fee.

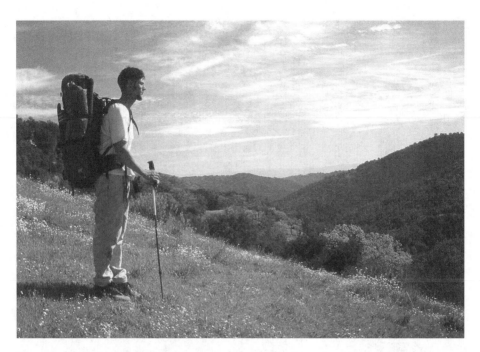

Above the Coyote Creek watershed

Description From the trailhead (0.0/940'), begin down wide Coit Rd. The route initially parallels the creek and quickly meets Grizzly Gulch Trail (your return route) on the right (0.1/960'). Continue on Coit Rd. as it begins a slow climb, passes a fenced cattle-loading enclosure, and encounters large, big-berry manzanita shortly before reaching a high point. You descend briefly past valley oak and a giant rusting water tank to reach Anza Trail on the right (1.0/1,090'), where an interpretive sign highlights the 1775–76 Spanish expedition. Nearby Woodchopper Spring is a dependable water source for much of the year.

Turn uphill on Anza Trail, following the singletrack path as it passes beneath bay trees and coast live oaks and switchbacks upward to reach Cullen Trail on the right (1.6/1,440'). Bear left to remain on Anza Trail, which now traverses open slopes flush with spring wildflowers to reach the junction with Jackson Trail (1.9/1,560')—turn right to head toward Kelly Lake.

Views expand as you ascend Jackson Trail. Looking north, Pine Ridge and the main park entrance area (Hike 10) are visible 6 miles away—the tall and distinctive ponderosa pines that give the ridge its name can be identified on clear days. Beyond, Lick Observatory can be spotted atop Mount Hamilton (4,213'). As the trail attains the Wasno ridgeline, views reach as far south as 3,171-foot Fremont Peak (Hike 8) and beyond to the Santa Lucia Range of Big Sur.

The trail passes two small ponds and reaches the junction for seasonally dribbling Elderberry Spring (3.3/2,360'), widening to become Jackson Rd. Hugging the ridgeline, the route passes a four-way junction for Rock Tower Trail (3.7/2,520') shortly before attaining the ridge's highest point (2,676'). Jackson Rd. now begins a slow descent past hidden Spring Trail on the left (4.2/2,630'), then banks sharply left to reach Wasno Rd. (4.7/2,420'). Turn right and briefly follow the road to Kelly Lake Trail on the left (4.9/2,420').

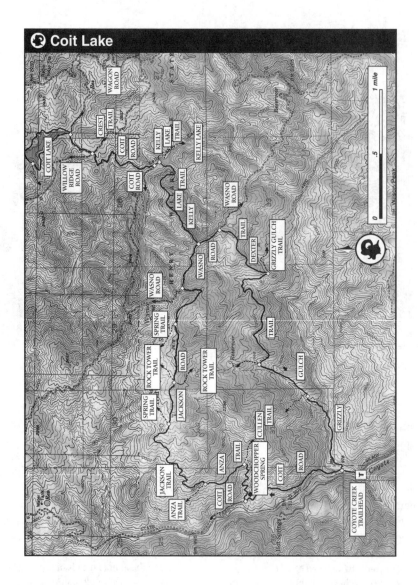

Coit Lake

Follow Kelly Lake Trail as it undulates through pleasant blue oak woodlands, then plummets down shadier slopes. The lake itself remains hidden from view until the very end, when the trail deposits you on the dam enclosing the northern shore. Steep and brushy slopes make accessing the lake difficult; try the area above the lake's south end.

Continuing on to Coit Lake, the route bears left at the northern end of the dam and then turns right on wide Coit Rd. by an outhouse

(5.9/1,880'). Coit Rd. climbs through a lush environment of oaks, bay trees, and buckeye and then traverses across more open chaparral slopes. You crest Willow Ridge between Kelly and Coit Lakes at a four-way junction with Willow Ridge Rd. (6.7/2,240'). From this point, you can look east across land singed by the 2007 Lick Fire. Continue straight on Coit Rd. as it descends to Coit Lake's reedy southern shore (7.0/2,080').

After savoring Coit Lake, retrace your steps back to Kelly Lake Trail and its junction with

Wasno Rd. (9.1/2,420'). Bear left on Wasno Rd. and then quickly turn right on Dexter Trail (9.3/2,420'), which descends through open blue oak woodlands and then drops steeply to reach the unsigned junction with Grizzly Gulch Trail (9.9/1,940'). Turn right on Grizzly Gulch Trail, traversing a moist creek gully and contouring across shady slopes to pass Rock Tower Trail on the right (10.9/1,740').

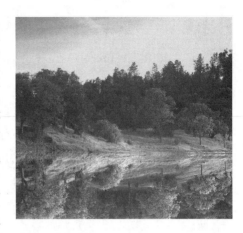

Contemplate Coe.

From here, Grizzly Gulch Trail descends above a narrow creek gully, where the moist environment nourishes lush valley oak, buckeye, and madrone. As you approach the canyon bottom, you pass the junction for indistinct Cullen Trail on the right (11.4/1,270'). After crossing Grizzly Gulch Creek, the trail ascends and contours the slopes, passing Spike Jones Trail on the left (12.1/1,060') and returning to Coit Rd. (12.3/960'). Turn left to return to the trailhead (12.4/940').

Nearest Visitor Center A self-service station at Hunting Hollow Trailhead is occasionally staffed on weekends. The main visitor center, 408-779-2728, is located at the park entrance at the end of East Dunne Ave. in Morgan Hill, a long drive from this trailhead. It is open Friday–Sunday 8 a.m.–4 p.m. year-round, with later hours during busy periods in spring and summer, and is open sporadically Monday–Thursday.

Backpacking Information A backcountry permit is required and can be obtained at the Hunting Hollow Trailhead. There is a permit fee of $5 per person per night and a parking fee of $8 per vehicle per night. Camping is prohibited within a half mile of the trailhead but is permitted everywhere else along this hike. Campfires are prohibited. A few established sites and outhouses can be found around Coit and Kelly Lakes. The park recommends leaving your vehicle at Hunting Hollow Trailhead; vandalism and theft have been reported at Coyote Creek.

Nearest Campground Coyote Lake–Harvey Bear Ranch County Park (73 sites, $24) is 5 miles from the trailhead on Gilroy Hot Springs Rd.; call 408-355-4201 for reservations or visit **parkhere.org**.

Additional Information www.parks.ca.gov, coepark.net

HIKE 10 Coyote Creek ⟳ 🚶

Highlights	Deep canyons and oak woodlands in Northern California's largest state park
Distance	12.1 miles
Total Elevation Gain/Loss	2,500'/2,500'
Hiking Time	6–10 hours
Agency	Henry W. Coe State Park
Recommended Maps	*Henry W. Coe State Park Trail and Camping Map* by Pine Ridge Association, USGS 7.5-min. *Mount Sizer, Mississippi Creek*
Best Times	February–May
Difficulty	★★★

HERE ARE GENTLE RIDGETOPS, steep canyons, gurgling creeks, 700 different plants, 137 species of birds, a radiant profusion of spring wildflowers, and immortal words etched on the monument to Henry W. Coe—"May these quiet hills bring peace to the souls of those who are seeking."

The largest state park in Northern California, Henry W. Coe State Park encompasses 85,000 acres (more than 130 square miles) and protects a diversity of plant and animal life, including coyotes, bobcats, foxes, black-tailed deer, feral pigs, mountain lions, and abundant birdlife. Complete checklists are available at the visitor center.

In September 2007, a large wildfire scorched 40,000 acres within Henry Coe, including most of the park's eastern half. Known as the Lick Fire, the conflagration reached the northern edge of this hike; evidence of the blaze is readily apparent today in several spots. The damage was not cataclysmic—most of the park's oak trees survived the blaze—but trails and large swaths of the landscape were significantly affected in the burned areas. Wildfires are a natural part of the park's ecosystem, and the backcountry is rapidly recovering, a process on full display in the areas north of Poverty Flat and Los Cruzeros Trail Camps.

The Hike begins from the main park entrance, cruises along diverse Pine Ridge, and then plummets more than a thousand feet to a year-round swimming hole in Coyote Creek. After winding through the Narrows, a thin creek-carved gap, the hike reaches idyllic Los Cruzeros Trail Camp along the babbling creekside. The journey returns via Poverty Flat Road, winding over the open hillsides of Jackass Peak, passing Middle Fork Coyote Creek, and then climbing steeply back up Pine Ridge. The hike can be shortened by more than 2 miles by using Creekside Trail between Poverty Flat and China Hole on Creekside Trail.

To Reach the Trailhead Take Hwy. 101 to Morgan Hill and take the East Dunne Ave. exit. Follow East Dunne Ave. east for 11 miles to the visitor center parking lot at the road's end. After leaving the residential area of Morgan Hill, the road is a narrow twisting ascent—RVs and trailers are not recommended. There is an $8 day-use fee.

Description The hike begins across from the visitor center on singletrack Corral Trail (0.0/2,650'). After crossing a small bridge, the trail contours above precipitous slopes in a lush world of black oak, bay trees, buckeye, snowberry bushes, and coast live oak. Soon you encounter the first big-berry manzanita of the trip. Dozens of manzanita varieties exist, but few approach the massive size of these specimens; their twisting, blood-red trunks are almost tree-like in girth. Chamise, toyon, and honeysuckle

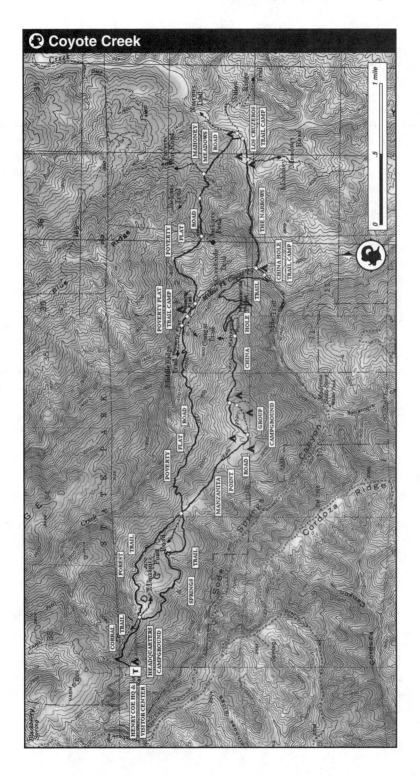

⊘ Coyote Creek

vines—common members of the park's chaparral community—appear alongside.

The path emerges onto open hillsides graced with large valley oaks and reaches a six-way junction at Manzanita Point Rd. (0.6/2,510'). Cross the wide road, grab an interpretive brochure from the post, and continue on Forest Trail. Numbered markers line the path and correspond to the brochure's descriptions of the park's flora. After contouring through this shady educational world, you rejoin Manzanita Point Rd. (1.8/2,330') at its junction with Springs Trail and Poverty Flat Rd.

Bear left on wide Manzanita Point Rd. and undulate along the ridgetop past valley oak and ponderosa pine. The road tours the pleasant Manzanita Group Camps and reaches the junction for China Hole and Madrone Spring Trails just past Sites 6 and 7 (2.6/2,260'). Turn left on China Hole Trail to begin the descent.

China Hole Trail contours below the last group sites (a spur trail splits right to Site 9) and then dives through a corridor of massive bigberry manzanita. You next emerge in an area burned by prescribed fire (a posted sign tells the story) where thick chamise and buckbrush thrive on the regenerating hillside. Good views open up of the Coyote Creek watershed and its multiple drainages below.

The trail encounters Manzanita Point and the junction with Cougar Trail (3.7/1,910'), where you continue straight on China Hole Trail to begin a series of long, descending switchbacks to the canyon bottom and the junction with Mile Trail (5.2/1,150'). China Hole Trail Camp and its year-round swimming hole await a short distance upstream. In summer and fall, this stream is the only reliable water source on the hike, so fill your bottles.

Continuing, proceed upstream to quickly reach the confluence of Coyote Creek's Middle Fork (left) and East Fork (right). Here Creekside Trail splits off to connect with Poverty Flat Trail Camp via the Middle Fork, a shorter return option. To complete the full loop, bear right up the East Fork and enter the lush world of the Narrows. There is no officially maintained trail through the Narrows, but a use path is generally obvious as it closely parallels the creek. This route requires crossing the stream in several places, and, depending on season and flow, this can be a rock-hop or knee-deep ford. In times of heavy rains the Narrows may become impassable—use caution.

Profuse spring wildflowers color the ground in this canyon environment, and soon you reach wide Mahoney Meadows Rd. and the start of Los Cruzeros Trail Camp near the confluence of East Fork Coyote and Kelly Creeks (6.2/1,230'). Bear left on Mahoney Meadows Rd. and cross the creek near the junction with Willow Ridge Trail (6.3/1,230'), a short distance upstream.

Follow wide Mahoney Meadows Rd. as it climbs steeply through open woodlands and then turn left onto broad Poverty Flat Rd. (6.8/1,620'). Remain on Poverty Flat Rd. as it ascends to reach Jackass Trail (7.0/1,790') before descending to a saddle below Jackass Peak (1,784'). A short side trip leads to the level summit and its near-360-degree views. Poverty Flat Rd. plummets past this point to meet Middle Fork Coyote Creek and Creekside Trail (8.2/1,150') arriving from China Hole. The wide streambed of sycamores is a pleasant backdrop to nearby Poverty Flat Trail Camp, which was used as a primary staging area during the Lick Fire.

Poverty Flat Rd. meanders among the camp's five sites and junctions for Cougar and Middle Ridge Trails, then begins a steady thousand-foot ascent along the flanks of Pine Ridge. Poverty Flat Rd. contours gently and ascends steeply for short, strenuous sections until an intense switchbacking climb at the end deposits you back atop Pine Ridge at the earlier junction with Manzanita Point Rd. (10.2/2,330'). Return to the trailhead on the road or via Springs Trail, which travels along the margin of open oak woodland and past several dribbling springs to reach Corral Trail (11.5/2,510') and the final section back to the visitor center (12.1/2,650').

Nearest Visitor Center The park visitor center, 408-779-2728, is open Friday–Sunday 8 a.m.–4 p.m. year-round with later hours during busy periods in spring and summer. It's open sporadically Monday–Thursday.

Backpacking Information Backcountry camping is permitted at China Hole, Poverty Flat, and Los Cruzeros Trail Camps. A permit is required and must be obtained the day of your departure. All permits are first come, first served—no reservations are accepted—though space is almost always available. There is a permit fee of $5 per person per night and a parking fee of $8 per vehicle per night. Campfires are prohibited.

Nearest Campgrounds Headquarters Campground (20 sites, $20) is below the visitor center and fills up most weekends in spring and summer. Large groups can also consider the Manzanita Group Camping Area (9 sites, $75), 2 miles from the visitor center. For reservations, visit **reserveamerica.com** or call 800-444-7275.

Additional Information www.parks.ca.gov, coepark.net

HIKE 11 Sunol Backpack Area ○ 🚶 🐕

Highlight	A hidden oak woodland oasis
Distance	5.9 miles
Total Elevation Gain/Loss	1,100'/1,100'
Hiking Time	3–5 hours
Recommended Maps	*Sunol Regional Wilderness Park Map* by East Bay Regional Park District, USGS 7.5-min. *La Costa Valley*
Best Times	February–May
Agency	Sunol Regional Wilderness, East Bay Regional Park District
Difficulty	★★

SHIELDED FROM VIEW behind landmark Mission Peak, peaceful Sunol Wilderness offers escape in beautiful rolling woodlands. An idyllic backcountry camping area is located at the hike's midpoint, a tranquil spot and a wonderful way to extend your visit.

The Hike explores the multifaceted character of Sunol Wilderness, passing through majestic oak woodlands, walking open hillsides, and pausing at substantial Alameda Creek as it rushes through a scenic section dubbed "Little Yosemite." This hike can be completed year-round, but spring is the time to come as

hillsides are carpeted green, wildflowers are in bloom, and temperatures are most ideal. Cows graze throughout the park, creating a pleasant manicured landscape full of cow-pie minefields. Crowds around Little Yosemite can be heavy, especially on weekends, but the rest of the trails are more peaceful. Poison oak and stinging nettle are ubiquitous and unfriendly companions on this hike—be watchful. Water is available at the trailhead.

To Reach the Trailhead Take Hwy. 680 east of Fremont to the Calaveras Rd. exit and proceed south on Calaveras Rd. for 4.3 miles to

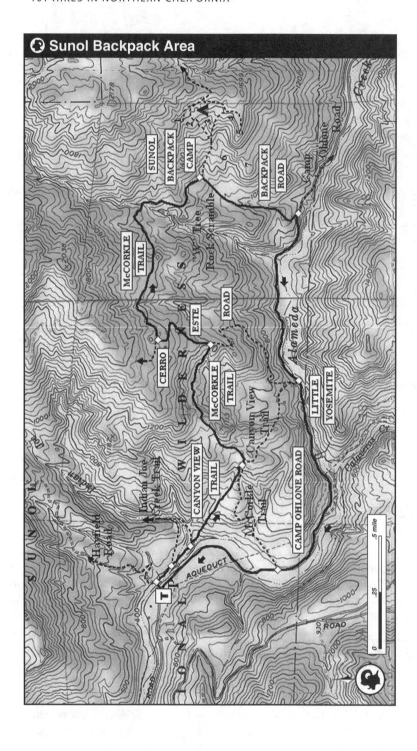

⊙ Sunol Backpack Area

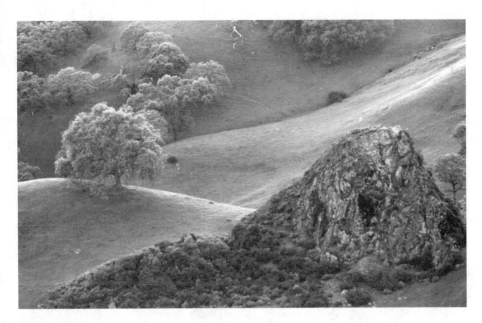

Sweet Sunol

Geary Rd. Turn left on Geary Rd., reaching the visitor center parking lot and trailhead in 1.9 miles. There is a day-use fee of $5 per vehicle, plus $2 per dog.

Description From the trailhead (0.0/410'), head to the wooden bridge over Alameda Creek and pause to admire the babbling waters. The largest watershed in the East Bay, Alameda Creek drains more than 700 square miles. Here it nourishes the mottled, smooth gray trunks and twisting branches of California sycamores, which line the streambed. With their broad leaves, sycamore trees can lose up to 50 gallons of water per day and grow only where such large volumes are available.

Cross the bridge, bear right on the wide path, and continue straight on Canyon View Trail as it quickly passes junctions on the left for Hayfield Rd., Indian Joe Nature Trail, and Indian Joe Creek Trail. Canyon View Trail soon climbs away from the creek and into a drier environment populated by blue oaks, the most drought-tolerant of all oaks. Easily recognized, their leaves are shallowly lobed with smooth margins. You pass through one of numerous

cattle gates to come (always leave them as you find them) and reach a four-way intersection with McCorkle Trail (0.7/700').

Turn left on McCorkle Trail and follow the overgrown path as it climbs the ridgeline and then turns east to traverse through chaparral. This low-lying and shrubby community flourishes in arid environments and is regularly seen throughout the hike. Its common constituents include coyote brush, toyon, sticky monkey-flower, bracken fern, coffeeberry, and plenty of poison oak. Valley oak also begins to appear along this section, identified by its 2- to 4-inch deeply lobed leaves.

The trail passes beneath some huge coast live oaks and reaches the junction with wide Cerro Este Rd. (1.7/1,180'). Bear left, make a steady uphill climb on Cerro Este Rd., and then bear right to return to singletrack McCorkle Trail (2.1/1,430'). Traversing steadily across open slopes, the route offers outstanding views of Mission Peak to the west, and south toward Calaveras Reservoir, the upper Alameda Creek watershed, and the more distant peaks of the Diablo Range. The trail makes a steep, switch-backing drop into the "W" Tree Rock Scramble and then continues its traverse to reach Backpack Rd. (3.4/1,150') and the gated edge of Sunol Backpack Camp. The camp's pleasant sites and potable water (above Site 3) make for a pleasant layover.

Continuing, follow wide Backpack Rd. as it steadily descends to Camp Ohlone Rd. (4.0/800'), where you turn right to begin your tour alongside nearby Alameda Creek. It's an easy cruise along this wide thoroughfare to Little Yosemite (4.5/450'). With a rushing river coursing through a small gorge over boulders blue and green, Little Yosemite is a pretty sight. From here, continue on level Camp Ohlone Rd. to rejoin the park road at the upper parking lot (5.5/420'). Watch for gray pine, California buckeye, and the reappearance of coast live oak and California bay along this final section. Walk the road to return to the visitor center (5.9/410').

Nearest Visitor Center The park visitor center is open Thursday–Sunday 10 a.m.–4 p.m. For general information, call 510-544-3249.

Backpacking Information Backcountry camping is permitted only in Sunol Backpack Area. Seven campsites ($5 per person per night and a one-time reservation fee of $8) are available and must be reserved at least 5 working days in advance by calling the East Bay Regional Park District reservation office at 888-327-2757, 8:30 a.m.–4 p.m. Monday–Friday. Fires and dogs are prohibited in the backpack area. Water is sometimes available depending on conditions.

Nearest Campground Sunol Wilderness has 4 drive-in campsites, but they are closed through at least 2016 while the Calaveras Reservoir is undergoing improvements. Check with the park for current information.

Additional Information ebparks.org/parks/sunol

Calaveras Reservoir is visible in the distance.

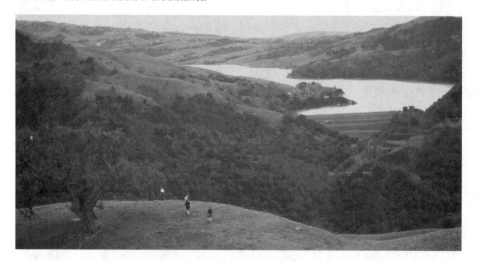

HIKE 12 Coyote Hills ⟳ ⛺ 🚶

Highlight	Shorebird paradise
Distance	2.5 miles
Total Elevation Gain/Loss	400'/400'
Hiking Time	1–2 hours
Recommended Maps	*Coyote Hills Regional Park* by East Bay Regional Park District, USGS 7.5-min. *San Leandro*
Best Times	December–May
Agency	Coyote Hills Regional Park, East Bay Regional Park District
Difficulty	★

A GRASSY SWELL IN the flatlands, Coyote Hills exists almost in the center of south San Francisco Bay. Protected marshlands enhance the unique perspective and offer a rich assortment of wildlife.

For thousands of years, the Ohlone Indians occupied the region around Coyote Hills, harvesting oysters, clams, mussels, cockles, and abalone from the extensive Bay mudflats; salmon, seals, sea lions, sea otters, and sturgeon from the water; and deer, elk, antelope, and rabbit from the surrounding hills. Using tule reeds from the vast marshlands, they constructed small boats for paddling in the bay. We know all this because four substantial middens still exist in Coyote Hills Regional Park. Middens—also referred to as shell mounds—are large piles of accumulated debris, the "kitchen wastes" of the Ohlone. Shells, bones, trinkets, and other discarded materials forming these large piles have shed a great deal of light on the Ohlone lifestyle.

With the arrival of the Spanish, it all came to an end. Disease and the mission system decimated the Indian population, and by the 19th century, salt evaporation ponds and ranch lands began to surround Coyote Hills, all but eliminating the vast marshlands. Having passed through various owners, the ranch land that included Coyote Hills and a large remaining segment of marsh was purchased by the East Bay Regional Park District in 1967. Today it provides an excellent opportunity to imagine the bay as it was before the Europeans came.

Wildlife still abounds in this ecological oasis. At least 210 species of birds have been spotted in the park, including a variety of herons, egrets, owls, pheasants, hawks, and shorebirds. More than 30 different mammals also exist in the park, mostly small rodents hunted by foxes, weasels, and raptors.

The Hike connects several short segments of trail to form a loop, passing first along the marsh before returning via Red Hill (291'). Expansive hilltop views can only be enjoyed immediately after a winter storm has cleansed the thick South Bay air; move fast—air quality begins to deteriorate within 24 hours. The hills are velvety green from January through May, turning brown in summer and fall when the skies fill with haze. Water is available at the trailhead.

To Reach the Trailhead Take Hwy. 84 to the east side of the Dumbarton Bridge and exit at Paseo Padre Pkwy. Head north on Paseo Padre for 1 mile and turn left onto Patterson Ranch Rd., following it for 1.5 miles to the visitor center at road's end. There is a $5 entrance fee per vehicle. The park opens at 8 a.m. and closes at sunset.

Description From the visitor center parking lot, go through the gate and take the paved Bayview Trail, skirting the edge of the marsh partly shaded by small willow and sycamore trees. A chittering of birds and croaking of frogs keep you company. The trail passes a few Monterey pines before reaching the junction for Lizard Rock Trail at the far end of the marsh—go right

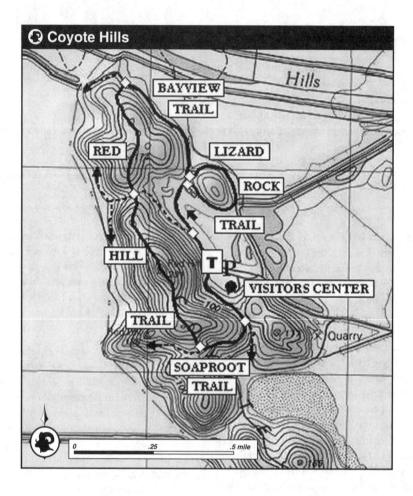

toward the red rock outcrop. This outcrop is Franciscan chert, formed from the silica-rich skeletons of microscopic sea creatures that collected on the ocean floor over millions of years. All of Coyote Hills is composed of this chert, which gains its red color from trace amounts of iron. Highly resistant to erosion, chert has withstood the elements while the surrounding area eroded and became covered with thick layers of mud and silt washed down from the hills. In a sea of mud, Coyote Hills is an isolated island of bedrock.

Stay by the marsh and loop east around the small hill before returning to Bayview Trail, passing a many-branched coast live oak along the way. Continuing on the paved path, you soon reach a junction where another paved trail splits right for the Alameda Creek Trail. Here you go left up dirt Red Hill Trail, climbing steeply to the top of the first hill before dropping down to a junction with Nike Trail, named for the Nike missile site that was situated on these hills between 1955 and 1959 to protect the United States from Communist invasion. Continuing straight, the trail ascends Red Hill, high point of the park, where your best views are had. Descending Red Hill, return to the visitor center by bearing left on Soaproot Trail and left again on wide Quail Trail.

Nearest Visitor Center Coyote Hills Visitor Center, 510-544-3220, is open Wednesday–Sunday 10 a.m.–4 p.m.

Additional Information ebparks.org/parks/coyote_hills

HIKE 13 Bob Walker Ridge ↻ 🐕

Highlight	Remote Diablo Range wandering
Distance	5.8 miles
Total Elevation Gain/Loss	850'/850'
Hiking Time	3–4 hours
Recommended Maps	*Morgan Territory Regional Preserve* by East Bay Regional Park District, USGS 7.5-min. *Tassajara*
Best Times	October–May
Agency	Morgan Territory Regional Preserve
Difficulty	★★

DEEP IN THE FURROWS of the Diablo Range, Morgan Territory Regional Preserve protects a little-trod landscape of rolling hills, oak-studded grasslands, and quality views. On many days, your only companions will be the looming massif of nearby Mount Diablo, the nodding blooms of spring wildflowers, and the many cows that graze the grassy woodlands.

The park gets its name from Jeremiah Morgan, an early pioneer who settled here in 1857 and hunted grizzly bears in the surrounding hills. The East Bay Regional Park District acquired the first parcel here in 1976, expanding its holdings during the 1980s and early 1990s to nearly 5,000 acres. Today old ranch structures belie the area's past; mountain lions, golden eagles, and a variety of other wildlife proclaim its future.

The Hike loops through the east half of the preserve, descending first along a shady creek corridor before circling around through oak woodland and open grasslands on a series of wide fire roads. The trip reaches its northernmost point below Bob Walker Ridge, where excellent views of Mount Diablo can be enjoyed from idyllic picnic spots. Water is available at the trailhead.

To Reach the Trailhead Take Interstate 580 to the North Livermore Ave. exit, head north on North Livermore Ave. for 4 miles, and turn right on Morgan Territory Rd., 0.5 mile beyond the point where North Livermore Ave. curves west and becomes Manning Rd. Follow twisting and one-lane Morgan Territory Rd. 5.5 miles to the signed trailhead on the right.

Description From the trailhead (0.0/2,030'), look for Mount Diablo to the north, your regular companion and landmark throughout the hike. To begin the journey, head out past the weathered ranch buildings and immediately bear left on singletrack Coyote Trail. The open grassland begins its transition to woodland and you soon pass the hike's first oak on your left. Parasitic clumps of mistletoe dangle from the branches of this large valley oak; recognize the tree by its large, deeply lobed leaves. Continue left on Coyote Trail as Condor Trail (your return route) splits off to the right (0.1/2,000').

The trail winds past a small pond and beneath twisting coast live oaks, which can be

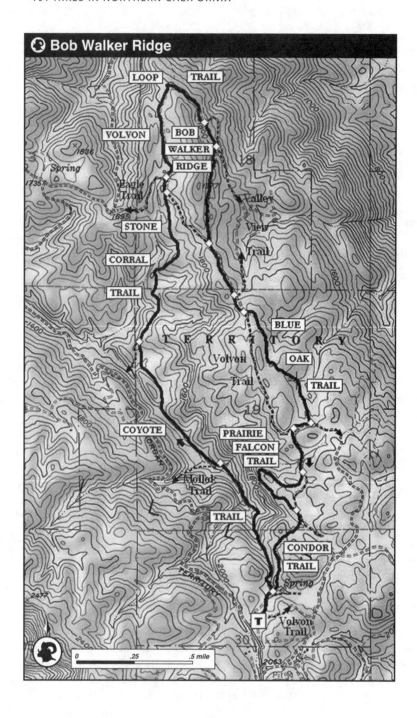

◔ Bob Walker Ridge

identified by their spiny leaves that bend under at the margins. The route drops steeply into a shady ravine populated by mossy bay trees and small oaks. Maidenhair ferns line the moist north-facing slopes. During the descent, you regularly cruise along the edge of two ecosystems. The drier world of blue oaks and manzanita is visible just above, while buckeyes, black oaks, and bigleaf maples grow in the lush environment below.

The occasional switchback leads you past Mollok Trail on the left (0.9/1,520'). Watch for baseball-sized buckeye seeds littering the ground as the gradient eases in the ever-wider drainage. Mature blue oaks cling to the hillside above you. Recognize these drought-deciduous trees by their smaller leaves and smooth, wavy leaf margins. The mottled trunks of a few sycamore trees appear in the creekbed below as the trail curves right to leave the drainage and crosses through a gate into open fields. The trail initially runs along a barbed wire fence but quickly becomes indistinct—traverse upward toward the right side of the field to reach Stone Corral Trail near the top (1.6/1,480').

Bear right on the wide dirt road and gently rise through blue oak woodlands, soon passing through another gate. You steadily traverse upward, passing numerous sandstone outcrops, before curving left to reach the junction with Volvon Loop Trail (2.3/1,780'). Follow Volvon Loop Trail, which immediately passes Eagle Trail on the left and then a small cattle pond ringed with cattails. The hike now cruises along the fields below Bob Walker Ridge; several use paths branch right to attain its rocky and tree-studded prow. A strong advocate for land protection, Bob Walker was a prolific photographer and played a major role in the expansion of Morgan Territory. He died in 1992 at the age of 40, but his 30,000 images of the East Bay region continue to inspire.

Near the end of the ridge, a pleasant knoll offers exceptional views northwest of the twin summits of Mount Diablo (Hike 14). The view northeast stretches toward the Delta area, where the Sacramento and San Joaquin rivers merge in a broad wetland area. The cities of

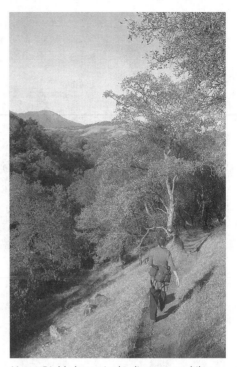

Mount Diablo looms in the distance as a hiker heads into Morgan Territory.

Antioch and Pittsburg line its shores. A collection of wind turbines marks the low rise of Grizzly Island near the confluence of these two mighty rivers.

Continuing, the trail wraps around the ridge, heads south, and crosses shadier, more tree-covered slopes. Intermittent views look southeast toward Los Vaqueros Reservoir. Remain on Volvon Loop Trail as Valley View Trail splits left (3.0/1,770'), followed shortly by a connecting path. The trail climbs briefly, levels out in nice blue oak woodlands, and reaches another junction (3.5/1,840'). Continue straight on Volvon Trail, which passes the south junction for Valley View Trail on the left (3.8/1,840') and then quickly forks. Bear left on Blue Oak Trail, which undulates through shady and mature forest punctuated by twisting snags and other crusty specimens. Bear right on Hummingbird Trail (4.5/1,960') to quickly return to Volvon Trail, where you turn left.

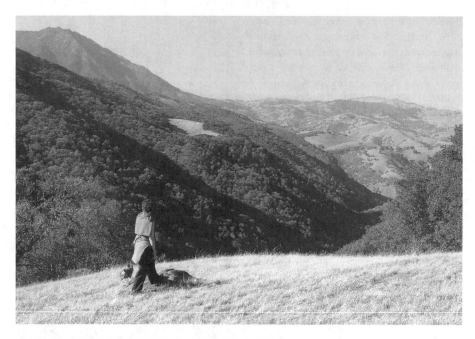

Looking north toward Mount Diablo and its eastern foothills

The trail now encounters a scrubby chaparral community, highlighted by the appearance of thick chamise, and soon reaches Prairie Falcon Trail on the right (4.8/1,960'). This short side loop is a worthwhile diversion, a singletrack path that winds over to a good vista down-valley before returning to Volvon Trail (5.3/1,970'). Bear right and quickly right again on Condor Trail, which rises briefly before descending to the earlier junction with Coyote Trail (5.7/2,000') by the trailhead.

Nearest Visitor Center This preserve doesn't have a visitor center. For general information, try 510-544-3060 or the visitor center at Black Diamond Mines Regional Preserve, 925-544-2750.

Nearest Campgrounds Mount Diablo State Park has 3 year-round campgrounds with a total of 56 sites. Juniper Campground, the largest, is along Summit Rd.; small Junction Campground is by park headquarters; and Live Oak Campground can be found on Mount Diablo Scenic Rd./South Gate Rd. (all campgrounds $30). Reservations are recommended for weekends; visit **reserveamerica.com** or call 800-444-7275.

Additional Information ebparks.org/parks/morgan

HIKE 14 Mount Diablo ⟳ 👫

Highlight	Viewpoint for much of Northern California
Distance	0.7 mile
Total Elevation Gain/Loss	100'/100'
Hiking Time	1 hour
Recommended Maps	*Mount Diablo, Los Vaqueros, and Surrounding Parks* by Save Mount Diablo, USGS 7.5-min. *Clayton*
Best Times	After storms
Agency	Mount Diablo State Park
Difficulty	★

DOMINATING THE landscape, Mount Diablo offers vistas from the Sierra Nevada to the Golden Gate in an all-encompassing sweep of Northern California. There is no other view like it.

Surrounded by encroaching development and connected to no greater mountain range, Mount Diablo is an oasis of both plant and animal life. Besides a variety of wildlife—and particularly birdlife—several plant species occur on the mountain that can be found nowhere else. Due to variations in elevation and precipitation, a variety of ecosystems are found here, and several can be explored on this short hike.

The Hike follows the Mary Bowerman Trail, an easy loop around the summit of Mount Diablo (3,849') offering spectacular vistas in every compass direction. An interpretive brochure and informative signs enhance the experience. The optimal time to come is immediately following a spring or winter storm when the air is cleanest, the views most far-reaching, and the landscape carpeted a vibrant green. Even then, a good breeze is necessary to blow away all lingering and newly forming clouds, which can hover around the mountain. Strong easterly winds during the spring can also push the haze away. While the hike is open year-round, haze and heat are thick throughout summer and fall. Water is available at the trailhead.

To Reach the Trailhead Take the Ygnacio Valley Rd. off-ramp from Hwy. 680 in Walnut Creek and proceed 3.8 miles east on Ygnacio Valley Rd. to Oak Grove Rd. Turn right on Oak Grove Rd. and then turn left onto North Gate Rd. in 1 mile. When you reach a junction with Mount Diablo Scenic Rd. at park headquarters 8 miles later, take Summit Rd. 5 miles farther to the summit. Park in the large lot where the lanes divide near the top. It is also possible to approach from the south by taking Diablo Rd. from Hwy. 680 in Danville east for 3 miles to Mount Diablo Scenic Rd. Turn left and proceed up the narrow, twisting road for 6 miles to the junction with Summit Rd., on which you continue 5 miles to the summit. There is a day-use fee of $10 per vehicle.

Description Be sure to pick up an interpretive brochure at the visitor center before you start. Beginning by the picnic tables across the road from the parking lot, the first half of the hike is paved and passes through a small sample of the oak woodland plant community, offering exceptional views north of distant Mount St. Helena (Hike 36) and northeast across the Sacramento Valley to the Sierra Buttes (Hike 72). Mount Shasta would be visible 240 miles away were it not blocked by the curvature of the earth. Closer to the north is nearby Eagle Peak (Hike 15). The rocks around you are greenstone and chert, the uppermost layers of what is known as an ophiolite suite, a group of rocks and minerals found close together wherever ancient seafloor is exposed.

The seafloor is composed of five layers. The bottom three form a surface that is essentially

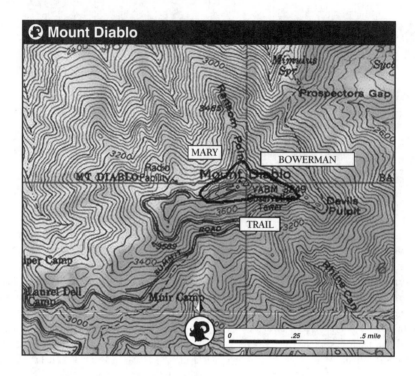

a solid piece of the earth's crust. The upper two layers are deposited underwater on this surface. At tectonic spreading ridges, liquid basalt is squeezed out onto the seafloor, piling up in distinctively shaped pillow basalts, which compose the first of the two upper layers. These are in turn covered by sediment settling from the ocean. Primarily made up of the microscopic skeletons of tiny sea creatures, this silica-rich upper layer takes millions of years to accumulate, gradually forming thin layers mixed with small bits of sand and mud. Altered by pressure and temperature, these two upper layers eventually become greenstone and chert. The Mount Diablo Ophiolite, as it is called, has been so heavily deformed and tilted that the sequence no longer lies flat. While its upper layers are visible at the summit, its lower layers are exposed

northwest at the Lone Star Quarry, where diabase, a constituent rock of the lower sequence, is used for roadbeds and foundations. Exactly how this piece of 165-million-year-old seafloor became emplaced in the young sediments ringing Mount Diablo remains a mystery.

As you hike into chaparral on the drier east slope of the mountain where the path becomes dirt, the peaks of Yosemite National Park (Hikes 85–90) can be identified. Let the gospel flow from atop Devil's Pulpit, a large outcropping of chert with a mildly precarious scramble to the top. Beyond it, the trail curves onto the south side of the mountain, where grassland replaces the chaparral ecosystem on this sunniest side of the summit. Coyote Hills (Hike 12) can be spotted to the southwest by the bay. The trail ends back by the parking lot.

Nearest Visitor Center The Summit Museum–Visitor Center, 925-837-6119, constructed on the actual summit of the mountain, is open daily year-round, 10 a.m.–4 p.m. For general information, call 925-837-2525.

Nearest Campground The park has three year-round campgrounds with a total of 56 sites. Juniper Campground, the largest of the three, is along Summit Rd.; small Junction Campground is by park headquarters; and Live Oak Campground can be found on Mount Diablo Scenic Rd./South Gate Rd. (all campgrounds $30). Reservations are recommended for weekends; visit **reserveamerica.com** or call 800-444-7275.

Additional Information mdia.org, savemountdiablo.org, and www.parks.ca.gov

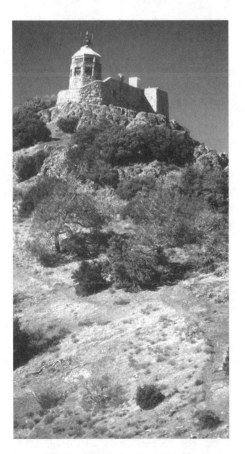

Summit Visitor Center atop Mount Diablo

HIKE 15 Eagle Peak ◐

Highlights	Flowers, oaks, and a secluded summit
Distance	4.0 miles
Total Elevation Gain/Loss	1,800'/1,800'
Hiking Time	3–4 hours
Recommended Maps	*Mount Diablo, Los Vaqueros, and Surrounding Parks* by Save Mount Diablo, USGS 7.5-min. *Clayton*
Best Times	February–May
Agency	Mount Diablo State Park
Difficulty	★★★

FROM A SEA OF rippling grassland rises Eagle Peak, a little-visited summit below the ramparts of Mount Diablo.

The Hike climbs to the summit of Eagle Peak (2,369') from the northern boundary of Mount Diablo State Park, ascending on Mitchell Rock Trail before returning via the Eagle Peak and Coulter Pine Trails. While the hike can be done year-round, spring is the time to come as the land is carpeted green, wildflowers bloom, and temperatures are most ideal. Sections of the trail are exposed, making sun protection crucial most of the year. Ticks and poison oak are of particular concern in the brush along much of the route. Crowds are minimal. Water is available at the trailhead.

To Reach the Trailhead Take the Ygnacio Valley Rd. off-ramp from Hwy. 680 in Walnut Creek and proceed 9 miles east on Ygnacio Valley Rd. to Clayton Rd. Turn right and in 1 mile turn right again on Mitchell Canyon Rd., proceeding 2 miles to the lot at the road's end. There is a day-use fee of $10 per vehicle.

Description From the parking lot (0.0/640'), begin by the fire gate and information sign and start up Mitchell Canyon Rd., bearing left onto Mitchell Rock Trail at the immediate junction. Stay on the wide trail as you pass two junctions for Bruce Lee Trail before turning right

on singletrack Mitchell Rock Trail (just past the second Bruce Lee intersection). In season, abundant wildflowers liven the ground here and throughout the hike—look for California poppies, yarrow, paintbrush, lupine, irises, orange bush monkeyflower, yerba santa, blue dicks, Ithuriel's spear, and the endemic Mount Diablo fairy lantern.

As you climb upward into thick forest, note the increasing number of pine trees. Two pines are found in this area, both producing massive cones with sharp hooks on the scales. Gray pine is the more common, abounding throughout California's foothills and easily identified by its wispy character. Its upper half, often drooping slightly to one side, tends to fork into a multitude of small branches with no clear center trunk. Its long grayish needles come in groups of three and give the tree its name. Coulter pine, on the other hand, is straight, stout, and considerably less common than gray pine, occurring only in the Coast Ranges from Mount Diablo south. They are at the northernmost limit of their range here and can be identified by their single trunk, long stiff needles (also in groups of three), stouter appearance, and gargantuan cones. Coulter pine cones are the largest known, giant loaves 12–14 inches long that easily weigh several pounds.

As you climb steadily, your views north of the creeping edge of suburbia continue to improve until you reach an open rock platform

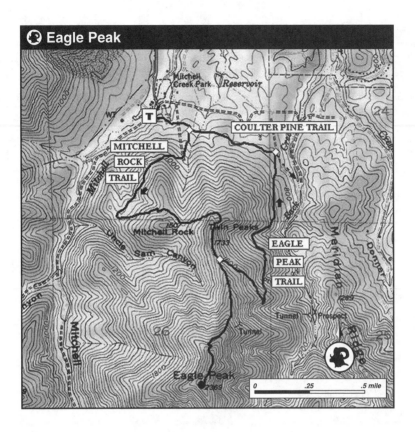

(0.6/1,080'). Directly across Mitchell Canyon, noisy Lone Star Quarry digs up diabase for use in roadbeds and foundations. Continuing up the trail, you ascend to a small saddle below Twin Peaks. As you traverse below Twin Peaks to attain the ridge, the Sacramento River Delta appears to the north and the broad expanse of the Great Central Valley peeks out east over the hills. An eagle eye can discern the confluence of the San Joaquin and Sacramento Rivers. Once on the ridgeline, views open up of the Mount Diablo massif—both North Peak (3,557') and the summit (3,849') are visible. From Twin Peaks (1.5/1,733'), Eagle Peak is clearly seen up the ridge.

Descending briefly, the trail passes a junction for Eagle Peak Trail (your return route) and then makes a steep, brushy, view-rich climb up the ridgeline to just below the summit, where a series of final switchbacks brings you to the top (2.3/2,369'). Bear right on Eagle Peak Trail on your downhill return from the summit to take a much steeper and more direct route to the bottom than Mitchell Rock Trail. Dropping above Back Creek canyon, the trail cuts sharply back before passing over a scree gully below Twin Peaks. As you continue to descend, an increase in pines and poison oak marks the approaching junction with the Coulter Pine Trail (3.4/780'). Bear left and enjoy the gentle ramble through flowers and oaks and rippling grass that returns you to the Mitchell Rock Trail and your trailhead.

Nearest Visitor Center Mitchell Canyon Ranger Station, near the end of Mitchell Canyon Rd., is open weekends 8 a.m.–4 p.m. during spring and summer, and 9 a.m.–3 p.m. in fall and winter. For general information, call 925-837-2525.

Nearest Campgrounds There are no park campgrounds accessible from the north side of Mount Diablo State Park, but 3 year-round campgrounds are accessible from the south side: Juniper Campground, the largest, is along Summit Rd.; small Junction Campground is by park headquarters; and Live Oak Campground can be found on Mount Diablo Scenic Rd./South Gate Rd. (all campgrounds $30). Reservations are recommended for weekends; visit **reserveamerica.com** or call 800-444-7275.

Additional Information mdia.org, savemountdiablo.org, and **www.parks.ca.gov**

HIKE 16 Cosumnes River ⟳ 👫

Highlights	Valley oak woodlands and wildlife
Distance	3.0 miles round-trip
Total Elevation Gain/Loss	10'/10'
Hiking Time	1–2 hours
Recommended Map	USGS 7.5-min. *Bruceville*
Best Times	October–April
Agency	Cosumnes River Preserve
Difficulty	★

COME EXPERIENCE California's great Central Valley as it used to be, a world of magnificent valley oaks flush with wetlands, wildlife, and wildflowers. The Cosumnes River flows through the preserve, the only remaining undammed river in the Central Valley. Migratory sandhill cranes flock here from November through February, for many the highlight of a spectacular birding destination year-round.

The Hike loops on easy level paths through the preserve, visiting ponds, meadows, riparian woodlands, and the banks of the Cosumnes River. The described hike meanders through much of the preserve, though it is also possible to make a shorter loop if desired. Open year-round, the preserve is best visited during the cooler months as summer temperatures can be scorchingly intense. Note that sections of trail can be flooded in winter following heavy rains.

To Reach the Trailhead Take I-5 to the Twin Cities Exit in Galt, turn east, and proceed 1.1 miles to Franklin Blvd. Turn right on Franklin Blvd. and continue 1.9 miles to reach the preserve entrance and main parking area.

Description The hike begins from the visitor center on the paved River Walk (0.0/20') and quickly proceeds into shady woods of young valley oak. Also present are prime examples of the many massive poison oak shrubs that grow throughout the preserve.

Recognize valley oak by its distinctive deeply lobed and rounded leaves. Once common throughout the central Valley, its population has been dramatically reduced by agricultural development. Today only a handful of locations still harbor portions of undisturbed valley oak habitat—this preserve is one of the best remaining examples.

You next cross a bridge over the Willow Slough floodplain, where a sign highlights the remarkable fact that here, more than 60 miles from San Francisco Bay, the elevation is a mere five feet above sea level and that tides cause the water here to rise and fall as much as five feet each day.

The path reaches a junction by wetlands (0.1/10'), where you turn right. The path winds by the edge of a pond and alongside wetlands thick with willow and oaks. It then travels atop a berm with wetlands on both sides, where you can see abundant "balls" hanging from many oak trees. These are striking examples of galls, which are created when insects lay their eggs on oak trees. This stimulates the tree to produce distinctive structures in response, which protect the young insects as they hatch. Hundreds of different types of gall-producing insects exist, each of which generates a different structure. A careful eye will find other varieties on leaves and branches throughout the preserve.

Urnlike barrels appear beside the trail as you continue. Part of the preserve's restoration efforts, they hold water to irrigate the plants along the berm. Turn left at the next junction (0.5/10'), where a short dead-end spur continues straight to a partial view of the Middle Slough.

At the next junction (0.7/10'), turn right to briefly parallel the railroad tracks on a dirt road, then go right again at the next junction (0.8/10') to remain on Nature Trail as it heads down toward the river. A grassy path now leads to a T-junction, where you turn left and attain a levee alongside a stand of riparian valley oaks. The large birdhouses you see, for wood ducks, mimic the large tree cavities the birds prefer.

The route curves left to return by the tracks, briefly runs along the base of a railroad trestle, and then bears right to pass underneath it (1.3/10'). You now enter a delightful example of valley oak savannah. Distinct from the moisture-rich river corridor, this ecosystem is populated by large and solitary oaks, their branches a dramatic canopy of twisting limbs and unique architecture.

You next reach a four-way junction (1.6/10'). Your return route heads left, but turning right

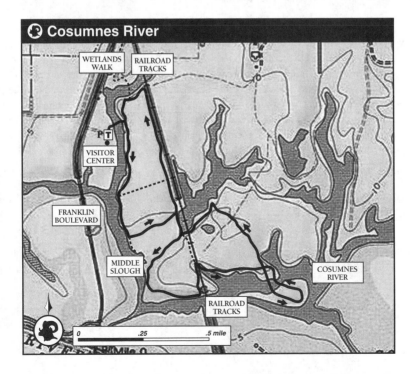

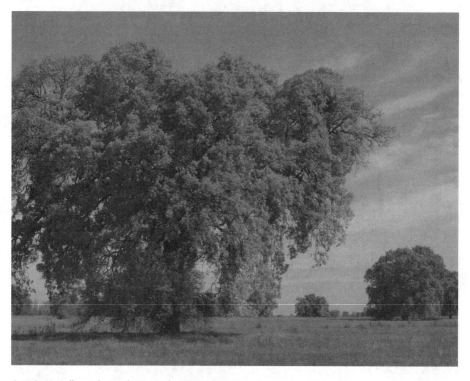

A majestic valley oak stands sentinel at Cosumnes River Preserve.

takes you on a worthwhile 0.4-mile side loop through the preserve's nicest section of riparian woodlands and past several scenic views of the adjacent river. Returning toward the trailhead, your route runs along the edge of beautiful oak savannah, crosses an access road, and continues on a grassy mowed path. You curve left near a magnificent oak tree, travel along the meadow's perimeter, and then bear right to pass under the tracks again and return to the access road, where you turn right (2.3/10').

The trail now runs parallel to the tracks past marshes and wetlands and then turns left as the tracks rise to attain an elevated trestle. You return to paved Wetlands Trail (2.8/10'), which quickly returns you to the visitor center (3.0/10').

Nearest Visitor Center Cosumnes River Preserve Visitor Center, 916-684-2816, a short walk from the main parking area, is open weekends 9 a.m.–5 p.m. September–June, and 8 a.m.–noon July and August; weekday hours vary depending on volunteer staffing availability.

Additional Information cosumnes.org

HIKE 17 Wildcat Peak ◯ 🐕

Highlight	East Bay escape with outstanding views of the Bay Area
Distance	7.0 miles
Total Elevation Gain/Loss	1,000'/1,000'
Hiking Time	3–5 hours
Recommended Map	USGS 7.5-min. *Richmond*
Best Times	Year-round
Agency	Tilden Regional Park
Difficulty	★★

A SURPRISING WORLD hides behind the East Bay Hills. Rolling hills, soaring raptors, and superlative views of the Bay Area highlight a peaceful oasis of nature.

The Hike runs through Tilden and Wildcat Canyon Regional Parks, passing along Wildcat Creek before returning via San Pablo Ridge and Wildcat Peak (1,280'). The excellent views from the open ridgetop are best in the morning and after storms. While the hike can be done year-round, the trails become thick with mud during the winter rainy season. As they have since European settlement of the region, cows graze on the open hillsides. People are common, especially along popular San Pablo Ridge, but quiet glades can usually be found. Water is available at the trailhead.

To Reach the Trailhead Take the Buchanan St. off-ramp from I-80 in Berkeley, and proceed east on Marin Ave. for 2 miles. Climb Marin above Marin Circle on the East Bay's steepest road, and turn left at the first stop sign onto Spruce St. Follow it to Grizzly Peak Blvd. Cross the intersection and take Canon Dr. steeply downhill to the visitor center and parking lot in Tilden Nature Center.

It is also possible to reach the trailhead by public transportation. AC Transit Bus 67 runs Monday through Friday every 40 minutes from the Berkeley BART station to the intersection of Spruce St. and Grizzly Peak Blvd. From the intersection, walk down Canon Dr. to the trailhead as described above. On weekends and holidays, Bus 67 runs every 45 minutes from the Berkeley

BART station and will drop you directly at the trailhead. Call 510-817-1717 for current schedule and fare information or visit **actransit.org.**

Description From the trailhead (0.0/530'), strike north from a small patch of redwood trees on wide Wildcat Creek Trail. Willow, California bay, coast live oak, coyote brush, California buckeye, poison oak, and introduced French broom line the trail as it parallels Wildcat Creek. Passing diminutive Jewel Lake, the trail soon crosses into Wildcat Regional Park. A wire fence lines the path below increasingly open hillsides. After nearly 2 miles of easy walking, you reach a gated junction for the Havey Canyon and Conlon Trails (2.3/490')—on your right immediately before reaching Rifle Range Road. Go through the gate and continue straight toward Havey Canyon. The trail climbs a lush, riparian valley flush with ferns, snowberry, and some unusually massive California bay before breaking out onto open slopes dotted with coyote brush. While cows are a common sight, more exciting are the raptors often seen overhead; red-tailed hawks, easily identified by their namesake tail feathers; and northern harriers, spotted by the distinctive white patch of feathers on their rump. As the trail curves north, distant Mount Tamalpais (Hike 31) becomes visible to the west. Soon, you go through another gate to reach paved Nimitz Way atop San Pablo Ridge (3.8/950')—bear right (south).

Views along the ridge are far-reaching, stretching from Vallejo in the north to Mount

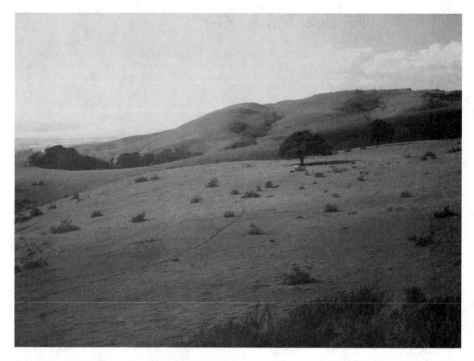

Escape to empty grasslands in Tilden Regional Park.

Diablo (Hike 14) in the east. The East Bay Hills' highest peaks rise from the ridge to the south, and San Pablo Reservoir lies below you. You reach another junction near Wildcat Peak (4.8/1,140')—leave the pavement and go straight up the rocky trail. After passing a few Monterey pine and Monterey cypress, you swing right along the wide path to descend the Conlon Trail. At this point, leave the trail to find a bench with incredible views of the Golden Gate (Hike 27) and central Bay Area. From the bench, bear left on a faint, barbed-wire-lined path, and cross through the fence at a small gap to continue up to Wildcat Peak's summit (5.4/1,280'). A stone platform crowns the summit and explains the purpose of the nearby Rotary Peace Grove. Savor the amazing views before dropping down to explore the grove of bushy giant sequoia, seemingly healthy despite being far removed from their native Sierra Nevada habitat.

To return to the trailhead, follow Peak Trail as it descends east from the summit, and take the singletrack trail branching right to quickly reach Laurel Canyon Rd. below. Alternatively, you can continue on Peak Trail to rejoin Nimitz Way—bear right and then right again upon reaching Laurel Canyon Rd.

Laurel Canyon is within the Tilden Nature Study Area, a designated area for protection of Tilden's unique flora and fauna. A maze of trails winds through it, each marked with a symbol. Laurel Canyon Rd. is the widest and easiest route, but any number of trail combinations will return you to the trailhead (7.0/530')—just keep bearing downhill.

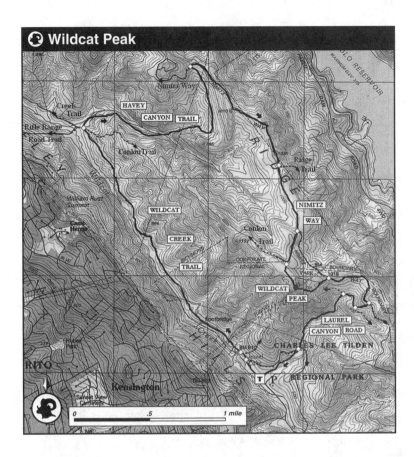

Nearest Visitor Center The Environmental Education Center and Visitor Center, 510-544-2233, at the trailhead, is open Tuesday–Sunday 10 a.m.–4:30 p.m.

Nearest Campgrounds There are 2 group campgrounds in the Tilden Nature Study Area. Reservations are required at least 1 week in advance and can be made by calling 888-327-2757, option 2.

Additional Information ebparks.org/parks/tilden

HIKE 18 Little Butano Creek Canyon Ω 🧍

Highlights	Canyon views, redwood forest, and knobcone pines
Distance	8.8 miles
Total Elevation Gain/Loss	2,100'/2,100'
Hiking Time	5–6 hours
Recommended Maps	*Butano State Park Map* by California State Parks, USGS 7.5-min. *Franklin Point*
Best Times	Year-round
Agency	Butano State Park
Difficulty	★★★

LITTLE BUTANO CREEK slices westward in a narrow defile almost completely protected within Butano (BOO-tah-no) State Park. Less than 4 miles long yet brimming with ecological diversity, the canyon contains an isolated and diverse world representative of the entire region. Extensive stands of redwoods thrive in the park's lush environment, including 315 acres of old-growth trees.

The Hike travels on seven different trails to complete a clockwise loop around the canyon. The trip can be completed year-round, with spring and fall offering the ideal combination of good weather and light crowds. Summer is foggy and people heavy, while winter and early spring are typically rainy, cool, and perpetually damp.

To Reach the Trailhead Take Hwy. 1 south of Half Moon Bay for 16 miles to Pescadero Rd. and turn left. In 2.5 miles, turn right on Cloverdale Rd. and proceed 4 miles to the park entrance on the left. Approaching from the south, take Hwy. 1 north of Davenport for 14 miles and turn right on Gazos Creek Rd., immediately north of the Beach House gas station. Follow Gazos Creek Rd. for 2 miles, turn left on Cloverdale Rd., and proceed 1 mile to the park entrance on the right. The posted trailhead is a half mile past the entrance station by a large turnout.

Description From the trailhead (0.0/230'), follow Mill Ox Trail across Little Butano Creek and quickly climb northeast to reach Jackson Flat Trail (0.2/430'). Redwoods, Douglas-firs, tanoaks, and huckleberry bushes surround you along this early section, joined intermittently by bigleaf maples, twisting madrones, sword and wood ferns, and the soft leaves of hazel bushes. Turn right on Jackson Flat Trail and begin a gradual rising traverse along the moisture divide between a damp redwood forest (a few large old-growth trees can be spotted) and drier mixed-evergreen forest.

Bear right on Canyon Trail (1.7/800') as Jackson Flat Trail curves left. You initially continue through thick redwood forest, but the woods soon transition to canyon live oak and madrone, then abruptly transform into an entirely different ecosystem. As the trail crosses the threshold of the Santa Margarita geologic formation—a sandstone layer poor in water and organic material—it encounters species uniquely adapted to these harsh conditions. Knobcone pines, spindly conifers that sprout their namesake cones everywhere, including from their branches and trunks, proliferate. Knobcones survive through serotiny—their cones open only from the heat of wildfires. This strategy populates the newly charred, nutrient-rich soil with a sudden, massive influx of seeds. Other members of the drier chaparral community grow alongside: manzanita, golden chinquapin (look under the leaves), toyon, scrub oak, and chamise.

The trail winds through this open community, passing views that reveal the depth of this diminutive canyon. The route momentarily banks left into a small tributary canyon and descends to cross a seasonally rushing creek (note

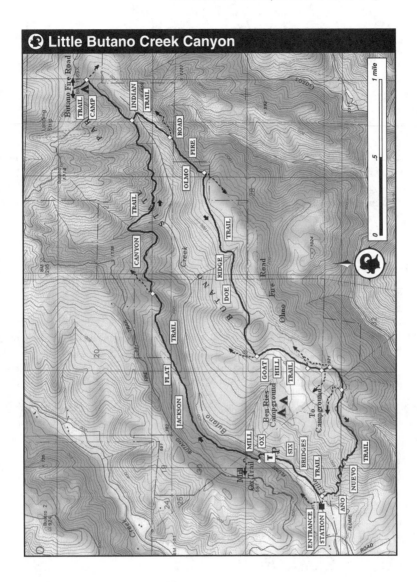

☉ Little Butano Creek Canyon

the bigleaf maples and change of ecosystem as moisture again increases). Several switchbacks then return you upward to the Santa Margarita Formation and its accompanying views and flora. The path contours around several small drainages, returns to thick forest, and reaches the posted junction for the park's trail camp (3.7/1,200'). (To reach the trail camp, bear left and head steeply uphill along the narrow trail for 0.5 mile to an unnamed fire road. The campsites are just uphill to your left.)

Remain on Canyon Trail as it continues briefly up the valley, crosses the headwaters of Little Butano Creek, and then curves right to start the return journey. Turn right upon reaching Olmo Fire Rd. (4.2/1,240') and follow the wide trail as it winds for 0.4 mile through private property owned by Ainsley Family Tree Farm. Please stay on the road in this section and enjoy glimpses south into the adjacent Gazos Creek drainage, the only views of the hike beyond Little Butano Creek.

You slowly descend to reach singletrack Doe Ridge Trail on the right (4.5/1,050'), which you follow to one of the hike's most idyllic stretches—old-growth redwoods stand tall above the level and nicely contoured path. You next turn left on Goat Hill Trail (6.0/840'), which proceeds through thick Douglas-fir forest recovering from recent logging. You pass a spur trail on the left (6.5/900') leading to adjacent Olmo Fire Rd., and then another spur quickly thereafter. Goat Hill Trail continues downhill from here toward the campground and offers a more direct and less strenuous

return route—just follow the park road from the campground to the trailhead.

To avoid the pavement, return to Olmo Fire Rd., turn right, and then bear left on Año Nuevo Trail (7.0/1,060'). The singletrack path contours briefly along a forested ridge, then banks right and heads down-canyon via a series of switchbacks. The foliage becomes thick with elderberry and blackberry, interspersed with airy views of the lower canyon. Upon reaching the bottom (8.3/220'), bear right on Six Bridges Trail and proceed along the banks of Little Butano Creek to return to the trailhead (8.8/230').

Nearest Visitor Center The park entrance station is staffed daily in summer and most weekends in the off-season. It's open sporadically the rest of the year. Call 650-879-2040 for general information.

Backpacking Information Backcountry camping is permitted only at the park's designated trail camp ($10), which features 8 primitive sites at the ridgeline headwaters of Little Butano Creek. No water is available at the camp, though there are nearby stream sources. Campfires are not permitted. Open seasonally, the trail camp is first come, first served. Register at the park entrance station upon arrival.

Nearest Campground Butano State Park Campground (38 sites, $35) is near the trailhead and open April–November. Reservations are recommended; visit **reserveamerica.com** or call 800-444-7275.

Additional Information www.parks.ca.gov

HIKE 19 Castle Rock ○ 🚶

Highlights	Wild rocks and airy views atop the Santa Cruz Mountains
Distance	5.2 miles
Total Elevation Gain/Loss	1,200'/1,200'
Hiking Time	3–4 hours
Recommended Maps	*Castle Rock State Park Map*, USGS 7.5-min. *Castle Rock Ridge*
Best Times	Year-round
Agency	Castle Rock State Park
Difficulty	★★

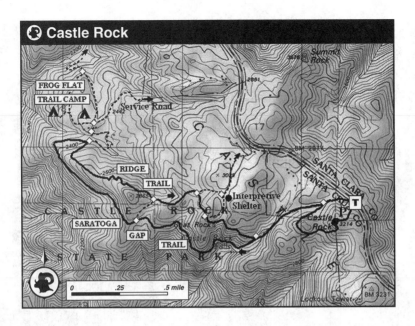

PERCHED ON the tallest ridgeline in the Santa Cruz Mountains, Castle Rock State Park provides towering views over the San Lorenzo River and Pescadero Creek watersheds. It also harbors a geologic wonderland of sandstone boulders, a powerful draw for climbers and gawkers alike.

The Hike traverses the upper tier of the Santa Cruz Mountains, running high along the western slopes en route to a pleasantly secluded trail camp. Summer fog can obscure the hike's incredible views and winter storms can be heavy, but there is no bad time to visit. Crowds on the trail are relatively light, but the intricate rock formations close to the park entrance usually attract large numbers of climbers on the weekends.

To Reach the Trailhead Take Hwy. 35 south of the Hwy. 9 junction for 2.5 miles. The posted entrance and parking area are on the west side of the road. There is an $8 day-use fee.

Description A small forest of signs marks the trailhead at the edge of the parking lot (0.0/ 3,070'). While the direct route proceeds straight on Saratoga Gap Trail, you should begin your trip among the park's boulders by turning left and heading toward Castle Rock.

Heavy precipitation (45–50 inches annually) falls upon the area's unusually hard sandstone outcrops, creating conditions ideal for some bizarre chemical weathering known as *tafoni*. Rainwater seeps inside the rocks and dissolves the thin matrix of calcium carbonate that binds the individual sand grains together. When dry conditions return, the moisture trapped inside the rocks is drawn back to the surface. Its evaporation leaves behind the calcium carbonate as a hard and intricate surface residue. Without the calcium carbonate "glue" to hold them together, the interior sand grains waste away and leave small cavities behind. Over time these cavities can become intricate catacombs, their puckered walls a fascinating honeycomb of pitted rock.

You quickly reach the first wild pile of stones on the left. From here a network of unsigned paths climbs past a variety of tafoni outcrops before reaching Castle Rock itself, an apartment-sized monolith deeply gouged by erosion. After

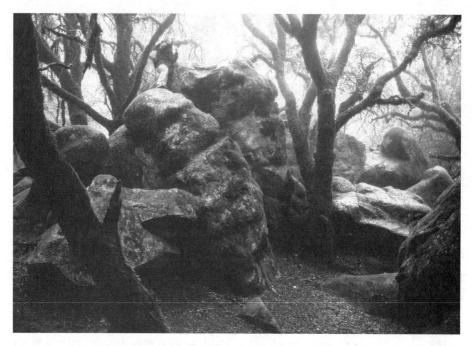

Jumbled geology in Castle Rock State Park

enjoying the geology, proceed to Saratoga Gap Trail and turn left (0.5/3,000').

The trail traverses downward along the flanks of the Kings Creek drainage, one of the uppermost headwaters of the San Lorenzo River. Mixed-evergreen forest covers the slopes, dominated by the drooping evergreen branches of Douglas-firs, the large spiny leaves of tanoaks, and the twisting trunks of madrones. Bigleaf maples flutter overhead, and thick clumps of sword ferns sprout along the moist creekbed. A trailside understory of blackberry and poison oak discourages a departure from the soft path.

Crossing the creek, the trail reaches the junction with Ridge Trail (0.9/2,730') and the beginning of the loop. Remain on Saratoga Gap Trail as it continues briefly along the creek, joined now by a few young redwoods, and reaches an overlook for the thin cascade of Castle Rock Falls (1.1/2,700'). From here Kings Creek plummets over a thousand vertical feet in less than a mile. The trail heads away from this drop and quickly passes onto drier slopes where coffeeberry, toyon, and fragrant California bay appear—plants better adapted to a world of less moisture.

Sandstone boulders protrude from the steep chaparral-cloaked slopes as you pass a connector trail on the right leading to nearby Ridge Trail (1.9/2,560') and reach the hike's first spectacular views. Looking south beyond the vast San Lorenzo River watershed on a clear day, you can see as far as the Monterey peninsula (a distance of more than 40 miles). To the west, the low ridge separating the San Lorenzo River and Pescadero Creek watersheds is apparent; the Skyline-to-the-Sea Trail follows this divide en route to Big Basin Redwoods State Park (Hike 20). Tall Bonny Doon Ridge hems the San Lorenzo River to the southwest, while Butano Ridge rises above Pescadero Creek to the west. The deep canyon of Pescadero Creek curves out of sight to the northwest.

Now gradually descending, you pass through chaparral thick with coyote brush and poison oak. The trail winds along sheer slopes and then turns sharply right to pass through a thick forest of tanoak and madrone and reach the junction with Ridge Trail (2.9/2,400'). (To reach nearby Frog Flat Trail Camp, bear left, and then left again on the wide fire road to reach the main area in 0.2 mile.)

Turn right and follow Ridge Trail as it climbs briefly through thick forest to emerge at another incredible viewpoint of the Santa Cruz Mountains. From here, the path returns to the woods, climbs along the north side of the ridge, and reaches the connector trail to Saratoga Gap Trail (3.7/2,700'). Continue on Ridge Trail as it climbs over a black oak-studded knoll and encounters a fork (4.0/2,900'). A left here leads to a nearby interpretive shelter, but you should bear right to remain on Ridge Trail. You pass a return trail from the shelter (4.2/2,960') and then reach the junction for exciting Goat Rock (4.3/2,920'). The rounded pinnacle of Goat Rock and its surrounding viewpoints can be accessed via numerous use trails and thrilling rock scrambles. After enjoying the most intense verticality of the hike, continue on Ridge Trail as it slowly descends along a narrow, rocky route to rejoin Saratoga Gap Trail (4.7/2,730') and the final climb back to the parking lot (5.2/3,070').

Nearest Visitor Center This park doesn't have a visitor center, but the entrance station is occasionally staffed on busy weekends. For general information, call 408-867-2952.

Backpacking Information Camping is permitted at Frog Flat Trail Camp (20 sites, $15 per site, maximum 6 people per site) on a first-come, first-served basis. Space is always available. Water is available, and campfires are permitted outside of wildfire season (typically June–November). Register at the park entrance station upon arrival.

Nearest Campgrounds The closest option is Big Basin Redwoods State Park, 30–45 minutes away on Hwy. 236. The park offers 4 campgrounds: Huckleberry (33 sites, 25 tent cabins), Blooms Creek (54 sites), Sempervirens (32 sites), and Wastahi (27 sites). Sites cost $35 per night; tent cabins are $79. Reservations are essential Memorial Day–Labor Day and for weekends in spring and fall; visit **reserveamerica.com** or call 800-444-7275.

Additional Information www.parks.ca.gov, thatsmypark.org

HIKE 20 Berry Creek Falls ⟳ 🚶

Highlights	Continuous old-growth redwood forest and waterfalls
Distance	9.0 miles
Total Elevation Gain/Loss	3,200'/3,200'
Hiking Time	6–8 hours
Recommended Maps	*Big Basin Redwoods State Park* by Bored Feet Press, USGS 7.5-min. *Big Basin* and *Franklin Point*
Best Times	Year-round
Agency	Big Basin Redwoods State Park
Difficulty	★★★★

A CONTINUOUS FOREST PRIMEVAL, laced with gurgling streams, Big Basin State Park is a green blaze of life. Yes, the park is popular and the waterfalls are a common destination. And yes, it's worth it.

Established in 1902, Big Basin was the first state park created to protect old-growth redwood forest in the Santa Cruz Mountains. In fact, the 3,800 acres initially set aside as parkland were the very first to protect coast redwoods anywhere. The park holdings have since expanded and the total park area now exceeds 19,000 acres, stretching from the Pacific Ocean at the mouth of Waddell Creek to the heart of the Santa Cruz Mountains. The old-growth redwood forest is extensive and unmatched in total area for hundreds of miles up the coast.

The Hike is a full-day adventure loop through substantial redwood forest to three waterfalls: Silver Falls, Golden Falls, and photogenic Berry Creek Falls. Fog may be present in the summer and rain might fall heavy in the winter, but there is no bad time to come here. Just be prepared for some very wet trail conditions if you arrive after a winter storm, and be ready for mud year-round. No matter what day you come, other people will be on the trail. Weekend crowds can be especially thick. A fall, winter, or spring weekday is the best bet for some solitude. Water is available at the trailhead.

To Reach the Trailhead Take Hwy. 236 west from one of its two junctions with Hwy. 9.

Approaching from the north on Skyline Blvd. (Hwy. 35), the turnoff is 6 miles south of the junction with Hwy. 9. From this turnoff, Hwy. 236 is a one-lane twister that reaches the visitor center in 9 miles—RVs and trailers are not recommended. Approaching from the south, the turnoff from Hwy. 9 is located in Boulder Creek. This more easily driven section of Hwy. 236 reaches the visitor center in 10 miles. Park in the large lot across from the visitor center. There is a day-use fee of $10.

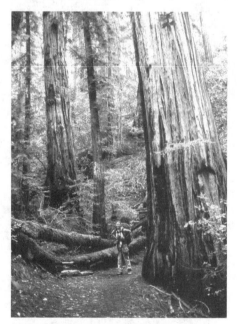

Old-growth redwoods dwarf a passing hiker in Big Basin.

Berry Creek Falls

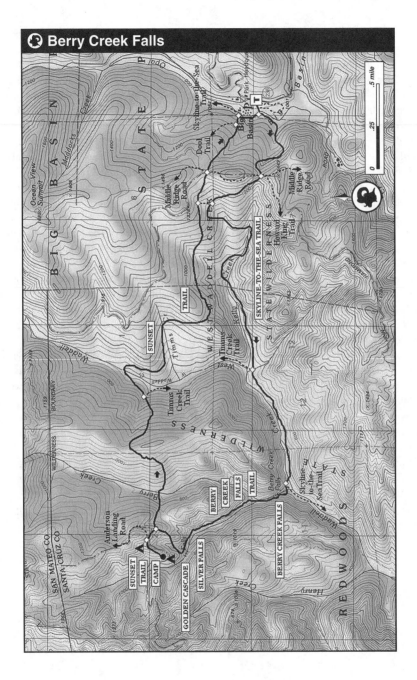

Description Beneath some particularly large redwoods, take broad Redwood Trail from the trailhead (0.0/990') beyond the restrooms and across Opal Creek to your junction with the Skyline-to-the-Sea Trail. Your return trail joins from the right but you head left, passing some large Douglas-firs and many tanoaks, whose toothed leaves wave everywhere. Continue toward Berry Creek Falls at the next junction and begin a steady climb out of the East Waddell Creek drainage. As you crest into the West Waddell Creek drainage (0.7/1,320'), a sign warns of the strenuous hiking ahead.

As you pass a connector to Sunset Trail, your trail drops rapidly down to Kelly Creek. The hike passes through dense stands of large redwoods, encrusted green by the moist environment, before reaching Timms Creek Trail (2.4/560'), another shortcut to Sunset Trail. Continuing, you descend to reach the junction with Berry Creek Falls Trail (3.8/350'). Turn right toward the falls, leaving the Skyline-to-the-Sea Trail that continues to the ocean, less than 6 miles away.

Unless a recent winter storm has swollen the waters, Berry Creek Falls are thin and drop in small cascades that mist the surrounding greenery. Passing near the bottom of the waterfall, the trail then climbs left above the falls and crosses Berry Creek. The muddy track stays close to the water and soon reaches Silver Falls, a small cascade falling over exposed sedimentary rock representative of the Santa Cruz Mountain geology.

The bedrock of the Santa Cruz Mountains is granite formed some 100 million years ago near the location of today's southern Sierra Nevada. When the San Andreas Fault became active, this piece of land began moving slowly northwest, becoming submerged beneath the sea as it went. Sand and mud settled from the ocean on this underwater surface, forming thick layers of loosely consolidated sandstone and mudstone. Within the past 4 million years, a change in the geometry of the San Andreas Fault thrust these layers above ground, folding them into the Santa Cruz Mountains and exposing the muddy layers to your boots. These loosely consolidated rocks create the huge landslide problems associated with this area today.

After climbing above Silver Falls, you soon reach Golden Falls and its series of three distinct cascades. Wooden steps and the odd switchback lead past this final waterfall to the junction with Sunset Trail (4.7/850'). Sunset Trail Camp is 0.2 mile straight uphill from here, but you turn right to begin the return journey.

Crossing Berry Creek on a solid wooden bridge, the trail then weaves slowly over a small divide between West Waddell and Berry Creeks. Fleeting views of both drainages open up before the trail descends to the Timms Creek Trail junction (5.9/680'). A long undulating traverse from here along the Sunset Trail returns you to the earlier junction with the Skyline-to-the-Sea Trail. Go left on the short Redwood Trail to the trailhead.

Nearest Visitor Center Park visitor center, 831-338-8860, is open daily 8:30 a.m.–4 p.m. (extended hours during the summer months).

Backpacking Information Backcountry camping in Big Basin State Park is allowed only at the park's designated trail camps, which are only open May–October. Sunset Trail Camp is the only option on this hike, above the waterfalls. Reservations are required and can be made by calling 831-338-8861 Monday–Friday 9 a.m.–5 p.m. There is an $8 reservation fee, and each site costs $15 per night for up to 6 people. Campfires are prohibited, and water is unavailable at the camp.

Nearest Campgrounds There are 4 park campgrounds: Huckleberry (33 sites, 25 tent cabins), Blooms Creek (54 sites), Sempervirens (32 sites), and Wastahi (27 sites). Blooms Creek is closest to the trailhead, but all are nearby. Sites cost $35 per night, tent cabins are $79. Reservations are essential Memorial Day–Labor Day and for weekends in spring and fall; visit **reserveamerica.com** or call 800-444-7275.

Additional Information www.parks.ca.gov

HIKE 21 **Purisima Creek** Ⓠ

Highlights	A secluded redwood forest and open ridgeline
Distance	7.0 miles
Total Elevation Gain/Loss	1,200'/1,200'
Hiking Time	3–5 hours
Recommended Map	USGS 7.5-min. *Woodside*
Best Times	Year-round
Agency	Purisima Creek Redwoods Open Space Preserve
Difficulty	★★★

JUST SOUTH OF Half Moon Bay, Purisima Creek slices quickly and deeply to the sea, with the northernmost redwood forest on the peninsula in its protected headwaters. So close to the urban mania yet hidden well enough to receive only light use, Purisima is a perfect place to quickly, easily, and totally get away from it all.

The rugged character of Purisima Creek Canyon proved challenging to early logging efforts. While readily accessible from the coast, the sheer walls at the creek's headwaters made shipping lumber directly east to the Bay Area difficult. Despite the uncooperative topography,

virtually all of the old-growth redwoods had been cut by the early 1900s, and seven different mills operated along Purisima Creek over the years. Today the forest has rebounded, with impressive second-growth redwoods now lining Purisima Creek. While no old-growth redwoods can be found along the trails, a few ancient trees are reputed to exist in the most inaccessible corners of the preserve.

The Hike follows Purisima Creek upstream through a substantial second-growth redwood forest before returning along Harkins Ridge. The open ridgetop offers excellent views of the

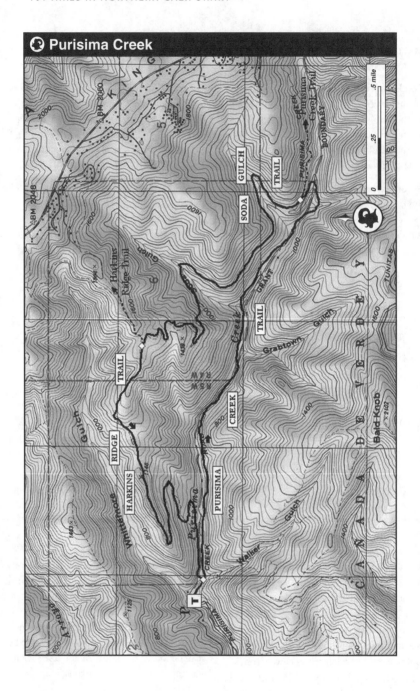

Purisima Creek

valley, visible from mountain to sea. Fog may be thick in the summer and rains might fall heavily in the winter, but there is no bad time to come here. While the main approach to the preserve is from Hwy. 35, this hike begins from the lower boundary, accessible only from the coast. Crowds are consequently light, although you will definitely see other people on the weekends. No water is available at the trailhead.

To Reach the Trailhead On Hwy. 1 drive 5 miles south of the intersection with Hwy. 92 in Half Moon Bay to Verde Rd. Turn left (east) and continue straight on Purisima Creek Rd. for 0.3 mile where Verde Rd. curves right. The small parking lot is 4 miles farther at the road's deepest penetration into the valley. It is also possible to reach the trailhead on longer and twistier Higgins–Purisima Rd., which joins Hwy. 1 next to the new Half Moon Bay fire station, 1.5 miles south of the Hwy. 92 intersection.

Description From the parking lot (0.0/420'), head up the wide path to quickly reach an information sign, where a bathroom is located and free maps are usually available. Your return trail crosses the creek on the left, but the hike continues straight on Purisima Creek Trail. As you go upstream, blackberry, hazel, thimbleberry, stinging nettle, poison oak, dogwood, deer fern, sword fern, five-finger fern, and bracken fern cover the surrounding slopes beneath the overhanging redwood trees. In addition to the redwoods, trees on this trail include the moss-coated trunks of alders, tanoaks, and bigleaf maples. Remain on Purisima Creek Trail as

you pass the junctions for Borden Hatch Mills Trail and Grabtown Gulch Trail, slowly gaining elevation on the gentle gradient. When the trail switchbacks and reaches the junction with Soda Gulch Trail (2.3/1,040'), go left.

Briefly joining the Bay Area Ridge Trail as you ascend on Soda Gulch Trail, the now singletrack path initially winds around a small stream gully. (The Bay Area Ridge Trail is a network of paths that traverse the Bay Area's ridgelands and will eventually be approximately 550 miles long.) Look for the good-sized Douglas-fir above the trail immediately before crossing the small stream, easily identified by their rougher, unfurrowed bark so distinct from that of redwoods. Continuing, a few tantalizing glimpses of upper Purisima Canyon can be had as the vegetation changes into that of the drier, sunnier upper slopes. Tanoak is still found here, but is now mixed with coast live oak and California bay. After traversing around substantial Soda Gulch, the trail suddenly bursts out into open fields of coyote brush and poison oak. Views are at their best here, as virtually the entire drainage of Purisima Creek can be seen curving west to the ocean.

Turning away from this excellent viewpoint, the trail climbs four quick switchbacks to reach the wide road of Harkins Ridge Trail (4.9/1,540'). Go left to descend along the ridgetop with Higgins Creek drainage briefly visible to the north. Your views are obscured when the trail reenters thick vegetation, descending on four long, lazy switchbacks to Purisima Creek and the earlier junction.

Nearest Visitor Center This preserve doesn't have a visitor center. For more information, call the Midpeninsula Regional Open Space District at 650-691-1200.

Nearest Campground Half Moon Bay State Beach Campground, 650-726-8819, is closest, just west of town in southern Half Moon Bay (52 sites, $35–$50 depending on site). Reservations are essential in summer and for weekends year-round; visit **reserveamerica.com** or call 800-444-7275.

Additional Information openspace.org/preserves/pr_purisima.asp

HIKE 22 Devil's Slide 🐾 🐕 👥

Highlights	Eye-popping coastal cliffs and scenery
Distance	2.6 miles round-trip
Total Elevation Gain/Loss	370'/370'
Hiking Time	2–3 hours
Recommended Map	USGS 7.5-min. *Montara Mountain*
Best Times	Year-round
Agency	San Mateo County Parks
Difficulty	★

DEVIL'S SLIDE IS THE moniker given to a sheer coastal bluff more than a mile long and 800 feet high. For decades Hwy. 1 traced a sinuous route upon its face, but the slope's loose rock was always vulnerable to slides, especially during the rainy winter months, which would periodically close this crucial coastal artery to traffic. To eliminate this risk, the state constructed a new 4,200-foot tunnel (the second longest in California) that punched a hole through Montara Mountain and avoided the entirety of Devil's Slide. Following the opening of the tunnel in 2013, the section of Hwy. 1 along Devil's Slide was converted into a broad, paved, multiuse path that today offers some of the most dramatic and accessible coastal scenery in the Bay Area.

The Hike visits the length of the trail, which connects a northern and southern trailhead on either side of the tunnel. While it is possible to begin from either direction, the described hike begins from the southern trailhead. Though paved and smooth, the trail is not a level walk; several steep climbs provide plenty of heart-pumping exercise.

The more significant challenge, however, is parking. The two trailhead parking lots offer only limited space and routinely fill, especially on weekends. Arrive early or visit on weekdays if possible, or consider utilizing the free weekend shuttle service that runs from Pacifica or SamTrans Route 17 (see below). Also be aware that fog is a regular visitor to this area in the summer months, which can completely obscure the many spectacular views. Bicycles are allowed; a designated bike lane runs the length of the trail.

To Reach the Trailhead Take Hwy. 1 south to Pacifica. From the junction with Hwy. 1 and Linda Mar Blvd. (the last stoplight in Pacifica), continue 1.0 mile south to the northern trailhead turnoff, on the right just before the highway curves left to cross the bridge toward the tunnel. To reach the southern trailhead, proceed through the tunnel and take an immediate right on the other side.

If the lots are full, do not be tempted to leave your car in areas marked no parking. The area is regularly patrolled and tickets routinely issued. The city of Pacifica runs a free weekend shuttle bus, which makes six trips over the course of the day and stops at multiple locations en route. One of the most convenient is the Linda Mar Park and Ride, just inland from the Hwy. 1 on Linda Mar Blvd. For a current schedule and more information, visit **cityofpacifica.org.**

SamTrans Route 17 also makes stops at both trailheads on its route between Half Moon Bay and the Linda Mar Park and Ride in Pacifica. It runs hourly on weekdays and every other hour on weekends. For more information, go online at **samtrans.com** or call 800-660-4287.

Description This route begins from the southern trailhead (0.0/260'). As you walk from the parking area, you can pause to look inland down the length of the adjacent Tom Lantos tunnel or toward the ocean, where the crashing surf has cut deep gashes into the slopes below. Pampas grass waves above you on the hillsides,

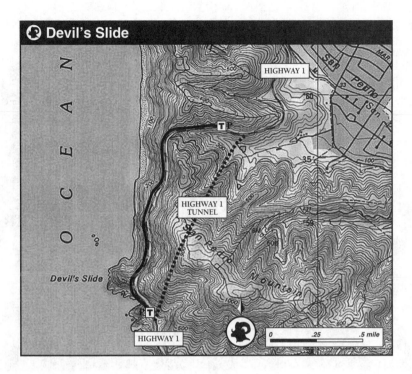

easily recognized much of the year by their tall and distinctive tufts. An invasive species native to South America, it thrives on the coastal bluffs throughout the region.

The trail begins through a deep gash in the slopes. Look to the slopes on the right here, where you can identify crumbly and deeply weathered granite. Formed approximately 80 million years ago in Southern California, this granite has since been forced hundreds of miles north by the San Andreas Fault system. Lands west of the fault, including Montara Mountain and all of Pacifica, are currently moving north at an average rate of 1–2 inches per year. Over millennia, the exact position of the San Andreas Fault has shifted in response to various geologic forces, and the San Andreas Fault once ran along the base of Montara Mountain on what is known today as the Pilarcitos Fault. During this period, the rocks along the fault were crushed into sediment, which easily eroded away to form San Pedro Valley after the San Andreas Fault shifted to its present course. Ancient movement along Pilarcitos

Fault brought the rocks of Montara Mountain and Devil's Slide into contact with those found north of San Pedro Valley. Beyond their current proximity to each other, the two rock groups are totally unrelated.

Continuing, you soon encounter open views of the frothy ocean below. Look again to the slopes on your right, where the geology has shifted from weathered granite to distinctive bands of light and dark rock. These are turbidites, a distinctive geologic structure that composes much of Devil's Slide. Turbidites are formed by massive submarine landslides along the continental shelf. As sediment flows into the ocean from locations inland, it steadily piles up along the shallow continental margin until it abruptly releases in an underwater landslide that pours down steep slopes into deeper water. As the landslide settles, the heavier grains of sand settle first to form a light-colored band. The smaller, finer particles settle next to form a darker band of mudstone. As this pattern repeats itself over geologic time, it forms deep deposits of distinctive bands. In some places,

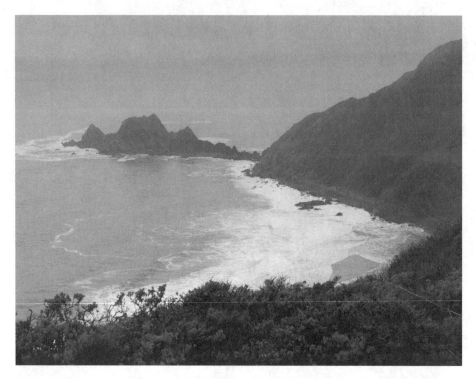

The jagged teeth of Pedro Point jut into the Pacific north of Devil's Slide.

such as here at Devil's Slide, tectonic activity ultimately heaved and tilted them upward to expose them once again on land.

Continuing, you can soon spot landmark Pedro Point extending out to sea, a jagged incisor formed entirely of vertically tilted turbidite layers. Farther in the distance, you can spot Mount Tamalpais (Hike 31). Behind you to the south, decaying and off-limits steps lead upward to an old radar station high on the bluffs; an interpretive sign details the location's interesting history.

As you continue, take time to pause at one of the many excellent viewpoints and look at the slopes below you and to the north, where you can spot a few remaining sections of the railroad bed once used by the Ocean Shore Railroad. A coastal rail line intended to connect San Francisco with Santa Cruz, the Ocean Shore Railroad began construction in 1905 but was never completed, reaching only as far as Tunitas Creek south of Half Moon Bay before service was discontinued in 1921. In this section, the rail line traveled through a tunnel (now collapsed) just inland from Pedro Point and then traversed across the steep slopes of Devil's Slide to points south.

The trail next makes a steady and sustained climb, passing numerous interpretive signs and viewpoints on its way to a large seating area at the crest (0.6/410'). This is a good spot to look west for the Farallon Islands, a linear series of small rocky islets stretching 8 miles northwest from the principal island cluster. With a summit 348 feet high, the largest and most commonly sighted member of the group is Southeast Farallon, at the far southern end of the chain. Eight miles northwest, a smaller group of rocky pillars known as the North Farallons jut from the water, ranging in elevation from 78 to 112 feet. Between the two groups is the lonely pinnacle of Middle Farallon, a single rock 50 feet wide standing 22 feet above the sea. *Farallon,* Spanish for "rocky promontory rising from the ocean," was a generic appellation that over the course of time became exclusively associated with these islands.

Continuing, you next tackle the steepest section of the hike, ascending a 9% grade past a wind-pruned Monterey cypress and increasingly apparent turbidite layers. Catch your breath at the top (0.8/510') and enjoy views south toward the coastal community of Montara. From here, you soon leave the ocean views behind as you descend and curve inland past a striking exposure of turbidites to reach the northern trailhead (1.3/410).

Return the way you came.

Nearest Visitor Center The Pacifica Chamber of Commerce runs an excellent visitor center in partnership with the Golden Gate National Recreation Area. Near the south end of Pacifica at 225 Rockaway Beach, it's open Monday–Friday 10 a.m.–5 p.m. year-round, and 11 a.m.–3 p.m. on weekends in summer. For information call 650-355-4122.

Nearest Campground Francis Beach Campground, 650-726-8819, is open year-round at the south end of Half Moon Bay State Beach, just west of Hwy. 1 on Kelly Ave.; the turnoff is 0.3 mile south of Hwy. 92 (52 sites, $35–$50 depending on site). Reservations are essential in summer and for weekends year-round; visit **reserveamerica.com** or call 800-444-7275.

Additional Information devilsslidecoast.org

HIKE 23 Montara Mountain ↗

Highlights	A dominating mountain and Montara Beach
Distance	5.4 miles round-trip
Total Elevation Gain/Loss	1,650'/1,650'
Hiking Time	4–6 hours
Recommended Map	USGS 7.5-min. *Montara Mountain*
Best Times	Spring and fall
Agency	San Pedro Valley County Park
Difficulty	★★★

MONTARA MOUNTAIN is a solid block of granite towering over Pacifica, a landmark peak forgotten by the Bay Area. Views are tremendous.

The Hike climbs Montara Mountain (1,813') from San Pedro Valley County Park in southern Pacifica. Fog envelops the mountain during the summer, obscuring views and making for a potentially chilly hike. Winter views between storms can be spectacularly clear, but strong winds are often a problem on the exposed mountain. Bring a warm sweater and windbreaker year-round. Water is available at the trailhead.

To Reach the Trailhead Take Hwy. 1 South from San Francisco to Linda Mar Blvd. in Pacifica and turn left (east)—the intersection is located at the southernmost stoplight in Pacifica. Proceed 1.7 miles to Oddstad Blvd. and turn right. The entrance is immediately on your left. Park in the Trout Farm Picnic Area lot to the right of the visitor center. There is a $6 day-use fee.

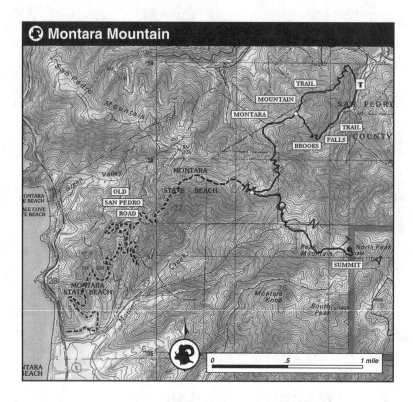

Description The trail begins in the Trout Farm Picnic Area lot by the restrooms (0.0/220') and follows Montara Mountain Trail for the first half of the hike. Both poison oak and stinging nettle grow nearby and are a hazard throughout the day. Ticks are common in the brush as well—stay on the trail. The trail reaches an immediate fork as you begin—bear right and continue on Montara Mountain Trail. To the left is Brooks Falls Trail, an alternate route that rejoins Montara Mountain Trail in 0.8 mile. Crossing a road, the trail begins switchbacking through dense eucalyptus before breaking out onto increasingly open slopes.

The vegetation of Montara Mountain is primarily coastal scrub composed of coyote brush, manzanita, and other low-lying brush highlighted with a seasonal display of wildflowers. Irises, lupine, buttercups, wild radishes, monkeyflowers, California poppies, and horse nettles are but a few of the varieties found here. Coast live oak, California bay, and Monterey cypress grow in more sheltered locations. Raptors—especially red-tailed hawks—can often be seen overhead hunting for unlucky rodents. Quail, bobcats, gray foxes, and deer roam the hillsides. The rarely seen mountain lion is known to live here as well.

Passing a bench with a good view north of nearby Sweeney Ridge, the trail continues its steady ascent. The towers of the Golden Gate Bridge (Hike 27) and the headlands of distant Point Reyes National Seashore (Hikes 33–35) can be picked out north-northwest on clear days. The view becomes ever more expansive as the trail gets rockier on the steep upper flanks of the mountain. A steep, switchbacking climb brings you to the ridge and an intersection with the broad road leading to the summit (1.7/1,460'). It's possible to head to Montara Beach from here. To do so, bear right and follow the road 0.5 mile to the junction with Old San Pedro Rd., a wide trail that drops down the southern flanks of Montara Mountain to ultimately reach the north end of Montara Beach. To continue to the summit, bear left and follow the gradual trail 1.0 mile to the top.

The rocks of Montara Mountain are granite and can be found exposed in places along the upper sections of trail. Formed approximately 80 million years ago in Southern California, the granite has since been forced hundreds of miles north by the San Andreas Fault system. You can trace this fault as it travels underwater northwest from Mussel Rock (just offshore north of the Pacifica Pier) and continues through the low gap between Point Reyes National Seashore and Mount Tamalpais. Lands west of the fault, including Montara Mountain and all of Pacifica,

are currently moving north at an average rate of 1–2 inches per year. Over millennia, the exact position of the San Andreas Fault has shifted in response to various geologic forces, and the San Andreas Fault once ran along the base of Montara Mountain on what is known today as the Pilarcitos Fault. During this period, the rocks along the fault were crushed into sediment, which easily eroded away to form San Pedro Valley after the San Andreas Fault shifted to its present course. Ancient movement along Pilarcitos Fault brought the rocks of Montara Mountain and landmark Pedro Point into contact with those found north of San Pedro Valley. Beyond their current proximity to each other, the two rock groups are totally unrelated.

Nearest Visitor Center The San Pedro County Park Visitor Center, 650-355-8289, is open weekends approximately 10 a.m.–4 p.m.

Nearest Campground Francis Beach Campground, 650-726-8819, is open year-round at the south end of Half Moon Bay State Beach, just west of Hwy. 1 on Kelly Ave.; the turnoff is 0.3 mile south of Hwy. 92 (52 sites, $35–$50 depending on site). Reservations are essential in summer and for weekends year-round; visit **reserveamerica.com** or call 800-444-7275.

Additional Information parks.smcgov.org

HIKE 24 San Andreas Fault 🐕 👫

Highlights	The San Andreas Fault and fossils on a forgotten beach
Distance	3.5 miles one-way
Total Elevation Gain/Loss	50'/50'
Hiking Time	2–3 hours
Recommended Map	USGS 7.5-min. *San Francisco South*
Best Times	September–May
Agency	Golden Gate National Recreation Area
Difficulty	★

AFTER COVERING 500 miles overland, the San Andreas Fault dives northwest from the bluffs of Daly City into the Pacific Ocean. North of this tectonic landmark, a beach of surprising seclusion runs for more than 3 miles below cliffs of mud, sand, and fossils.

Approximately 2 million years ago, the geography of the Bay Area differed radically. The Point Reyes Peninsula sat directly west of today's Golden Gate, partially enclosing a shallow basin between itself and the mainland. Sediments poured in from the surrounding landmasses, filling the basin with thick layers of sand, mud, and gravel. In all, a deep reservoir of sediment more than a mile thick was deposited. Layers formed during periods of shallow water include thick beds of fossils—crushed

Slip-sliding along

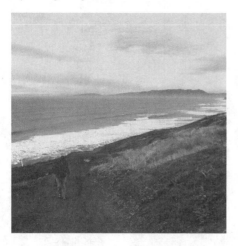

shells make up the bulk of the material, but entire preserved sand dollars and clams can also be found. Within the past 300,000 years, changing geometry along the San Andreas Fault lifted the entire basin and tilted its beds gently north to expose it as today's Merced Formation. A small piece of the northern basin remained attached to the southeast corner of the Point Reyes Peninsula as it was wrenched into its current position; it is now exposed in the bluffs east of Bolinas, as explained by Ted Konigsmark in *Geologic Trips.*

The Hike follows the beach north from Mussel Rock in north Pacifica to Fort Funston in San Francisco. *This trip can become dangerous during high tides, when big waves can wash to the base of the bluffs and suck people out to sea. Do not venture onto the beach if you see waves reaching the bluffs. No tide tables are posted at the trailhead—check in advance.* The hike can be made into a round-trip by returning along the beach to the trailhead. Otherwise, car arrangements must be worked out for the return to Pacifica. For those unable to do the full hike, the general flavor and experience of the locale can be had in a short 1-mile round-trip from the trailhead. While the hike can be done year-round, fog is thick in the summer and makes for a cold, low-visibility day at the beach. Crowds are light compared to other area beaches. No water is available at the trailhead.

To Reach the Trailhead From San Francisco, follow Hwy. 1 south, take the first Pacifica exit at Manor Dr., and turn right on Palmetto Dr.

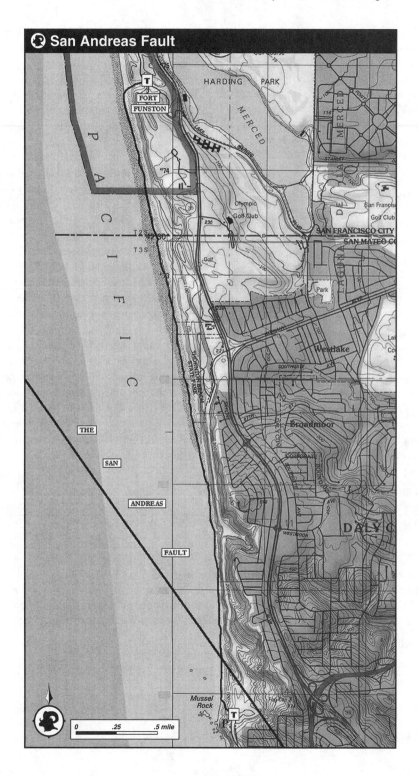

Go 0.8 mile and turn left on Westline Dr. Bear left toward the Mussel Rock Transfer Station (the dump), keep left again as the road forks right to the dump, and park in the large lot at the road's end. To reach Fort Funston, take Skyline Dr. (Hwy. 35) 4 miles north from Hwy. 1 in north Pacifica—the parking lot is on the left. Approaching Fort Funston from San Francisco, follow Skyline Dr. 0.8 mile south of the Great Hwy.

Description From the parking lot by Mussel Rock, walk through the opening in the fence and descend along roads leading down toward the beach. Looking above you to the west, notice the loose, unconsolidated slopes along the bluffs—the result of many landslides. The bluffs above the landslide area recede at a rate of up to 3 feet per year, undercutting houses that should never have been built or purchased in the first place. The edges of the landslide mark the rough boundaries of the San Andreas Fault Zone, an area approximately a half mile wide. The loose slopes mask any actual fault trace in the hillside, but it is definitely there—the great 1906 San Francisco earthquake had its epicenter immediately inland from this location.

Walking north on the beach, notice the northward tilt of the layers in the bluffs. Deposited sequentially, these layers represent a chronology of the former basin environment; they become progressively younger as you go north. Fossil beds can be identified by the white, linear exposures of crushed shells contained in a matrix of mudstone. The views north include most of the Marin coast, and Point Bonita (Hike 28) can be picked out across the Golden Gate on clear days. Fort Funston can be identified near the northern end of the bluffs as they drop in elevation. Turning south, Montara Mountain (Hike 23) forms the skyline closest to the sea, plunging into the ocean at landmark Pedro Point.

Continuing north, you pass the deep gash that Woods Gulch makes in the bluffs. Because saturated slopes increase the risk of landslides and accelerate erosion, draining this threatened area is an attempt to slow the imminent destruction of its cliffside homes. The number of people increases as you approach the path that leads up to the viewing platform and parking lot at Fort Funston. A former military reservation developed at the turn of the century, Fort Funston is now part of the Golden Gate National Recreation Area. It's a popular site for hang gliders and parasailors between March and October, when strong west winds rise over the blufftop.

Nearest Visitor Center The Pacifica Chamber of Commerce runs an excellent visitor center in partnership with the Golden Gate National Recreation Area. Near the south end of Pacifica at 225 Rockaway Beach, it's open Monday–Friday 10 a.m.–5 p.m. year-round, and 11 a.m.–3 p.m. on weekends in summer. For information call 650-355-4122.

Nearest Campground Francis Beach Campground, 650-726-8819, is open year-round at the south end of Half Moon Bay State Beach, just west of Hwy. 1 on Kelly Ave.; the turnoff is 0.3 mile south of Hwy. 92 (52 sites, $35–$50 depending on site). Reservations are essential in summer and for weekends year-round; visit **reserveamerica.com** or call 800-444-7275.

Additional Information n/a

HIKE 25   San Bruno Mountain   ↗

Highlight	An island of nature in a sea of humanity
Distance	4.9 miles round-trip
Total Elevation Gain/Loss	700'/700'
Hiking Time	2–3 hours
Recommended Map	USGS 7.5-min. *San Francisco South*
Best Times	After storms
Agency	San Bruno Mountain State and County Park
Difficulty	★★

FOUR CITIES LAP AT the base of San Bruno Mountain, encircling it with the concrete bustle of the 21st century. Yet it stands, protected, an oasis of rare plant life, the hunting ground for dozens of soaring raptors, one of the premier viewpoints in the Bay Area.

Viewed from nearby freeways, San Bruno Mountain seems barren and almost lifeless. Yet this landmark ridge preserves a large native plant community akin to what once covered all the hills of San Francisco. Isolated as it is from surrounding mountain ranges, San Bruno harbors several species of plants found almost nowhere else today. At present, 14 species of rare or endangered plants exist on the mountain. In addition, four rare species of butterflies flutter over the slopes, including the endangered San Bruno elfin and Mission blue. Nonendangered rodents, prey for dozens of raptors, scurry through the thick brush.

As the tide of development reached the base of the mountain in the 1960s, efforts began to protect this unique natural feature and its native habitats. In 1978 the state purchased the core of the new park, and in 1982 the Habitat Conservation Plan was established with developers, allowing construction on some of the surrounding native habitat in exchange for funding to preserve and protect the ecosystem within the park. This unusual plan created the San Bruno Mountain Habitat Conservation Trust Fund, used to eradicate encroaching nonnative species such as eucalyptus and reestablish endangered, existing native plants.

The Hike follows the spine of San Bruno Mountain (1,314') from the central ridgetop parking lot to the eastern end above Hwy. 101, an easy hike with incredible views. The trail is entirely exposed to the elements. Wind is common and fog can envelop the mountain from May through September, so be prepared. Views are best immediately following a winter storm, hazing up rapidly in the days that follow. Despite the millions of people residing and working around the mountain, the trails are lightly traveled—especially on weekdays. No water is available at the trailhead.

To Reach the Trailhead It is possible to approach from both I-280 and Hwy. 101. From 101, take the Bayshore Blvd. exit and turn west on Guadalupe Canyon Pkwy., reaching the park entrance (on the north side of the road) in 1.6 miles. Approaching on I-280 from the north, take the Eastmoor Ave. exit, turn left on Sullivan Rd., then quickly left again on San Pedro Rd. to cross the freeway. As you continue on San Pedro Rd., it becomes first East Market St. and then Guadalupe Canyon Pkwy. before reaching the park entrance. Approaching on I-280 from the south, take the Mission St. exit, turn left on Junipero Serra Blvd., right on San Pedro Rd., and proceed as described above. From the parking lot at the park entrance, drive underneath Guadalupe Canyon Pkwy. and up Radio Rd. to the summit parking lot. There is a day-use fee of $6.

Description The trail begins at the east end of the parking lot, following a disused dirt road

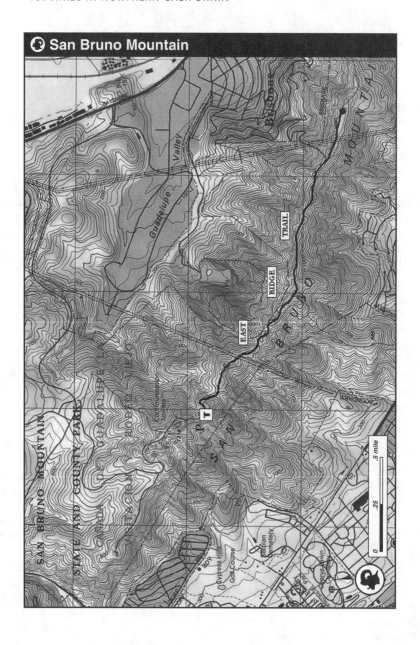

on an undulating route to East Peak. Yarrow, wild strawberry, poison oak, and other small plants hide among the skeletal fingers of the ubiquitous coyote brush. San Francisco International Airport is less than 5 miles away and continuously fills the skies with aircraft. Raptors soar in the more immediate air. The more common include red-tailed hawk, easily identified by its distinctive cry and orange-red tail; northern harrier, spotted by the large white patch on the rump; and American kestrel—the smallest raptor—identified by its small size, bandit black eye stripes, and constant tail twitching while in flight. While East Peak seems close throughout the hike, it takes longer to get there than you think. Where the slopes plummet down to Hwy. 101, you've arrived. Return the way you came, pondering this dramatic contrast between urban mania and Mother Nature.

Nearest Visitor Center This park doesn't have a visitor center. For general information, call 650-992-6770.

Nearest Campground Francis Beach Campground, 650-726-8819, is open year-round at the south end of Half Moon Bay State Beach, just west of Hwy. 1 on Kelly Ave.; the turnoff is 0.3 mile south of Hwy. 92 (52 sites, $35–$50 depending on site). Reservations are essential in summer and for weekends year-round; visit **reserveamerica.com** or call 800-444-7275.

Additional Information parks.smcgov.org

HIKE 26 San Francisco's Pacific Shore

Highlight	The wild, scenic, historic Pacific margin of San Francisco
Distance	5.5 miles one-way
Total Elevation Gain/Loss	500'/500'
Hiking Time	5–7 hours
Recommended Maps	USGS 7.5-min. *Point Bonita* and *San Francisco North*
Best Times	September–May
Agency	Golden Gate National Recreation Area
Difficulty	★★

HERE IS the power of the Pacific, breaking upon storied shores too rugged for development, punctuated by wild geologic exposures, immediate to the densest collection of humanity in California. Wander the urban wild of San Francisco.

The Hike follows San Francisco's Pacific shore from Ocean Beach to the Golden Gate Bridge, an all-day adventure completely accessible by public transportation. Cool ocean breezes make a warm sweater and/or windbreaker critical year-round. Avoid the summer months when fog envelops the Pacific shore, lowering the temperature and obscuring the spectacular views. A shuttle by bus or car is required to return to Ocean Beach at the end of the day. While no water is available at the trailhead, sources are plentiful along the way.

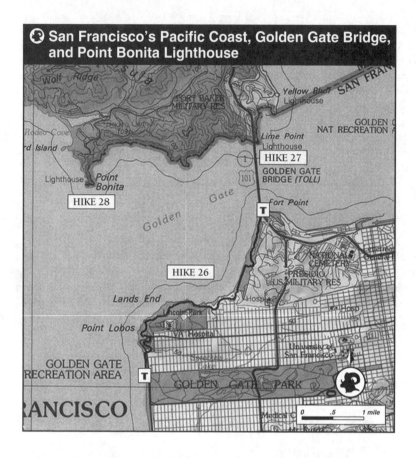

There is no safe swimming anywhere along this hike. The Pacific Ocean in San Francisco is dangerous, currents are strong, and waves can be powerful. People have been swept out to sea and drowned. Precarious cliffs are also a hazard. Respect the ocean and heed all warning signs.

To Reach the Trailhead Head to the north end of Ocean Beach at the western edge of Golden Gate Park and park in one of the large lots adjacent to the beach. Approaching from the Golden Gate Bridge, take Hwy. 1 south, turn right on John F. Kennedy Dr. and, when Kennedy Dr. ends, turn right again on Martin Luther King Jr. Dr. to reach the ocean. Approaching from the south on I-280, take the Hwy. 1/19th Ave. exit, go north on 19th Ave. to Kennedy Dr., turn left, and proceed as described above. Approaching from the Bay Bridge, take the Fell St. exit,

go west on Fell St. to Golden Gate Park, bear right on John F. Kennedy Dr., follow it through the park, and continue as described above. The northern end of this hike is located in the large tourist parking lot at the southern end of the Golden Gate Bridge, immediately east of the toll plaza.

Public transportation for this hike is provided by **Muni Bus 38** (service along Geary Blvd. to Point Lobos) and **Bus 28** (service from the Golden Gate Bridge with a stop at Geary Blvd.). Call 311 (within San Francisco) or 415-701-2311 for current schedule information, or visit **sfmta.com**.

Description From the parking lot at Ocean Beach, drop down a stairwell to the open sand. Four miles long, Ocean Beach is the largest beach in the Bay Area and stretches from Fort

Funston to the Cliff House, visible on the rocks immediately north. The Richmond and Sunset districts east of the beach were built upon a vast field of sand dunes, which covered most of northwest San Francisco and was once the fourth largest dune complex in California. All this sand originated between 10 and 15 thousand years ago during the last ice age when sea level was approximately 200 feet lower. San Francisco Bay was dry land, and the shoreline was roughly 20 miles west of its current location—you could have walked to the Farallon Islands! Instead of dropping its sediment in the bay as it does today, the Sacramento River flowed beyond the Golden Gate, depositing sand in a broad alluvial fan that was blown onshore by prevailing northwesterly winds to form Ocean Beach and the vast dune fields. Most of the sand here actually originated in the Sierra Nevada.

After enjoying Ocean Beach, walk north toward the Cliff House, head up Stairway 4, cross the Esplanade to the corner of Balboa and La Playa, and climb the stairs toward Sutro Heights on Sutro Dunes Path, which visits a 3.3-acre remnant of the dunes that once covered this area. As is true throughout this hike, numerous use paths diverge in all directions as you proceed. Continue generally north through eucalyptus and Monterey cypress to reach the top of Sutro Heights, where an open area of grass and unusual trees can be found. The tall, straight-trunked trees sporting strange wand-like foliage here are monkey puzzle trees, a type of araucaria native to Chile and Argentina.

To understand the history of Sutro Heights and its surrounding landmarks requires a brief biography of Adolph Sutro. A native of Prussia, Sutro immigrated to California in 1850 and in 1869 began constructing a tunnel designed to access and ventilate the rich mines of Nevada's Comstock Lode. Completed in 1878, the Sutro Tunnel was a huge financial success, earning Sutro a tidy fortune when he sold his shares in 1879. Returning to San Francisco, he acquired vast amounts of real estate for the future structures of Sutro Heights, the Cliff House, and the Sutro Baths. At one point, he owned one-eleventh of all city land. Over the next 20 years, Sutro helped build San Francisco, even serving

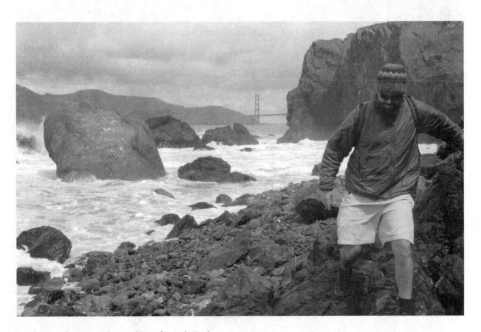

Exploring the rugged coastline of Lands End

as mayor from 1895 to 1897. After his death in 1898, the sights and wonders he created slowly fell into disrepair, leaving little but memories and the photographs so well preserved by the National Park Service today.

Acquired by Sutro in 1881, Sutro Heights was an open blufftop with little vegetation. With the help of 11 full-time gardeners, he transformed it into an exotic plant and flower garden with a substantial greenhouse. A popular tourist destination while in operation, the structure was torn down in 1939. South from the large viewing platform, you can see the long stretch of Ocean Beach and distant Montara Mountain (Hike 23) terminating in the ocean at Point San Pedro. Visible on clear days are the Farallon Islands to the west and Point Reyes to the northwest.

From Sutro Heights, head down to the Lands End Lookout parking lot—the dirt path splits north from the paved trail by the small gazebo. Cross Point Lobos Ave. and make the quick side trip down to the Cliff House. The current Cliff House is the third structure occupying this precarious site. The first was an unassuming structure known as Seal Rock House, purchased by Sutro in 1881, that catered to San Francisco's elite. Destroyed by fire in 1894, Seal Rock House was replaced by the opulent Victorian Cliff House, an eight-story marvel styled after a French chateau, which survived the 1906 earthquake only to be destroyed by fire in 1907. Constructed in 1909 by Sutro's daughter, the third and current Cliff House is a less-exciting neoclassic building. Immediately offshore from the Cliff House sit Seal Rocks, named for the California and Steller's sea lions (once considered seals) that have historically used the rocks as a safe haven and bark boisterously into the

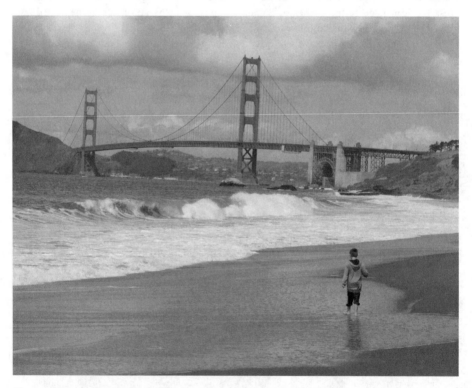

The gentle sands of Baker Beach offer an exceptional view of the Golden Gate.

wind. Today, Seal Rocks are much quieter as most of the sea lions seem to be congregating near Fisherman's Wharf at Pier 39.

From the Cliff House, walk back up Point Lobos Ave. to the Lands End Visitor Center, which provides excellent interpretive displays of the area's fascinating history and geology. After savoring the information overload, head down to the ruins of Sutro Baths.

Opened to the public in 1896, the Sutro Baths complex covered more than 3 acres and was enclosed by 100,000 square feet of glass. In addition to one freshwater pool, 1.685 million gallons of seawater filled 6 separate saltwater swimming tanks that could be flushed in less than an hour by the incoming tides. There were 9 springboards, 7 toboggan slides, 3 trapezes, 1 high dive, 30 swinging rings, 20,000 bathing suits, 40,000 towels, 500 private dressing rooms, a 5,300-seat amphitheater, 3 restaurants, natural-history exhibits, art galleries, and a jungle of exotic plants. Up to 1,600 bathers could swim at once, the main room had a capacity of 15,000, and more than 25,000 people could visit in a single day. Following Sutro's death, the baths slowly fell into disrepair; they were destroyed by fire in 1966. Today the trail leads past the remaining foundation to a large concrete platform, which was the site of two-gun Battery Lobos during World War II. Also worth a visit is the nearby tunnel, which penetrates into the rock slopes, booms with the crash of pounding waves, and terminates at an ocean-swept pile of rocky coast.

The hike continues uphill on a stairway to rejoin the broad Coastal Trail. Bear left on the Coastal Trail, the former roadbed of the Ferries and Cliff House Railroad. Continue north where a wide trail joins from the right; you will soon see the entire Golden Gate Bridge (Hike 27) through the surrounding Monterey cypress. As the large building of the Veterans Administration Hospital appears south over the bluffs above you, look left for the trail leading down to the ocean at Mile Rock Beach and Lands End. A small promontory offering views of a San Francisco coastline as wild as any in California, Lands End is a side trip not to be missed.

The main trail now heads east, visiting incredible views as it passes off-limits Painted Rock Cliff and undulates up and down before reaching the immaculate greens of Lincoln Golf Course. Follow signs toward Eagle's Point, where you can peer down to Dead Man's Point, a gnarly surf break that attracts surfers willing to brave this inhospitable spot.

You next reach El Camino del Mar, where you go left (east) down the sidewalk, bearing left at all intersections to reach the posted access for China Beach (via a hard left leading to parking above the small sandy beach). From this intersection, continue on Sea Cliff Dr. to its eastern end, turn left on 25th Ave. N., and follow the path down to Baker Beach.

Named for a prominent San Francisco lawyer killed in the Civil War, Baker Beach was the site of San Francisco's only shark attack, a fatal incident that occurred in 1959. Walk north along the beach and make the sandy, exhausting ascent up the stairway to Lincoln Blvd. Turn left and walk parallel to Lincoln Blvd. for approximately 100 yards to a trail heading left for Battery Crosby, one of 22 coastal batteries constructed in and around the Presidio. The majority of these, including Crosby, were built and manned between 1895 and 1945 as a defense against potential invasion. From here, a maze of trails winds north on the bluffs above the ocean. While the main trail continues along Lincoln Blvd., it is possible to follow any number of the use paths—just keep heading north.

The distinctive green bluffs here are composed of serpentine, an unusual rock that produces soils inhospitable to most plants. Consequently, unique ecosystems have developed on serpentine outcrops around the state, which harbor many rare and endangered species found nowhere else. Please respect the signs and fences along this section—they are designed to protect and rehabilitate this rare San Francisco ecosystem. The heavily sheared, landslide-prone bluffs here can be closely examined by scrambling down to the secluded rocky shoreline at their base, an exciting side trip.

Continuing north past Batteries West (armed with 12 cannons and operational 1873–1898),

Godfrey (3 guns, 1896–1943), Boutelle (2 guns, 1898–1917), Marcus Miller (3 guns, 1899–1920), and Cranston (2 guns, 1898–1943), the maze of trails meets a paved bike path that leads underneath the Golden Gate Bridge to the large parking lot and tourist center by the toll plaza.

Nearest Visitor Center The Lands End Visitor Center, 415-426-5240, is just north of Cliff House on Point Lobos Ave. It's open weekdays 9 a.m.–5 p.m., and weekends 9 a.m.–7 p.m.

Nearest Campgrounds Group campsites are available in the Marin Headlands at Kirby Cove (4 sites, $25; open April–October). Reservations are essential and can be made up to 3 months in advance; visit **recreation.gov** or call 877-444-6777. There is also a free walk-in campground at Bicentennial near Battery Wallace (3 sites, maximum 3 people per site, open year-round). Reservations are required and can be made up to 30 days in advance by calling the visitor center at 415-331-1540. Permits must be picked up at the visitor center, on Bunker Rd. in Rodeo Valley and open daily 9:30 a.m.–4:30 p.m.

Additional Information nps.gov/goga

HIKE 27 Golden Gate Bridge ↗ 🚶

Highlights	The bridge. The view. The experience.
Distance	2.4 miles round-trip
Total Elevation Gain/Loss	60'/60'
Hiking Time	1–2 hours
Recommended Map	USGS 7.5-min. *San Francisco North*
Best Times	September–May
Agency	Golden Gate National Recreation Area
Difficulty	★

(See map on page 96.)

A GRACEFUL SWEEP of perfection, the Golden Gate Bridge is the defining landmark of Northern California. It is a marvel of human ingenuity that spanned an impossible gap across a violent strait, an engineering masterpiece famous the world over.

The Hike covers the length of the Golden Gate Bridge and explores its location, history, and construction. While the round-trip hike can be completed from either end, the description below begins from the south. It is usually cold and windy on the bridge with summer months bringing dense fog to the mix, obscuring the incredible views, and making the rest of the year preferable for a visit. A warm sweater and windbreaker are recommended items year-round. Tourists are thick on the bridge and the wide diversity of countries represented is entertaining. The bridge is closed to pedestrians after dark and reopens at 5 a.m. Water is available at the trailhead.

To Reach the Trailhead Take Hwy. 101 to the southern end of the bridge and park in the main tourist lot immediately east of the toll plaza. To reach the trailhead by public transportation, take **Muni Bus 28.** Call 311 (within

San Francisco) or 415-701-2311 for current schedule information, or visit **sfmta.com**.

Description The hike begins by the statue of Joseph Strauss, chief engineer of the Golden Gate Bridge from inception to completion. An engineer whose college graduation thesis was a bridge design for spanning the 50-mile-wide Bering Strait between Alaska and Russia, Strauss was a man of intense vision, purpose, and ingenuity. By the time construction began in early 1933, he had completed more than 400 bridges around the world and was considered by many to be the only man capable of realizing such an ambitious project. It would be his final and greatest work.

From here, head to the bridge itself, passing the rotunda gift shop to get to the east sidewalk near a barrage of signs and regulations. As you begin walking across the bridge, contemplate the fury beneath your feet. The Sacramento River drains more than 59,000 square miles (40% of the entire state), pouring into shallow San Francisco Bay from the northeast. The bay has only one outlet—the Golden Gate—a narrow 1-mile-wide channel to the sea that is affected twice daily by the changing tides. During incoming tides, the rising waters pour into the bay and impound the freshwater brought in by the Sacramento River. As the tides reverse, an unbelievable volume of water rushes out the narrow entrance. Every 12 hours, the bay disgorges one-sixth of its entire volume through the Golden Gate at a rate of roughly 2.3 million gallons per second. Moving at a speed of between 4.5 and 7.5 knots, the average flow is seven times that of the Mississippi River. Add to that powerful winds capable of reaching 60 miles per hour and the fury of nature here is readily apparent.

Savor the views as you walk toward the south tower. Southeast, Coit Tower and downtown San Francisco are apparent, connected to the East Bay via the Bay Bridge. Looking east across the bay, the summit of Mount Diablo (Hike 14) can be seen crowning the East Bay Hills, and downtown Berkeley is visible beyond nearby Alcatraz Island. Northeast is substantial

Angel Island and the Tiburon peninsula. While views west are somewhat obscured by the far railings, the jagged spit of Point Bonita (Hike 28) juts from the north. Fort Point is directly beneath you, a pre–Civil War fort built during the 1850s to safeguard America's newfound western possession. In designing the bridge, Strauss recognized that preservation of this important historical landmark was imperative; he built the distinctive rainbow arches above to frame it visually. The many emergency phones along the sidewalk are to help prevent potential suicides—to date, more than 1,000 people have leapt to their deaths from the bridge.

Reaching the south tower, look up its fluted form. Tapering as it rises to its peak of 746 feet above sea level, this tower proved to be one of the greatest engineering challenges of the bridge. Its concrete foundation pier sits more than 1,100 feet offshore on a sloping underwater ledge between 60 and 80 feet deep, fully in the brunt of waves and tidal current. To build it required construction of a precarious trestle from shore to site, building fenders around the pier site, blasting a foundation hole to a level depth of 100 feet below sea level, extending the fenders from surface to bottom, and then dewatering (pumping out the water from) the entire thing. The trestle and fenders were destroyed by waves during early construction and had to be rebuilt prior to pouring the concrete. The north pier foundation proved less difficult; it was built close to shore on a flat, shallow ledge a mere 20 feet below the surface.

The massive steel towers sit on top of these concrete piers, each constructed of 43 million pounds of steel designed to support 85 million pounds of dead weight. Surprisingly, they are not solid, constructed instead of hollow cells 42 inches square by 35 feet high, which allow each tower to move laterally up to 13 inches and to bend 18 inches toward the channel and 22 inches toward the shore, as the cables expand and contract with the temperature. In driving the 600,000 rivets required to put each tower together, workers had to scramble inside and through the honeycombed boxes. Remarkably,

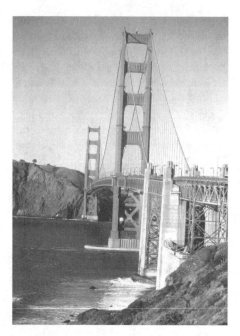

The Golden Gate Bridge

the entire south tower was constructed in a scant 101 days.

The distance between the two towers is 4,200 feet; as you walk it, admire the catenary curve of the two main bridge cables. These huge cables measure 36.5 inches in diameter, are 7,650 feet long, and weigh 7,125 tons each. They attach to the earth at four massive concrete anchors buried 12 stories deep in the ground and capable of withstanding 63 million pounds of pull each. Essentially spun in place,

each cable is composed of 27,000 strands of thin wire, which were individually strung from anchorage to tower to tower to anchorage and back again. Approximately 80,000 miles of this pencil-thin wire were used, enough to wrap around the equator three times.

The Golden Gate Bridge is a suspension bridge. That is, the roadway is suspended from cables supported by towers. Once the cables were complete, construction of the 90-foot-wide roadway began. Strauss was farsighted enough to build a bridge six lanes wide, a width considered somewhat excessive at the time—the traffic around you today probably would have surprised him. Construction began from both towers simultaneously and the roadway was joined in November 1936. Paving the roadway followed; it resulted in the main fatalities of the construction process. An innovative safety net had been rigged beneath the expanding and precarious roadway, saving fallen men from plummeting to their death. (Those so saved by the net formed a small "Halfway to Hell" club.) Unfortunately, in February 1937, a platform supporting a work crew detached, ripping through the net and killing 10 men. An earlier crane accident had claimed the bridge's first victim, making a final count of 11 fatalities. Yet construction proceeded, and on May 27, 1937, the $35 million bridge opened to the public amid great fanfare. Joseph Strauss died the following year.

Continue to the viewing platform at the north end of the bridge and admire this masterpiece before returning.

Nearest Visitor Center The Golden Gate Bridge Gift Center, on the southeast side of the toll plaza, is open daily 9 a.m.–6 p.m., with extended hours during the summer.

Nearest Campgrounds Group sites are available in the Marin Headlands at Kirby Cove (4 sites, $25; open April–October). Reservations are essential and can be made up to 3 months in advance; visit **recreation.gov** or call 877-444-6777. There is also a free walk-in campground at Bicentennial near Battery Wallace (3 sites, maximum 3 people per site, open year-round). Reservations are required and can be made up to 30 days in advance by calling the visitor center at 415-331-1540. Permits must be picked up at the visitor center, on Bunker Rd. in Rodeo Valley and open daily 9:30 a.m.–4:30 p.m.

Additional Information goldengatebridge.org

HIKE 28 Point Bonita ◢ ╱ 🛉

Highlights	The jaws of the Golden Gate and the legacy of "wickies" and "surfmen"
Distance	1.0 mile round-trip
Total Elevation Gain/Loss	50'/50'
Hiking Time	1 hour
Recommended Map	USGS 7.5-min. *Point Bonita*
Best Times	September–May
Agency	Golden Gate National Recreation Area
Difficulty	★

(See map on page 96.)

TAKE A SHORT STROLL to the farthest edge of the Bay Area. Perched on a naked fin of rock jabbing into the ocean, Point Bonita Lighthouse is a lonely sentinel with extraordinary views.

The Hike follows an easy paved path through a tunnel and over a unique suspension bridge to the lighthouse. Unfortunately, the lighthouse path is only open Saturday through Monday from 12:30 to 3:30 p.m.; otherwise, it is closed at the tunnel. While the hike to the tunnel is pleasant, it cannot rival the full lighthouse experience. Prepare for wind—lots of wind—as Point Bonita is always blustery. Timing is important— fog blankets the point for days on end during the summer months, making the rest of the year better for a visit. The lighthouse may be closed if wave and weather conditions are too severe.

To Reach the Trailhead Take Hwy. 101 to the Alexander Ave. exit, the first off-ramp north of the Golden Gate Bridge. Following signs to the Marin Headlands, quickly turn left to pass through the one-lane tunnel. A mile past the tunnel turn left onto McCullough Rd., follow it uphill, and then turn right onto spectacular Conzelman Rd., which becomes a narrow one-lane road that drops precipitously to a T-junction by a YMCA. Go left and park in the posted Point Bonita lot.

Public transportation to Point Bonita is available from San Francisco on weekends and some holidays aboard **Muni Bus 76X,** which departs once an hour from downtown. For current schedule information, **sfmta.com.**

Description From the parking area, follow the paved path below a stand of Monterey cypress. Dropping toward the tunnel, you reach an informative placard detailing the story of the Point Bonita Lifesaving Station and the "surfmen" who manned it. According to a 1908 *San Francisco Chronicle* article describing the surfmen, "Every man enlisted in this daring work must have had at least three years of experience as a sailor. He must be an expert boatman and physically perfect. He is not allowed to drink while in uniform, and to be caught intoxicated means immediate dismissal. As a matter of course he must be courageous. The discipline is very strict."

As you approach the tunnel, the first views north open up and Point Reyes and Bolinas are visible beyond the pounding surf. The shark fin of rock through which the tunnel passes is composed of pillow basalt, a rock highly resistant to erosion. It is formed on the ocean bottom when liquid magma is extruded from the seafloor. As the molten rock encounters seawater, its outer shell is instantly cooled to form a distinctive pillow shape. Liquid magma remains inside, however, and as it is squeezed out again, another pillow is formed on top, creating large stacks of these distinctive formations.

Before you enter the tunnel, notice the odd, large-leafed plants clinging to cracks in the

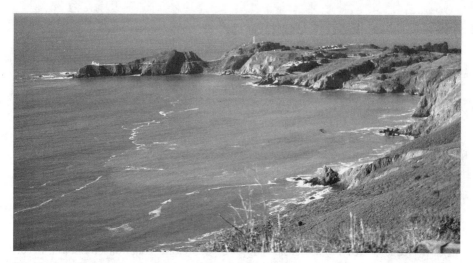

Point Bonita Lighthouse perches on the tip of a jagged peninsula.

rock. These are feral cabbages, escaped from the gardens of past lighthouse keepers and now uniquely adapted to survive the hostile environment of Point Bonita. On the other side of the tunnel, railings protect you from the drop to the rocks below. When you reach the suspension bridge, please observe the five-person limit.

When Point Bonita Lighthouse opened in 1855, it was the third lighthouse constructed on the West Coast, built in response to the more than 300 ships that had run aground near the Golden Gate during the Gold Rush period. The original Fresnel lens, constructed in France, was capable of bending 70% of radiant light onto a horizontal plane. Its original light was the flame on an oil-fed wick, tended by resident lighthouse keepers known as "wickies." Incredibly, the same lens is still in use today, sending a beam of light visible for 18 miles. In 1980 the lighthouse was the last in the United States to become automated, and today a single 1,000-watt bulb provides the light. The lighthouse building is open to the public, but light itself is off-limits.

Nearest Visitor Center The Marin Headlands Visitor Center, 415-331-1540, 1 mile from Point Bonita on Bunker Rd. in Rodeo Valley, is open daily 9:30 a.m.–4:30 p.m. year-round.

Nearest Campgrounds Group campsites are available in the Marin Headlands at Kirby Cove (4 sites, $25; open April–October). Reservations are essential and can be made up to 3 months in advance; visit **recreation.gov** or call 877-444-6777. There is also a free walk-in campground at Bicentennial near Battery Wallace (3 sites, maximum 3 people per site; open year-round). Reservations are required and can be made up to 30 days in advance by calling the visitor center. Permits must be picked up at the visitor center during open hours.

Additional Information nps.gov/goga

HIKE 29 Gerbode Valley ↻ 🚶

Highlights	Wildflowers, wildlife, and wild land—so close, yet so far away
Distance	6.1 miles
Total Elevation Gain/Loss	1,500'/1,500'
Hiking Time	3–5 hours
Recommended Maps	Tom Harrison's *Mount Tamalpais,* USGS 7.5-min. *Point Bonita*
Best Times	September–May
Agency	Marin Headlands, Golden Gate National Recreation Area
Difficulty	★★

IT IS AS IT WAS. Rolling hills cleft by valleys, split by ridges, battered by the sea; a land of sweeping vistas, vibrant life, and dramatic geology in a natural world protected from the bustle of the Bay Area. The Marin Headlands await.

The Hike loops around broad Gerbode Valley in the central Headlands, offering far-reaching views of sea, slopes, and city from the heart of this protected landscape. The clear skies and abundant wildflowers of spring are optimal for a visit, though the sunny days of fall and crystalline air of winter are also pleasant. Summer brings fog and windy conditions. The area's immediate proximity to San Francisco draws regular crowds, and you'll likely encounter dozens of hikers and mountain bikers, especially on weekends. No water is available at the trailhead.

To Reach the Trailhead From the south, take Hwy. 101 to the Alexander Ave. exit (the first off-ramp north of the Golden Gate Bridge) and follow signs toward the Marin Headlands, turning left to pass through the one-lane tunnel and then continuing straight on Bunker Rd. for approximately 2 miles to the visitor center. Bear right toward Fort Cronkhite, reaching the trailhead on the right in a quarter mile.

Approaching from the north, take the last Sausalito exit immediately before the Golden Gate Bridge, turn left at the stop sign, bear right up steep Conzelman Rd., and continue on Conzelman Rd. for 3 miles to the intersection by Battery Alexander. Turn right, continue 0.5 mile

to the visitor center, and turn left toward Fort Cronkhite.

Description From the trailhead (0.0/20'), begin on broad Miwok Trail as it passes through open grassland punctuated by coyote brush, blackberry brambles, and a seasonal display of lupine, poppies, paintbrush, checkerbloom, irises, and other wildflowers. As you proceed, watch for quail and jackrabbits in the brush, black-tailed deer and the elusive bobcat in open clearings, and red-tailed hawks and other raptors overhead.

The trail briefly enters a small riparian alley filled with willows, stinging nettle, wild cucumber vines, horsetail, elderberry, dogwood, bracken fern, vetch, and other moisture-loving plants, a marked contrast to the surrounding dry slopes. You pass a feeder trail on the right from nearby Bunker Road (0.4/20') and then quickly reach Bobcat Trail (your return route) on the right (0.5/30'). Remain on Miwok Trail as it turns toward the valley slopes and steadily climbs toward the ridgeline. Enjoy views north into adjacent Tennessee Valley as you pass Wolf Ridge Trail on the left (1.6/600') and briefly undulate along the ridge. Downtown San Francisco peeks over the hills to the south and the long spine of Mount Tamalpais slowly rises to the north. Miwok Trail narrows to single-track shortly before reaching Old Springs Trail (1.9/640').

Continue straight on Miwok Trail as it climbs steeply toward the Federal Aviation Administration (FAA) facilities atop Hill 1041, offering stratospheric views across the Bay Area. To the

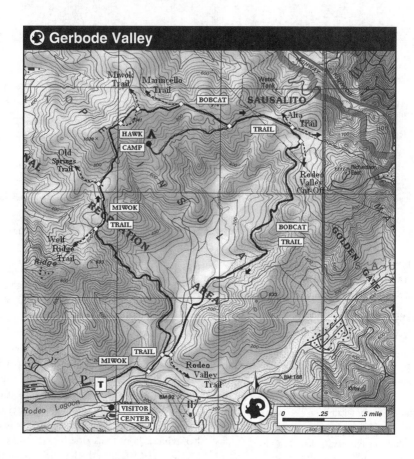

Gerbode Valley

south are the Golden Gate Bridge, downtown San Francisco, antenna-lined San Bruno Mountain (Hike 25), and distant Montara Mountain (Hike 23). To the east are Mount Diablo (Hike 14), the Bay Bridge, Oakland, Berkeley, and the entire East Bay hills. To the north, Mount Tamalpais (2,571') dominates above Mill Valley, the Tiburon peninsula, and Angel Island. To the west is the vast Pacific Ocean, pimpled with the Farallon Islands on clear days.

The trail splits and rejoins around the fenced-off FAA facilities. Past the FAA hilltop, continue straight on Bobcat Trail as Miwok Trail splits left to descend into Tennessee Valley (2.5/ 1,000'). Descending briefly, Bobcat Trail quickly reaches the junction with Marincello Trail (2.8/ 900'). This is an appropriate point to marvel at the protected world of Gerbode Valley, a world almost lost to development.

Imagine 30,000 people living in the valley below, with hundreds of homes lining Wolf Ridge and 19 high-rise buildings towering over schools, churches, shopping centers, and light industry. During the 1960s, it almost happened. A master development plan for a town named Marincello was drawn up for the privately owned valley and an access road (Marincello Trail) was built to facilitate construction. Financial and bureaucratic delays slowed the project, however, and a key court decision in the late 1960s ultimately stopped it altogether. The Nature Conservancy later purchased the land for $6.5 million and bequeathed it to the National Park Service, forever protecting it for public enjoyment.

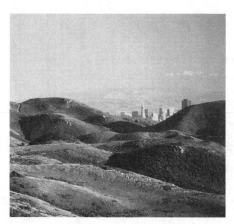

So close, so far away—San Francisco peeks over the hills of the Marin Headlands.

Bear right on Bobcat Trail, soon passing the junction for Hawk Camp (3.1/780') on the right. A small copse of trees marks the camp location a half mile away. Continuing, Bobcat Trail dips beneath power lines and passes junctions on the left for Alta Trail (3.6/730') and Rodeo Valley Cut-Off Trail (3.7/720'). As you begin the slow downward traverse back toward the trailhead, note the different vegetation in the adjacent north-facing gullies—bay, hazel, coast live oak, elderberry, and the occasional Douglas-fir flourish in these moist pockets. Bobcat Trail passes Rodeo Valley Trail on the left (5.5/50') shortly before reaching the earlier junction with Miwok Trail (5.6/30') and the final return stretch to the trailhead (6.1/20').

Nearest Visitor Center The Marin Headlands Visitor Center, 415-331-1540, is open daily 9:30 a.m.–4:30 p.m. year-round.

Backpacking Information Backcountry camping is allowed at Hawk Camp (3 sites, free). Each site accommodates a maximum of 4 people. An outhouse and picnic tables are provided, but water is not available. Reservations can be made up to 30 days in advance by calling the visitor center; unreserved sites are available at the visitor center on a first-come, first-served basis.

Nearest Campgrounds Group campsites are available in the Marin Headlands at Kirby Cove (4 sites, $25; open April–October). Reservations are essential and can be made up to 3 months in advance; visit **recreation.gov** or call 877-444-6777. There is also a free walk-in campground at Bicentennial near Battery Wallace (3 sites, maximum 3 people per site; open year-round). Reservations are required and can be made up to 30 days in advance by calling the visitor center. Permits must be picked up at the visitor center during open hours.

Additional Information nps.gov/goga

HIKE 30 Ring Mountain ↻ 🐕 👫

Highlights	Bay-sweeping views and cathedral oaks
Distance	3.2 miles
Total Elevation Gain/Loss	600'/600'
Hiking Time	2–3 hours
Recommended Map	USGS 7.5-min. *San Quentin*
Best Times	Year-round
Agency	Ring Mountain Open Space Preserve, Marin County Open Space District
Difficulty	★★

RING MOUNTAIN BULGES upward from the shores of San Francisco Bay, a bald hillock offering exceptional 360-degree views of the northern Bay Area. A few ancient live oaks line the ridges, twisting in gnarled and fantastic form. Add in some unusual rock outcrops and you've got a full array of natural highlights.

The Hike loops to the summit of 602-foot Ring Mountain from the north, winding upward to meet a series of fire roads near the top. After a visit to hulking Turtle Rock and the nearby summit, you loop downward past several enormous live oaks. The hike can be completed year-round, though wet conditions make for muddy walking at times. The far-reaching views are the primary attraction; aim for a fog-free day. No water is available at the trailhead.

To Reach the Trailhead Take Hwy. 101 to the Paradise Dr. exit and follow Paradise Dr. east for 1.5 miles to the signed trailhead on the south side of the road. Park by the roadside.

Description From the trailhead (0.0/10'), the wide path strikes out past coyote brush, toyon, and young bay trees. You quickly reach a junction, where you bear right on Phyllis Ellman Trail (you'll return from the left on Loop Trail). The singletrack trail winds upward past blackberry vines and abundant rock outcrops, evidence of the site's unusual geology.

As a tectonic plate is forced beneath an adjacent continent—or *subducted*—it descends 10–30 miles into the earth's mantle, where

temperatures are hot enough to melt all rocks. However, since the diving plate is cool and warms slowly, not all of it may melt. Instead, portions are altered into new rock forms by extreme pressure, reemerging much later to indicate the site of the former subduction zone. Subduction occurred along the coast of California for approximately 150 million years, until the San Andreas Fault became active roughly 28 million years ago. On Ring Mountain, these telltale rocks include blueschist, a

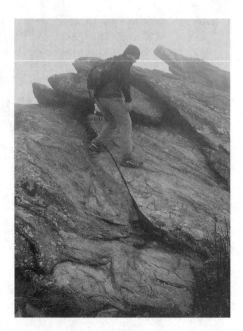

The Turtle suffers no fools.

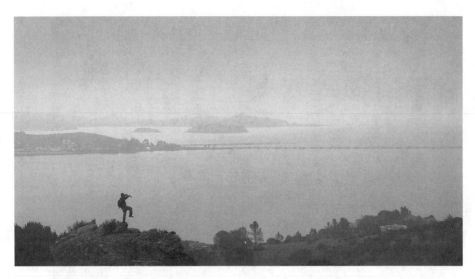

Step into the ring.

vibrantly dark-blue stone; and waxy-green serpentine, California's state rock.

Views steadily expand as you ascend, peering north toward the San Rafael Bridge and San Quentin Prison on its western end. Two unnamed side paths soon split off to the right—remain left to begin traversing up the hillside. The route switchbacks above a small ravine, where your return route on Loop Trail is visible on the opposite side.

The trail soon forks again. Stay right on the posted trail to quickly crest at a copse of ancient live oaks (0.6/340'). From here, the trail widens and becomes steeper as it ascends the grassy flanks to Ring Mountain Fire Rd. (0.9/460'). Views now open south toward the spires of San Francisco and the central San Francisco Bay. Bear left, passing Loop Trail on your left (1.0/520') and hulking Turtle Rock—a popular bouldering spot—on your right. Less technical climbers can easily scramble atop its shell from behind.

The trail crests and drops briefly to Taylor Fire Rd. (1.2/540'). Turn right on the asphalt path, then quickly bear left on an unpaved road that wanders over to Ring Mountain's highest point on the east end of the broad hilltop (1.4/602'). A small grove of wind-sculpted bay trees marks the spot. From here, enjoy some of the hike's most expansive views. Paradise Cay and the swanky shoreline homes of Tiburon lie below you to the southeast. The Oakland–Berkeley hills line the eastern horizon; the pyramidal summit of Mount Diablo (Hike 15) peeks over the top on clear days. To the west, the flanks and summit of Mount Tamalpais (Hike 32) loom, while the rolling hills of the Marin Headlands (Hike 30) hide just out of sight to the southwest. San Francisco pincushions the sky farther south.

Retrace your steps to the earlier junction with Loop Trail (1.8/520') and turn right to begin your downward journey. The singletrack trail steadily drops down a small ridgeline intermittently shaded by bay trees. You pass another incredible coast live oak along the way (2.8/420') whose elephant leg branches extend far down the hillside. Enjoy continuous views north as you descend past numerous use paths crisscrossing the hillside; the main path is obvious and marked by a series of numbered interpretive posts. As you approach the preserve boundary, the trail curves left into the adjacent gully, crosses its ephemeral rivulet, and reaches the earlier junction with Phyllis Ellman Trail (3.1/60'). Turn right to return to the trailhead.

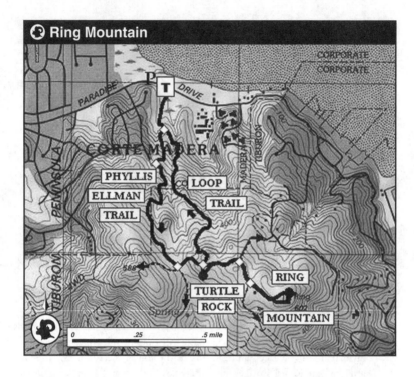

Nearest Visitor Center This preserve doesn't have a visitor center. Call the main Marin County Open Space District office at 415-499-6387 for general information.

Nearest Campgrounds Nearby Mount Tamalpais State Park has Pantoll Campground, by Pantoll Ranger Station (16 first-come, first-served sites); and Bootjack Campground, on Panoramic Hwy. (15 first-come, first-served sites). Both are $25/night and require a short 100-yard walk-in and usually fill by afternoon. Steep Ravine Environmental Campground, on a marine terrace 1 mile south of Stinson Beach on Hwy. 1, has 10 rustic cabins ($100/night) and 7 primitive campsites ($25). Reservations are essential months in advance for the cabins; visit **reserveamerica.com** or call 800-444-7275.

Additional Information marincountyparks.org

HIKE 31 Mount Tamalpais ◯

Highlights	A summit challenge with premier views of the Bay Area
Distance	6.8 miles
Total Elevation Gain/Loss	1,900'/1,900'
Hiking Time	4–6 hours
Recommended Map	USGS 7.5-min. *San Rafael*
Best Times	Year-round
Agency	Mount Tamalpais State Park, Marin Municipal Water District
Difficulty	★★★

VISIBLE THROUGHOUT the Bay Area, the long spine of Mount Tamalpais constantly beckons the hiker with a few recreational hours to spare. Read on for an excellent taste of all the mountain has to offer.

The Hike climbs steeply from Mountain Home Inn on Panoramic Hwy. directly to the summit of Mount Tamalpais (2,571'), before looping around the mountain's eastern flanks to return to the trailhead. With a maze of trails crisscrossing the mountain, the hike utilizes the following ones in this order: Gravity Car Grade, Old Railroad Grade, Vic Haun, Temelpa, Verna Dunshee, Eldridge Grade, Wheeler, and Hoo-Koo-E-Koo. The hike can be done year-round, with spring and fall offering the most idyllic weather. The stunning views are clearest following winter storms. Summer fog can be thick in the area, but even then views tend to remain dramatic. Water is available at the trailhead.

To Reach the Trailhead From Hwy. 101 in Marin City, take Hwy. 1 northwest toward Stinson Beach and bear right on Panoramic Hwy. at the posted Y-junction. Remain on Panoramic Hwy. for 5 miles following the ridgetop, and park in the lot across from Mountain Home Inn (at the edge of Mount Tamalpais State Park). If the lot is full, go down the small paved road across the highway and park at the side where it turns to dirt.

Public transportation is available on **West Marin Stagecoach Route 61,** which makes four runs daily to Bolinas from Marin City, stopping at Mountain Home Inn along the way (415-526-3239, **marintransit.org**).

Description From the trailhead (0.0/930'), Muir Woods' deep watershed is visible southwest below you and the summit towers due north above you. The trail begins across the highway on a small paved road that immediately brings you to a fork by a watershed boundary sign—bear right. Now on a dirt road, the trail soon crosses a gate. Beyond the gate, Douglas-fir, madrone, coast live oak, toyon, and tanoak all appear along the broad trail, as do abundant second-growth redwood trees. Tantalizing views of San Francisco and the Bay Area open up intermittently as you proceed, soon reaching an area where several wide roads intersect (0.8/1,100')—continue left toward East Peak on Old Railroad Grade.

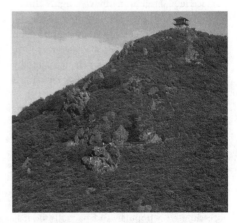

Exceptional views await atop the summit of Mount Tamalpais.

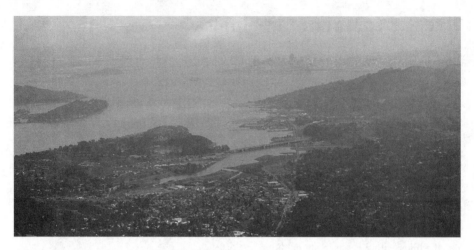

Looking south from the flanks of Mount Tamalpais

For the next 0.3 mile, you are walking on the old roadbed used by steam trains of the Mount Tamalpais and Muir Woods Railway between 1896 and 1930. While in operation, "the crookedest railroad in the world" journeyed 8.25 miles from Mill Valley to the summit on an estimated 281 curves. After making two of those curves, the roadbed reaches a posted junction with the wide Hoo-Koo-E-Koo Trail (1.1/1,200'), which heads east while Old Railroad Grade curves back west. Between these two wide paths, directly at the junction, the unposted singletrack Vic Haun Trail strikes almost directly uphill—take it!

Vic Haun Trail immediately begins climbing through a tunnel of manzanita and small redwoods before breaking out onto more open slopes with increasingly excellent views south. Large chinquapin bushes appear occasionally by the trail before it traverses east, crossing a small stream thick with California bay. When you reach the Temelpa Trail, your path continues steeply upward via numerous switchbacks to the paved Verna Dunshee Trail, which encircles the summit (2.3/2,320'). Go either left or right; either way gets you to the parking lot at the crowded summit. The fire lookout above you marks the top and is easily accessible by a popular and partially boardwalked trail.

The summit and spine of Mount Tam are composed of an unusual erosion-resistant tourmaline, formed by a reaction when sandstone becomes permeated with boron-rich water. Exposures are plentiful as you make the final push to the lookout. From the top you can see the heart of the Bay Area.

Back down at the parking lot, walk a short distance down the main paved road to find the posted gate for Eldridge Grade on the right. Drop down the wide rocky trail, noting the change in vegetation. California bay and madrone are common, joined by California nutmeg trees with pointy fir-like needles. Winding below the summit, the trail reaches an obvious spur on the left due north from the peak. This is a steep, singletrack shortcut to Inspiration Point that bypasses a long switchback on Eldridge Grade. From Inspiration Point (4.0/1,880'), continue descending east on Eldridge Grade until you reach a posted junction (4.6/1,580') at a large switchback—continue straight on singletrack Wheeler Trail.

Wheeler Trail is steep, descending rapidly through thick, young redwood forest and huckleberry bushes to reach the wide Hoo-Koo-E-Koo Trail (5.0/1,110'). Turn right and stay on Hoo-Koo-E-Koo Trail until you rejoin the Old Railroad Grade (5.7/1,200'). Retrace your earlier steps to the trailhead (6.8/930').

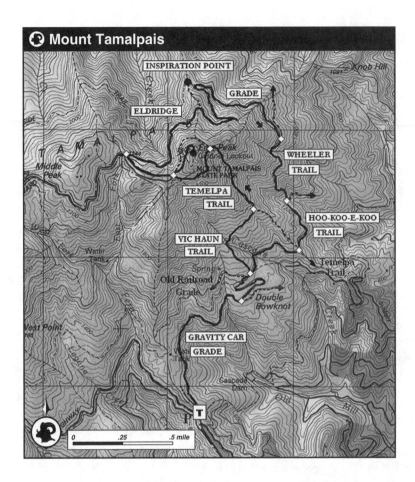

Nearest Visitor Center East Peak Visitor Center, by the summit parking lot, is open weekends approximately 11 a.m.–4 p.m. Also try Pantoll Ranger Station, 415-388-2070, 2.8 miles west of the trailhead on Panoramic Hwy.; it's open approximately 9 a.m.–6 p.m. daily in summer, with reduced hours (usually weekends only) in winter.

Nearest Campgrounds Pantoll Campground, near Pantoll Ranger Station (16 first-come, first-served sites), and Bootjack Campground, on Panoramic Hwy. (15 first-come, first-served sites), cost $25/night, require a short 100-yard walk-in, and usually fill by afternoon. Steep Ravine Environmental Campground, on a marine terrace 1 mile south of Stinson Beach on Hwy. 1, has 10 rustic cabins ($100/night) and 7 primitive campsites ($25). Reservations are essential months in advance for the cabins; visit **reserveamerica.com** or call 800-444-7275.

Additional Information www.parks.ca.gov

HIKE 32 Martin Griffin Preserve ⟳ 🏃

Highlight	Developing avian awareness at a major heronry
Distance	2.3 miles
Total Elevation Gain/Loss	700'/700'
Hiking Time	2–3 hours
Recommended Map	USGS 7.5-min. *Bolinas*
Best Times	April–mid-December
Agency	Audubon Canyon Ranch
Difficulty	★★

WITH DOZENS OF PAIRS of great egrets, great blue herons, and snowy egrets nesting in a perfectly visible treetop community, Audubon Canyon Ranch is a terrific draw. Add Bolinas Lagoon, a shallow mudflat alive with more than 60 species of birds, and an impressive oak forest, and the allure becomes difficult to resist. Together these two landmarks form the 1,000-acre Martin Griffin Preserve.

In the preserve, three small canyons cut down to the edge of a large, shallow mudflat and protect a rich array of life regenerating from past human influences. Logged to build 19th-century San Francisco and once used for dairy ranching, the landscape is recovering well. More than 90 species of birds can be sighted here, amphibians crawl its moist creek-beds, and steelhead trout once again swim its streams. The herons and egrets arrive by March, choose mates after elaborate courtship rituals, and then raise their young for 12 weeks in the heronry. Located in the upper canopy of a few redwood trees in lower Picher Canyon, the site provides shelter and ready access to the fish and crustaceans found in Bolinas Lagoon. From mid-June through mid-July, volunteers keep careful track of the nesting pairs, follow the development of the chicks, and then watch the entire community gradually disperse.

Note that in 2013 fewer nesting pairs returned than normal and none successfully raised any young—the first complete nesting failure since record keeping began in 1967. The cause of this decline is uncertain. The preserve is closely monitoring the situation and may close during future nesting seasons as part of an ongoing effort to help rehabilitate the heronry. Check ahead before planning a visit.

The Hike is a circuit around Picher Canyon on Griffin Trail, passing the overlooks of Bolinas Lagoon and the heronry early on. Telescopes are provided and friendly docents enrich the experience, making this one of the best sites in California to learn about birds. The preserve is open intermittently during the day (usually 10 a.m.–4 p.m.) from April through mid-December on some weekdays and many weekend days. Call ahead or check the preserve web site for the latest schedule.

While April and May have traditionally been the most eventful months in the heronry, a powerful telephoto lens is necessary to capture the scene on film. Crowds tend to concentrate at the overlooks, leaving the trails surprisingly empty. Water is available at the trailhead.

To Reach the Trailhead Drive 3 miles north of Stinson Beach on Hwy. 1—the posted turnoff has an open sign hanging if you've come at the right time. Volunteers usually greet you and tell you where to park. While there is no entrance fee, donations are strongly encouraged and help support Audubon Canyon Ranch, a private nonprofit managing this and three other nature preserves in Marin and Sonoma counties.

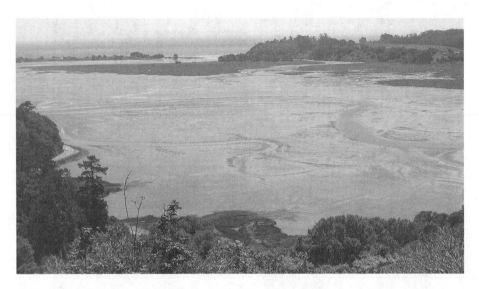

Bolinas Lagoon from Audubon Canyon Ranch

Reaching the trailhead by public transportation is challenging but possible. **West Marin Stagecoach Bus 61** goes to Audubon Canyon Ranch four to eight times daily from Marin City. Call 415-526-3239 for current schedule information, or visit **marintransit.org.**

Description Pick up a free map of the preserve from the visitor center before walking briefly back down the entrance road to the start of Griffin Trail (0.0/10'). The wide trail immediately starts climbing through California buckeye, live oak, and California bay to reach the first overlook. Depending on tides, Bolinas Lagoon may be filled with shallow water or exposed as fractal-patterned mudflats. Birdlife is always abundant, and the preserve's interpretive panels and telescopes are lots of fun.

Past the lagoon overlook, the trail forks—bear right toward the next overlook. Climbing through dense foliage, you soon reach another fork—bear right again and climb the short spur to Henderson Overlook (0.3/200'). Note the sign: QUIET—BIRDS NESTING. White splotches in the green canopy, enlarged and defined by powerful telescopes here, compose the heronry below you to the east. Learn all you can of these beautiful birds before returning to the main trail.

Back on Griffin Trail, you ascend the ridge. Look for redwood trees providing excellent examples of basal sprouting. Once cut, a redwood tree immediately sprouts a series of saplings from its root system, forming a roughly concentric circle around the stump known as a "fairy ring." Some rings here include more than a dozen trees. Where Zumie's Loop splits left at the junction near the top (0.8/720'), keep right on the Griffin Trail. After cresting out, the trail swings right and crosses the lush creek gully; then it continues on a level traverse through a dense alder thicket. The path gradually descends through a thick forest of redwood and Douglas-fir to an open ridgetop before beginning its steep descent to the trailhead.

Views of Stinson Beach, Bolinas Lagoon, and Olema Valley open up as you descend. The San Andreas Fault underlies these landmarks, and fault movement in the Olema Valley during the 1906 earthquake was more than 12 feet in places. One earth fissure reportedly swallowed an entire cow—except for the legs left protruding upward from the ground! The trail descends the ridgeline steeply to the visitor center, passing beneath some very impressive coast live oaks at the end.

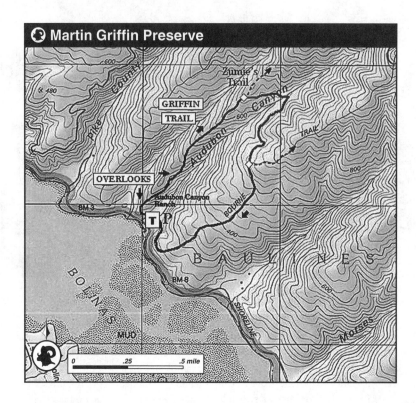

Nearest Visitor Center The Audubon Canyon Ranch visitor center and bookstore, 415-868-9244, among the old ranch buildings, is open when the preserve is open.

Nearest Campgrounds Privately owned Olema Ranch Campground (200 sites, $53–$65) is in Olema on Hwy. 1. Also try the campground in Samuel P. Taylor State Park (60 sites, $35), 6 miles east of Hwy. 1 on Sir Francis Drake Blvd. Reservations are recommended for Samuel P. Taylor April–October; visit **reserveamerica.com** or call 800-444-7275. Or try Pantoll Campground (16 sites) or Bootjack Campground (15 sites) in Mount Tamalpais State Park. These first-come, first-served sites require a short 100-yard walk-in and usually fill by afternoon ($25).

Additional Information egret.org

HIKE 33 Alamere Falls 🥾 🎒

Highlights	Mind-bending geology, ocean vistas, and a beachside waterfall
Distance	8.5 miles round-trip
Total Elevation Gain/Loss	900'/900'
Hiking Time	5–7 hours
Recommended Maps	*Point Reyes National Seashore and West Marin Parklands* by Wilderness Press, Tom Harrison's *Point Reyes National Seashore*, USGS 7.5-min. *Double Point*
Best Times	September–May
Agency	Point Reyes National Seashore
Difficulty	★★

ALAMERE FALLS is an accessible yet remote destination, where a small stream tumbles directly over coastal bluffs onto a sandy beach. The oceanside cliffs, Double Point view, and inviting freshwater lakes along the trail are all expressions of the unique geology of southern Point Reyes National Seashore.

The Hike follows the Coast Trail from Palomarin Trailhead to Alamere Falls, a fairly long day hike that can be extended to an overnight trip by continuing 1.5 miles past Alamere Falls to Wildcat Camp. Fog is common in the summer months and should be avoided. Swimming and fishing are possible in freshwater Bass Lake halfway to the falls, but ocean frolicking is not recommended due to the strong rip currents, undertow, and frigid water. This is not an isolated hike, especially on the weekends, and you can expect to see other people on the trail and at the waterfall. Poison oak, stinging nettle, and ticks are common hazards in the brush. No water is available at the trailhead, and there are no reliable sources before Alamere Falls.

To Reach the Trailhead Take Hwy. 1 north from Stinson Beach for 4.4 miles to the northern edge of Bolinas Lagoon and turn left onto Olema–Bolinas Rd. The turnoff is not posted, so keep your eye out. In 1.3 miles the road reaches a T-junction—go left, continuing on Olema–Bolinas Rd. for another 0.6 mile before turning right again on Mesa Rd. Follow Mesa Rd. 5 miles to the parking lot at the road's end, passing a Coast Guard radar station and the Point Reyes Bird Observatory along the way. The last 1.5 miles are unpaved.

Description From the trailhead (0.0/280'), the wide path immediately enters a thick eucalyptus grove where wild cucumber vines twine and a few enormous trees dominate—one huge Hydra-like specimen is by far the largest eucalyptus on any hike described in this book. Good views south open up next as the trail winds along open bluff tops, and the Farallon Islands are visible southwest on a clear day. The trail turns inland, crossing two small creek gullies choked with brush, horsetail, watercress, monkeyflower, and ferns before resuming

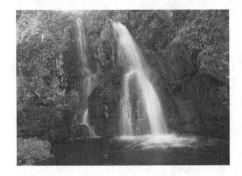
Upper Alamere Falls

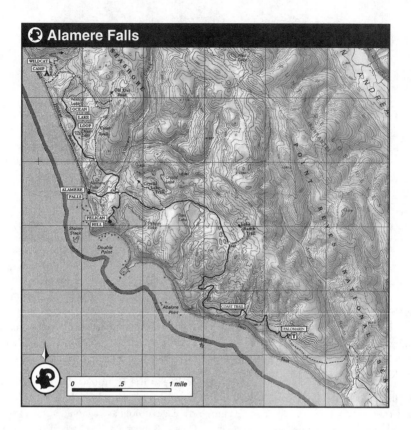

ocean views. At the third significant creek gully, the trail continues inland, climbing over a small divide to the Lake Ranch Trail (2.2/570') junction. Continuing ahead on the Coast Trail, you meander through a dense forest of Douglas-fir, the conifer common throughout this hike. The trail passes several swampy ponds full of lily pads before Bass Lake comes into view. Gradually descending along its northern shore, the path leads to a short spur trail and an open space excellent for a break on hot days. Beyond the lake, the trail soon passes a junction for unexciting Crystal Lake before traversing above beautiful Pelican Lake. Point Reyes and the long curving arc of beach and coastal bluffs appear north.

Descending, you reach a spur junction on your left (4.0/290') immediately after views north are hidden by coastal bluffs. This small trail leads 0.3 mile to the top of Pelican Hill

(380') and the north end of Double Point, a spectacular, recommended side trip. Besides far-reaching views south and north from the summit, the inaccessible cove beach below is often filled with hundreds of hauled-out seals. This is also a good vantage point to contemplate the geologic forces that created this landscape.

The rock of this area is called the Monterey shale, a sequence of sedimentary layers up to 8,000 feet thick that were deposited on top of the granite bedrock of Point Reyes National Seashore over the past 20 million years. In the region around Double Point, this shale has become involved in a huge landslide nearly 4 miles long and at least a mile wide. As this huge block of land slips slowly toward the sea, as explained by Alan Galloway in *Geology of the Point Reyes Peninsula,* depressions are formed that fill with freshwater lakes such as Pelican and Bass lakes.

Immediately past the junction for Pelican Hill, another unposted spur trail splits left. This overgrown and brushy path leads down to Alamere Falls, unseen until the very end, where some scrambling is required to reach the stream and its series of cascades. A final section of challenging and precarious scrambling will take you down to the beach via a rocky chute. The bluffs are impressive, and the tilted, exposed layers of Monterey shale are spectacular south of the falls.

From here, it is possible to hike 1.3 miles north along the sands of Wildcat Beach to Wildcat Camp. Note, however, that sections of the beach can be impassable during high tides and heavy surf, and that there is *no exit* from the beach between the falls and camp. The narrow beach section immediately north of the falls is a good indication of the route's feasibility—if waves are reaching the cliff base, do not proceed.

To continue inland, return to Coast Trail and head north into the watershed of Alamere Creek. Contouring around the creek, Coast Trail next reaches the junction with Ocean Lake Loop (4.2/240'). While both trails lead equidistantly to camp, bear left on more scenic Ocean Lake Loop Trail (perhaps returning on Coast Trail for variety).

The singletrack trail drops gently to bank around marshy Ocean Lake and then climbs abruptly to a bench with great views of Wildcat Beach. You next descend past brush-lined Wildcat Lake and reach Coast Trail joining from the right (5.3/220'). Bear left to quickly reach the bluff top views from Wildcat Camp (5.5/70').

Alamere Falls tumbles directly onto Wildcat Beach.

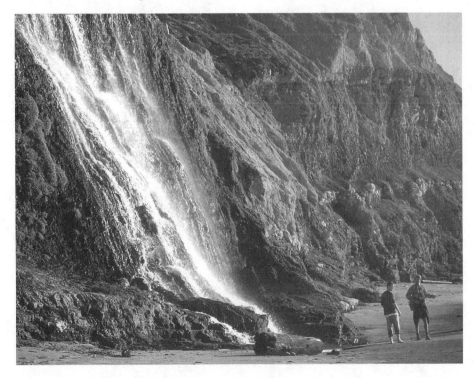

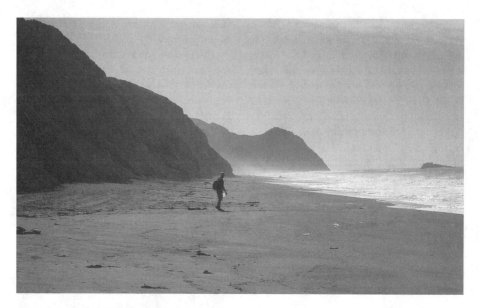

The remote sands of Wildcat Beach

Nearest Visitor Center Bear Valley Visitor Center, 415-464-5138, on Bear Valley Rd. just west of Olema, 8 miles north of the turnoff for Olema–Bolinas Rd., is open weekdays 10 a.m.–5 p.m. (until 4:30 p.m. in winter) and 9 a.m.–5 p.m. weekends and holidays year-round.

Backpacking Information Backcountry camping at Wildcat Camp is by permit only. Eight sites are available, including 3 group sites. Reservations are essential and can be made up to 6 months in advance; visit **recreation.gov** or call 877-444-6777. Weekends fill far ahead of time, especially May–October; weekdays are often available on shorter notice.

Note that you must make a reservation at least 2 days in advance of your departure; same- or next-day reservations are not available. Walk-in registration is possible for same-day departures on the rare occasion when sites are available. Permits cost $20–$50 per night, depending on group size, and must be picked up at the Bear Valley Visitor Center prior to leaving on your trip. After-hours pickup is allowed—permits are placed in a wooden box by the information board in front of the visitor center. Wood fires are prohibited.

Nearest Campgrounds There are no drive-in campgrounds within Point Reyes National Seashore. The closest campgrounds are Pantoll and Bootjack Campgrounds in Mount Tamalpais State Park, near Pantoll Ranger Station on Panoramic Hwy. (31 first-come, first-served sites that require a short 100-yard walk-in and usually fill by afternoon; $25), and privately owned Olema Ranch Campground (200 sites, $53–$63), in Olema on Hwy. 1.

Additional Information nps.gov/pore

HIKE 34 Sky and Coast Trails ○ 🥾

Highlights	Old-growth ridgeline and wave-swept coastline
Distance	10.8 miles
Total Elevation Gain/Loss	1,800'/1,800'
Hiking Time	5–7 hours
Recommended Maps	*Point Reyes National Seashore and West Marin Parklands* by Wilderness Press, Tom Harrison's *Point Reyes National Seashore*, USGS 7.5-min. *Double Point*
Best Times	September–May
Agency	Point Reyes National Seashore
Difficulty	★★★

THIS LOOP HIKE explores the full spectrum of Point Reyes National Seashore, from the lush forest atop its highest ridges to the sculpted promontories above its salty shore. Along the way, you'll tag the peninsula's tallest point, stand atop a wave-tunneled bluff, and savor abundant views of the cerulean sea.

The Hike directly ascends 1,407-foot Mount Wittenberg from Bear Valley Visitor Center and then descends Sky Trail to the ocean, winding through verdant mixed-evergreen forest and past open viewpoints en route to the coast. The journey then heads south on Coast Trail to striking Arch Rock, returning inland beneath the majestic trees of Bear Valley Trail.

To Reach the Trailhead Take Hwy. 1 to Olema and head west on Bear Valley Rd.; the turnoff is immediately north of the intersection of Hwy. 1 and Sir Francis Drake Blvd. In 0.5 mile, turn left to reach the Bear Valley Visitor Center and trailhead parking.

Public transportation is available Monday through Saturday on **West Marin Stagecoach Route 68,** which makes eight runs daily to Inverness from San Rafael, stopping at Bear Valley Visitor Center along the way (call 415-526-3239 or visit **marintransit.org**).

Description From the trailhead (0.0/80'), follow Bear Valley Trail past Rift Zone and Woodpecker Trails to reach Mount Wittenberg Trail by a stand of coast live oaks and a massive bay tree (0.2/80'). Bear right and ascend Mount Wittenberg Trail beneath the arcing branches of fragrant bay trees. The shady woodlands slowly transition into a mixed-evergreen forest of Douglas-fir, hazel bushes, and sword ferns, interspersed with the occasional buckeye and tanoak tree.

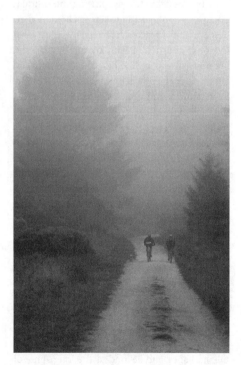

A foggy day on Sky Trail

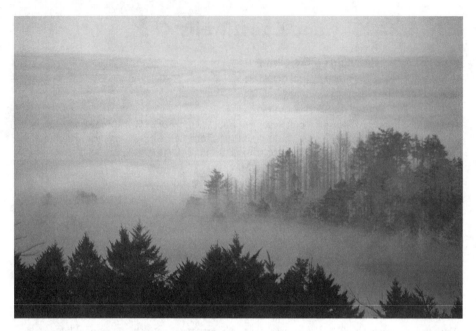

A sea of fog washes the terrain below Sky Trail.

The trail rises steadily, passing intermittent glimpses of Bolinas Ridge across Olema Valley. You eventually reach a clearing ringed by coast live oaks and dotted with coyote brush—you are now halfway up the hill. The trail narrows, climbs three steep switchbacks, and levels briefly to contour around a small drainage. Upon cresting Inverness Ridge, you are rewarded with northwest views toward Limantour Beach, Drakes Estero, and Point Reyes itself. Z Ranch Trail and the spur to Wittenberg's summit lie just ahead (2.0/1,260').

This spot marks the boundary of the 1995 Vision Fire, a human-caused conflagration that scorched 12,000 acres of the seashore. Its effects can be seen in the regular size and age of the young, regenerating Douglas-firs in the area, as well as the burned trunks of nearby fire survivors. From here it's a short 0.4-mile round-trip to the top of Mount Wittenberg (1,407'), the highest point in Point Reyes National Seashore. The summit is ringed by young Douglas-firs, but a few tantalizing glimpses peek south to Olema Valley and beyond to the long spine of Mount Tamalpais.

Continue on Mount Wittenberg Trail as it curves down past a shrubby undergrowth of yerba santa and bracken fern and reaches the junction with Sky and Meadow Trails (2.4/1,120'). Sky Camp is 0.6 mile away to the north but your continuing journey heads left, following Sky Trail into the woods. Douglas-firs tower overhead and strain moisture from the fog, keeping the environment green year-round. Moss-bearded branches and tree-bound ferns droop above abundant elderberry, huckleberry, blackberry tangles, and sword ferns. In September, the huckleberry bushes dangle with abundant—and deliciously edible—blue-black berries.

Sky Trail passes Woodward Valley Trail on the right (3.1/890'), climbs briefly to pass Old Pine Trail on the left (3.4/1,020'), and then gently descends. The surrounding environment transitions to low-lying coastal scrub as you crest a small rise and reach the junction with Baldy Trail (4.8/870'). Continue your descent on Sky Trail toward the increasingly visible ocean. The route passes a few burnt snags—more remnants of the Vision Fire—and makes a final drop via two switchbacks to reach Coast Trail (6.3/130').

A right turn leads in 0.2 mile to an enormous eucalyptus by the access point for Kelham Beach, a remote strand of cliffs and sandy solitude. The continuing hike heads left (south) on wide Coast Trail, which quickly leads to Bear Valley Trail and the nearby promontory of Arch Rock (6.8/110'). Take the time to visit the open bluff top of Arch Rock and its excellent views, which stretch north along adjacent Kelham Beach to Point Resistance and beyond. On the south side of Arch Rock, a well-worn but precarious path descends into the mini-gorge of Coast Creek. At low tide, you can walk north through the arch to access Kelham Beach. To the south, a small pocket beach stretches a short distance to Millers Point.

You now leave the ocean behind and head inland on wide and well-traveled Bear Valley Trail, which quickly returns to thick woods alongside alder-choked Coast Creek. The curving branches of massive bay trees shade your journey past Glen and Baldy Trails (7.7/180')

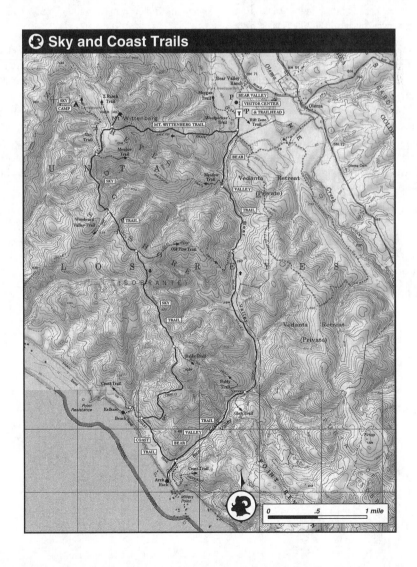

and onward to Divide Meadow (9.2/320'). Ringed by coast live oaks, the meadow sits on the divide between the Olema Valley and Coast Creek watersheds and is the only low-elevation gap through Inverness Ridge. A hunting lodge owned by the Pacific Union Hunting Club of San Francisco once sat in the northwest corner; it served as a backcountry base for pursuing bears and mountain lions from the 1890s until the Great Depression. The lodge has long since been removed; two huge introduced Monterey pines and a few patches of exotic pink flowers are all that remain.

Continuing on Bear Valley Trail, you enter one of the seashore's most majestic forests. California bay, alders, and tanoak thrive. Mighty Douglas-firs rise above, each unique in form and character. On your way out, you pass Meadow Trail (10.0/150') and Mount Wittenberg Trail just before returning to the trailhead (10.8/80').

Nearest Visitor Center Bear Valley Visitor Center, 415-464-5100, is on Bear Valley Rd. just west of Olema and open weekdays 10 a.m.–5 p.m. (until 4:30 p.m. in winter) and 9 a.m.– 5 p.m. weekends and holidays year-round.

Backpacking Information Backcountry camping at Sky Camp is by permit only. Twelve sites are available, including 1 group site. Reservations are essential and can be made up to 6 months in advance; visit **recreation.gov** or call 877-444-6777. Weekends fill far ahead of time, especially May–October; weekdays are often available on shorter notice.

Note that you must make a reservation at least 2 days in advance of your departure; same- or next-day reservations are not available. Walk-in registration is possible for same-day departures on the rare occasion when sites are available. Permits cost $20–$50 per night, depending on group size, and must be picked up at the Bear Valley Visitor Center prior to leaving on your trip. After-hours pickup is allowed—permits are placed in a wooden box by the information board in front of the visitor center. Wood fires are prohibited.

Nearest Campgrounds There are no drive-in campgrounds within Point Reyes National Seashore. The closest campgrounds are Pantoll and Bootjack Campgrounds in Mount Tamalpais State Park, near Pantoll Ranger Station on Panoramic Hwy. (31 first-come, first-served sites that require a short 100-yard walk-in and usually fill by afternoon; $25), and privately owned Olema Ranch Campground (200 sites, $53–$63), in Olema on Hwy. 1.

Additional Information nps.gov/pore

HIKE 35 Tomales Point ↗

Highlights	A herd of tule elk and prairie blufftops above pounding surf
Distance	9.0 miles round-trip
Total Elevation Gain/Loss	1,300'/1,300'
Hiking Time	4–5 hours
Recommended Maps	*Point Reyes National Seashore and West Marin Parklands* by Wilderness Press, Tom Harrison's *Point Reyes National Seashore*, USGS 7.5-min. *Tomales*
Best Times	September–May
Agency	Point Reyes National Seashore
Difficulty	★★★

HERE IS A HIKE of sweeping coastal views along an elevated, granite peninsula, covered by an open grassland famous for its wildflowers and tule elk. The Point Reyes Peninsula is a migrant piece of land. Its deepest bedrock is granite, formed in southern California approximately 100 million years ago.

When the San Andreas Fault became active roughly 28 million years ago, pieces of North America west of the emergent fault began slowly migrating north at a rate of 2–3 centimeters per year, traveling hundreds of miles over the ensuing millenia. The granite of Point Reyes Peninsula was one of these pieces and became covered by thick, waterborne sediments while submerged beneath the sea for almost 10 million years on its journey north. Roughly 4 million years ago, a slight change in the geometry of the San Andreas Fault system increased compression between the rocks on either side of the fault, pushing Point Reyes Peninsula— and most of the Coast Ranges—above sea level. Erosion then began stripping away the overlying sediment, once again exposing the erosion-resistant granite on today's Inverness Ridge and the bluffs of Point Reyes itself. Today, Tomales Point is a solid piece of granite battered by the seas into sheer cliffs of solid rock, a striking contrast to the loose slopes found most places on the California coast.

The Hike goes to land's end at Tomales Point from historic Pierce Point Ranch, a chilly trip

that is almost always rainy, windy, foggy, or some combination of the three. The trail is entirely exposed and offers no shelter from the elements, making a good sweater and windbreaker crucial year-round items. Fog is consistent during the summer months, obscuring views and making a visit at some other time more desirable. While you will almost surely see other people, crowds are generally light. No water is available at the trailhead or anywhere en route.

To Reach the Trailhead Take Sir Francis Drake Blvd. west from Point Reyes Station on Hwy. 1 for 6.7 miles to the turnoff for Pierce Point Rd. Bear right on Pierce Point Rd. where Sir Francis Drake Blvd. curves left, and proceed 9 miles to the parking lot by the white buildings of historic Pierce Point Ranch.

Description The trail begins from the west side of the parking lot by an informative sign, and for most of its length the hike follows an old lane—now a broad and friendly path—to the former site of lower Pierce Point Ranch. Passing between the still operational buildings of upper Pierce Point Ranch and a linear windbreak of Monterey cypress, the wide trail shortly breaks out into open fields of bush lupine and coyote brush where wild cucumber wraps its tendrils through the brush. Raptors— especially red-tailed hawks—are a common sight as they soar over the open fields, hunting

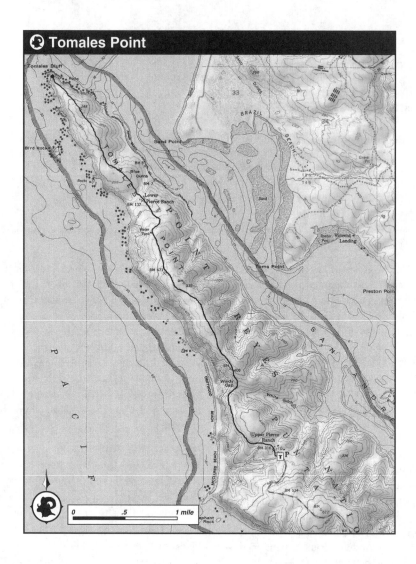

for small prey. As you continue on the undulating route, keep an eye out for the herd of tule elk that wanders these bluffs, reintroduced in 1978 by the National Park Service. Numbering in the hundreds, these impressive creatures are a memorable and photogenic sight.

To the east the San Andreas Fault underlies Tomales Bay, a trough formed when the rocks along the fault were ground into easily eroded sediment. The fault continues northwest toward Bodega Head (Hike 39), the small peninsula immediately north of Tomales Point. Similar to Point Reyes Peninsula, Bodega Head

is another piece of granite covered by sediment, separated from the mainland by the San Andreas Fault, and slowly moving northwest. Northeast, the highest peak visible is Mount St. Helena (Hike 36). Looking south, the long sandy stretch of Point Reyes Beach terminates at rocky Point Reyes itself.

A long, undulating traverse more than 300 feet above the breaking waves eventually leads to a steady descent that ends in a grove of trees, the former site of lower Pierce Point Ranch. From here, the trail gets sandier and less distinct as it passes through fields

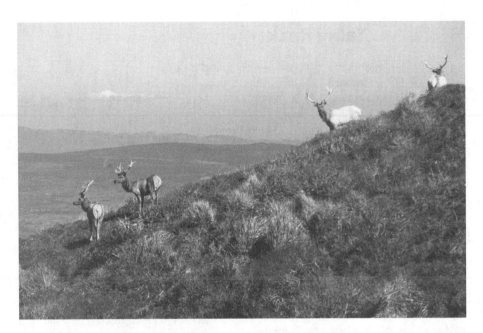

A herd of tule elk roams Tomales Point.

thick with irises, climbing first before dropping down to the precipitous granite cliffs of Tomales Point itself. Bird Rock, just offshore to the west, is a rookery for numerous seabirds and a major pupping area for harbor seals. Great white sharks are commonly sighted in the waters around Tomales Point and have attacked divers in the past. You can get close, but the ocean remains out of reach less than 30 feet below. Be respectful of the dangerous cliffs as you explore the point. Return the way you came.

Nearest Visitor Center Bear Valley Visitor Center, 415-464-5138, on Bear Valley Rd. just west of Olema, 8 miles north of the turnoff for Olema–Bolinas Rd., is open weekdays 10 a.m.–5 p.m. (until 4:30 p.m. in winter) and 9 a.m.–5 p.m. weekends and holidays year-round.

Nearest Campgrounds There are no drive-in campgrounds within Point Reyes National Seashore. The closest campgrounds are Pantoll and Bootjack Campgrounds in Mount Tamalpais State Park, near Pantoll Ranger Station on Panoramic Hwy. (31 first-come, first-served sites that require a short 100-yard walk-in and usually fill by afternoon; $25), and privately owned Olema Ranch Campground (200 sites, $53–$63), in Olema on Hwy. 1.

Additional Information nps.gov/pore

HIKE 36 Table Rock ⬈

Highlights	Distant views and dead-drop cliffs
Distance	4.4 miles round-trip
Total Elevation Gain/Loss	1,400'/1,400'
Hiking Time	3 hours
Recommended Map	USGS 7.5-min. *Detert Reservoir*
Best Times	Year-round
Agency	Robert Louis Stevenson State Park
Difficulty	★★★

OVERLOOKING CALISTOGA VALLEY, beneath dominant Mount St. Helena, on the lip of sheer volcanic cliffs, the view from Table Rock is something to remember.

The Hike travels to Table Rock, an unusual volcanic formation within a delightful pocket of hidden wilderness. Much of the hike is exposed, making sun protection imperative most of the year. Because the cliff edge is unprotected and a fall would be fatal, this is not a good location for children. Robert Louis Stevenson State Park is little known and has few amenities. No water is available at the trailhead.

To Reach the Trailhead Take sinuous Hwy. 29 north from Calistoga for nearly 8 miles to the divide below Mount St. Helena. Park in the lot east of the road exactly at the divide. Approaching from the north, take Hwy. 29 south from the junction of Hwys. 29 and 53 in Lower Lake for 26 miles to the divide.

Description From the posted trailhead (0.0/ 2,300') the trail gently climbs among Douglas-fir, tanoak, madrone, ponderosa pine, California bay, and black oak, while you get increasingly better views of Mount St. Helena (4,343'). In the summer of 1880, author Robert Louis Stevenson spent a month-long, cash-strapped honeymoon squatting in an old cabin on the slopes of Mount St. Helena, penciling notes later incorporated into his novels. *The Silverado Squatters* and *Treasure Island* both include descriptions of the surrounding landscape.

As the trail winds briefly along northern slopes, views north down Collayomi Valley appear and Snow Mountain (7,056') can be seen capping the skyline beyond the valley's end. You'll see wispy gray pines and get ever more distant views beyond Mount St. Helena as the trail traverses back around to the southern exposure.

After a very brief climb, the trail reaches a junction (0.7/2,550')—go right, toward Table

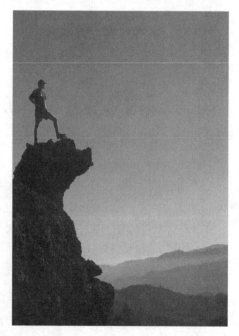

Riding the Rhino

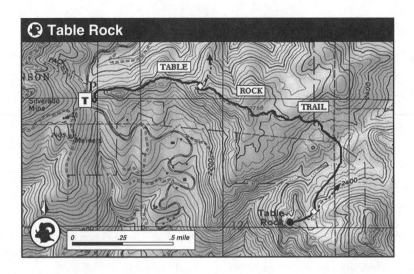

Rock. As the trail begins to descend, tantalizing views south transform into sweeping panoramas at Devils Sofa, an exposure of large, rounded, volcanic boulders. Napa Valley's rich tapestry trends southeast toward the distant massif of Mount Diablo (Hike 14). Looking east on a clear day, the Sierra Nevada can be seen beyond linear Blue Ridge. West, the sea is just beyond the farthest visible hills.

From here, the trail descends among thick chaparral before climbing to regain the open slopes and reach the posted junction (2.0/ 2,350') for nearby Table Rock, a short 0.2 mile away. Fantastical formations will delight you as you walk toward the cliff edge. Look for the Rhino. Thrill to a hair-raising view down a vertical cliff face. Contemplate the geology as you savor the view.

Over the past 28 million years, the ever-shifting geometry between the Pacific and North American tectonic plates has created a vast system of faults, associated with the greater San Andreas Fault system. These faults have ripped apart this region and formed the distinctive linear valleys and ridges visible here. Between 13 and 2.7 million years ago, some large fissures created by this activity allowed liquid magma to rise to the surface and spill across the landscape, covering it with thick layers of volcanic rock. Over time, erosion weathered the hardened basalt to form the sheer cliffs below you. Return the way you came.

Nearest Visitor Center This park doesn't have a visitor center. For general information, call Bothe–Napa Valley State Park at 707-942-4575.

Nearest Campground Bothe–Napa Valley State Park Campground (50 sites, $35) is 5 miles north of St. Helena on Hwy. 29. Reservations are recommended in summer; visit **reserve america.com** or call 800-444-7275.

Additional Information www.parks.ca.gov

HIKE 37 East Austin Creek ↻ 🧍

Highlight	The remote valleys of the northern Coast Range
Distance	9.1 miles
Total Elevation Gain/Loss	1,150'/1,150'
Hiking Time	5–7 hours
Recommended Maps	*Austin Creek State Recreation Area Map* by California State Parks, USGS 7.5-min. *Cazadero*
Best Times	Year-round
Agency	Austin Creek State Recreation Area
Difficulty	★★★

A HIDDEN, WILD world lurks in the rumpled Coast Range just north of the Russian River. Closely packed ridges rise more than 1,000 feet above narrow canyons barely 200 feet above sea level. The nearby San Andreas Fault has shaped the area, squeezing it upward, riddling it with smaller faults. Heavy rainfall then dissects the terrain, eroding the folded landscape into today's convoluted topography.

Within this tortured geography, Austin Creek State Recreation Area straddles an ecological divide between lush coastal redwood forest and drier oak woodland. Only 10 miles from the ocean, yet guarded from summer fog by several intervening ridges, the area receives significant precipitation in the winter months (more than 50 inches) yet bakes during the summer in temperatures that can approach 100°F. The results are perennial streams in lush canyons, open grasslands of twisting oaks and spring wildflowers, chaparral-cloaked southern slopes, and surprising pockets of redwood forest.

The Hike descends steeply from ridgeline to lush valley bottom, visits four mellifluous streams, and tours a wide diversity of ecosystems. This is a year-round destination. Even during the heat of summer, the park's deep valleys provide shelter from the intense sun. Winter and fall are nice, but spring is the optimal time for a visit, when wildflowers carpet the hillsides, crowds are light, and the weather is pleasant. Note that you must ford unbridged East Austin Creek at the hike's midpoint, a

potential challenge during rainy spells. Water is available near the trailhead in adjacent Bullfrog Pond Campground.

To Reach the Trailhead Take Hwy. 116 or River Rd. west from Hwy. 101 to Guerneville and turn north on Armstrong Woods Rd.; the turnoff is 0.1 mile west of the Russian River Bridge. In 2.5 miles you reach the Armstrong Redwoods State Natural Reserve entrance and visitor center. A thrilling 2.5 miles later you reach the East Austin Creek Trailhead and parking area at Vista Point. This final 2.5 miles of road is narrow and twisting, with several steep sections (12% grade) and multiple 5-mile-per-hour hairpin turns. Vehicles longer than 20 feet are not permitted.

Description From the trailhead (0.0/1,400'), savor the sweeping view across the rolling terrain. Note the varied ecosystems that thrive here. Coyote brush, manzanita, and several species of oak (coast, Oregon, and black) grow on the drier, sun-exposed west-facing slopes; bay trees, willow, buckeye, and poison oak are nourished by the moist shelter of nearby gullies; and water-loving Douglas-fir and redwoods flourish on shady north- and east-facing slopes. Descending on East Austin Creek Trail, you soon pass a spur trail on the right (0.2/1,150') joining from lower Bullfrog Pond Campground. The slopes are flush with seasonal wildflowers. Baby blue eyes, shooting stars, and brodiaea are particularly abundant on the descent. Also look

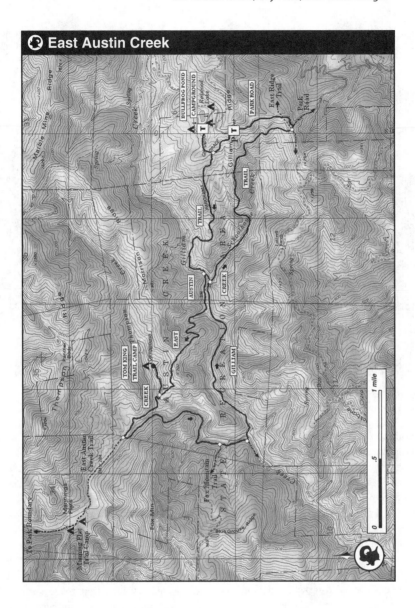

East Austin Creek

for evidence of wild pigs; they regularly root up the hillside in search of edible roots.

Near the canyon bottom, the trail curves right and descends into a thickening mixed-evergreen forest. You briefly travel above crystalline Gilliam Creek, then reach it near a bridge and junction for the short spur trail that leads to nearby Gilliam Creek Trail (1.5/340'). Those fortunate to be here in March may witness

orange-bellied newts congregating by the dozens to mate in these waters.

Cross the bridge over Gilliam Creek and continue on wide East Austin Creek Trail as it climbs briefly up a small, unnamed drainage flush with bigleaf maple, peeling madrone, and giant chain ferns (the state's largest fern). You then emerge above it all on open oak hillsides with exceptional views. The small linear valley

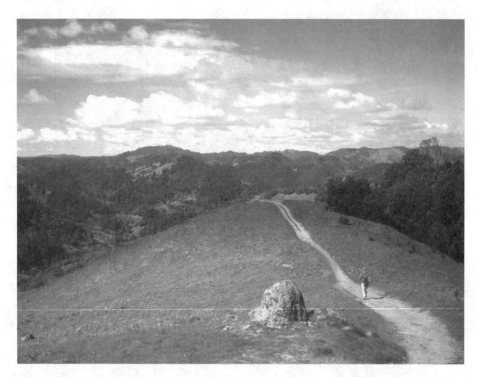

Trailhead view above the Austin Creek watershed

of Thompson Creek is visible to the north and the deep drainage of East Austin Creek twists southwest toward the Russian River. The route crests near some coast live oaks (2.5/750') and descends to the junction with Tom King Trail (2.9/450'). If you're looking for an idyllic picnic spot, turn right here and proceed a gentle 0.3 mile to the camp.

To continue, remain on East Austin Creek Trail as it switchbacks twice and crosses Thompson Creek. Old-growth redwoods appear across the stream as the wide trail parallels East Austin Creek to reach unsigned Gilliam Creek Trail (3.5/190'). Manning Flat Trail Camp lies 0.7 mile ahead, but you turn left to ford unbridged East Austin Creek and follow Gilliam Creek Trail onto shadier east-facing slopes. Climbing briefly, the trail winds well above the rushing stream and its narrow

canyon before descending to pass Fox Mountain Trail on the right (4.6/290').

Bear left at the next junction (4.8/290') to remain on Gilliam Creek Trail and descend to the confluence of East Austin and Gilliam Creeks. Ford East Austin Creek once more to immediately reach the former site of Gilliam Creek Trail Camp, in a large grassy field near the creek. Beyond camp, the trail winds through a narrow canyon, briefly climbs a short distance above the creek, then drops to cross and recross the creek nine times over the next mile. The stream crossings are not always obvious (only a few are signed) but the trail is apparent; if you find yourself on a disappearing track, retrace your steps. At Schoolhouse Creek you encounter the unposted junction for the short connector to East Austin Creek Trail (6.5/360') and the most direct route back to the trailhead.

This hike continues straight on Gilliam Creek Trail, which crosses the creek three more times and then climbs steeply along a small feeder creek to an open, oak-studded ridge. Manzanita, toyon, and chamise line the trail as it steadily ascends the ridgeline, levels out, and banks right to traverse the upper Schoolhouse Creek drainage (passing through several nice redwood groves en route). The trail alternately contours gently and ascends steeply to reach the junction with East Ridge Trail and the park road (8.5/1,300'). Savor the beautiful vistas one last time as you bear left (north) and hike along the park road to return to the trailhead (9.1/1,400').

Nearest Visitor Centers Armstrong Redwoods Visitor Center, 707-869-2958, is open daily 11 a.m.–3 p.m., with longer hours in summer. The park entrance station, 707-869-2015, is staffed in summer Monday–Thursday 8:30 a.m.–4 p.m. and Friday–Sunday 10:30 a.m.–4:30 p.m.; it's open weekends only in spring and fall and sporadically in winter. Note that hours may vary depending on staffing availability. Also try the office of the Stewards of the Coast and Redwoods, 707-869-9177, in Armstrong Reserve near the picnic area.

Backpacking Information Backcountry camping is allowed at Manning Flat (2 sites) and Tom King Trail Camps (2 sites) on a first-come, first-served basis. A permit is required and must be obtained from the entrance station. There is a fee of $25 per site. Picnic tables, fire rings, and outhouses are provided; water is available from the adjacent creeks. Campfires are not allowed during fire season (typically late July–October).

Nearest Campground Bullfrog Pond Campground (24 sites, $35), near the trailhead, has 7 sites available on a first-come, first-served basis; the remainder can be reserved online at **hipcamp.com.**

Additional Information www.parks.ca.gov

HIKE 38 Cache Creek 🥾🧍🐕

Highlights	Oak woodland, bald eagles, and tule elk
Distance	10.0 miles round-trip
Total Elevation Gain/Loss	1,100'/1,100'
Hiking Time	4–6 hours
Recommended Map	USGS 7.5-min. *Lower Lake*
Best Times	December–April
Agency	Cache Creek Wilderness, Bureau of Land Management
Difficulty	★★

GNARLED OAKS twist skyward in a rolling landscape flushed green by winter rains. Cache Creek ripples through placid pools, a herd of tule elk wanders the area, and a population of bald eagles winters here. Come for a taste of the low-lying foothills ringing the Great Central Valley.

The Hike follows Redbud Trail over a low divide to Baton Flat on the banks of Cache Creek and then continues into 27,245-acre Cache Creek Wilderness to visit Wilson Valley, a broad area of oaks and meadows alongside Cache Creek. The hike is open year-round, but summer months are scorching and fall is extremely dry. Winter rains usually begin

Blue oaks thrive in the Cache Creek drainage.

in December, coinciding with the arrival of the first bald eagles. Cache Creek can be difficult to ford after heavy storms (no bridge is provided) and the Yolo County Conservation District schedules agricultural water releases from Clear Lake during the summer with only 24-hour advance notice—these can also render the creek impassable.

A herd of tule elk wanders the area, best viewed from October through April. Note that portions of the Cache Creek area may be closed from April through June to protect the elk during calving season; call ahead if you are planning a visit during this period. Bald eagles also overwinter here; look for them from late November through March. No water is available at the trailhead.

To Reach the Trailhead Take Hwy. 20 east from the intersection of Hwys. 53 and 20 near Clear Lake for 5.4 miles. The turnoff is just west of the Cache Creek highway crossing. Approaching from the east on Hwy. 20, the turnoff is 7 miles past the junction with Walker Ridge Rd.

Description From the parking lot (0.0/980'), the hike begins along a gravel road, which crosses a meadow to reach a wash gully. Veer right where the trail enters the trees and begin looking for the two types of oak that exist here: valley oak and blue oak. Blue oak is the most drought-resistant oak and can be identified by its smaller (1–3 inches) leaves that have wavy margins and shallow lobes. Adapting to the intense heat and dry conditions found in

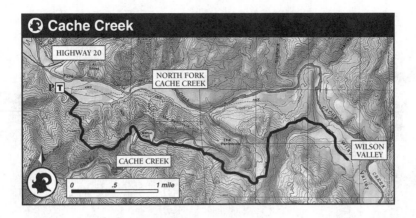

California at low elevations, the blue oak reinforces its leaves with cellulose, and drops them entirely in times of severe drought. Found on drier hillsides, they develop a bluish cast in the late summer and fall. Valley oak is deciduous and can be identified by its larger leaves (2–4 inches) that are deeply lobed. Requiring more water than blue oak, it is found along valley bottoms. Among the oak are gray pines, wispy trees that generate substantial cones.

As you slowly climb above North Fork Cache Creek, keep an eye out for elk tracks and the animals that made them. The sandstone badlands across the river contain sediments deposited over the past 5 million years, when sea-level fluctuations submerged this low-lying region for long periods and coated it with thick layers of sand and mud. More recent tectonic compression has molded it into these rolling foothills. As you crest the ridge (1.0/1,450'), the drainage of Cache Creek opens up.

Cache Creek drains Clear Lake, a large body of water formed within the past few thousand years when a large landslide dammed the headwaters of Cold Creek and blocked the westward flow of water into the Russian River drainage. Water impounding behind the new barrier filled the level valleys, creating an enormous lake. It found an outlet east in Cache Creek, draining into the Sacramento River.

As you descend toward Cache Creek, note on the opposite south slope the continued presence of gray pine but the total absence of oak.

This is due to the nutrient-poor serpentine soil found there. Oaks are unable to survive in such deficient soils, but gray pines continue to thrive.

A gradual, occasionally switchbacking descent brings you to the banks of Cache Creek near a delightful swimming hole at Baton Flat (1.7/1,000'). Campsites are located on both banks and the creek is fun to explore in both directions.

Cross Cache Creek and continue on the path as it briefly climbs and descends. The trail cruises gently over the next mile through thick blue oak woodland with intermittent access to Cache Creek, then climbs steeply up the slopes to reach a dense chaparral corridor of chamise, yerba santa, toyon, and buckbrush. You next attain a broad ridgeline, which you follow for just under a mile. Views of upper Wilson Valley open up near the northern end of the ridge, where the trail curves right to descend toward the pleasant oasis. Scrubby chaparral transitions back to gray pine and oak woodlands as you approach the bottom. The trail crosses Rocky Creek (4.7/930') and enters the gentle terrain of Wilson Valley, where a mature blue oak savannah populates the open landscape.

Campsites are abundant throughout the mile-long valley, though Cache Creek can only be accessed at its northern and southern ends (steep cutbanks prevent access elsewhere). Explore the heart of this delightful landscape (5.0/980'), then return the way you came.

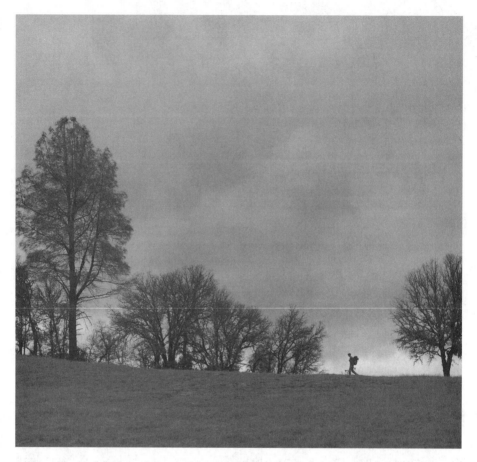

A hiker walks through blue oak savannah in Wilson Valley.

Nearest Visitor Center There are no visitor centers nearby. The area is managed jointly by the Bureau of Land Management (BLM) in Ukiah, 707-468-4000, and the California Department of Fish and Game in Yountville, 707-944-5500.

Backpacking Information Backcountry camping is permitted throughout this hike. A campfire permit is required. Cache Creek can be impassable after heavy winter storms since no bridge is provided. Campfires are allowed only in designated sites during certain times of the year and are prohibited when fire danger becomes extreme. Call the BLM office for current information.

Nearest Campground There's nothing close. Try Clear Lake State Park, on the lake's south shore near Kelseyville.

Additional Information ca.blm.gov/ukiah

HIKE 39 Bodega Dunes ⟲ 👫

Highlights	Dune fields and barefoot beach hiking
Distance	2.2 miles
Total Elevation Gain/Loss	50'/50'
Hiking Time	1–2 hours
Recommended Map	USGS 7.5-min. *Bodega Head*
Best Times	Year-round
Agency	Sonoma Coast State Beach
Difficulty	★

A CHUNK of granite spearheading the tectonic migration northwest, Bodega Head is backed by massive sand dunes and the longest beach on the Sonoma County coast. The fun of hiking barefoot is enhanced by distant views north up the rugged coastline.

The Hike explores the world of Bodega Dunes and the geology of Mussel Point before returning along Salmon Creek Beach. The entire hike is on loose sand that makes walking arduous but shoes unnecessary. Fog is common during the summer months, eliminating views and chilling the air. Fall offers the most consistent weather, winter the clearest views (between storms), and spring a profusion of flowering bush lupine. Crowds are heaviest in the summer months, dwindling to only the local surfers

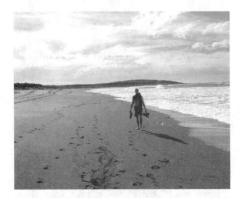

Barefoot along Bodega Dunes

in the winter. Monarch butterflies overwinter in the park campground, making December and January an exciting time to visit. No water is available at the trailhead.

To Reach the Trailhead Take Hwy. 1 north from the town of Bodega Bay for 6.5 miles—the posted turnoff is on the west side of the highway. Approaching from the north, the turnoff is 9 miles south of the junction of Hwys. 1 and 116. Past the entrance station, turn right on Beach Rd. and follow it to the substantial parking lot and picnic area at the road's end. An $8 day-use fee is charged.

Description The trail begins at the gate by the parking lot entrance and immediately enters dune world. As is evident from the beginning, paths crisscross the dunes throughout this hike. The actual trail is generally obvious and parallels the beach behind the front line of dunes—please try to stay on this main trail in order to prevent erosion of the fragile environment.

The trail initially parallels a line of scrubby Monterey cypress and conspicuous flecks of white are everywhere in the sand around them. These are shell fragments, part of a midden used by the native inhabitants of the area prior to European settlement. Regularly harvesting shellfish from the ocean for food, the Coast Miwok would deposit the accumulated shell debris in large piles, an ancient "trash can" they also filled with discarded bones, artifacts, and tools. Built up over hundreds of years, they are

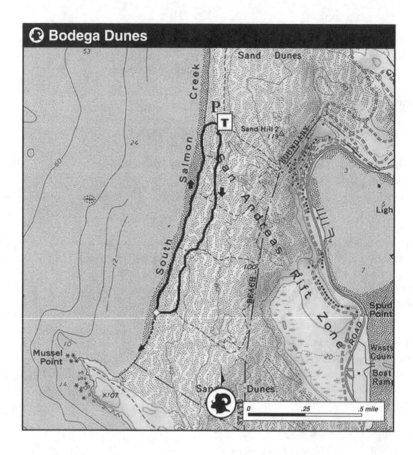

now covered by drifting sand, the scattered fragments on the surface their only indication.

As you continue through the dune fields, you are gradually surrounded by a world of sand, bush lupine, and beach grass. The larger dunes here approach 150 feet in elevation, somewhat stabilized by the European beach grass planted after cattle grazing had dangerously denuded existing native vegetation. Foxes, weasels, and black-tailed deer roam the dunes. Northern harriers and red-tailed hawks scan the ground below for the mice, voles, and jackrabbits that scurry through the undergrowth.

Although several trails split left back to the campground, continue to parallel the hidden beach at all junctions. Posted Jackrabbit and Scrub Jay spur trails on your right head to the beach, providing quicker access for those unexcited about continuing through the dunes. The

last beach access point is at the posted junction for Westshore Regional Park—bear right toward the ocean.

Once on the broad beach, views of the coastline north open up dramatically. Between you and the north end of Salmon Creek Beach, the San Andreas Fault slices underground and travels just offshore before briefly touching land again 15 miles north near Fort Ross. A keen eye can pick out Goat Rock and the mouth of the Russian River 9 miles up the coast.

Continue south along the beach to its terminus at Mussel Point, which is also the northern end of Bodega Head. A surprising outcrop of granite is exposed beneath a thin layer of sandstone here. Bodega Head is the northernmost exposure of the Salinian Block, a large piece of granite bedrock torn from Southern California and thrust northwest by actions of the San Andreas Fault. Significant in size, the Salinian Block stretches from here out to the Farallon Islands and south down the entire California coast, but its granite heart is exposed in few places. At the north edge of the Salinian Block, the rocks at Mussel Point are the northernmost outcrop of granite on the California coast. Return along the beach, enjoying the views north, and reach the parking lot via the obvious wooden platform and walkway.

Nearest Visitor Center There are no visitor centers in the park—call 707-875-3483 for general information. Try the visitor center along Hwy. 1 in Jenner, which is open weekends approximately 10 a.m.–4 p.m. Also try the park ranger station, 0.7 mile north of the park turnoff on Hwy. 1.

Nearest Campground Bodega Dunes Campground (97 sites, $35) is by the park entrance. Reservations are essential in summer; visit **reserveamerica.com** or call 800-444-7275. Monarch butterflies congregate in the upper loop during December and January.

Additional Information www.parks.ca.gov

HIKE 40 Fort Ross and Sonoma's Lost Coast

Highlights	A 200-year-old Russian outpost, a wild and nearly inaccessible coastline
Distance	2.2 miles round-trip, plus up to 6 miles of extreme coastal adventure
Total Elevation Gain/Loss	150'/150'
Hiking Time	1–2 hours, 4–6 hours one-way for Lost Coast section
Recommended Maps	*Fort Ross State Historic Park Map,* California State Parks; USGS 7.5-min. *Fort Ross* and *Arched Rock*
Best Times	Spring and fall
Agency	Fort Ross State Historic Park
Difficulty	★ to Reef Campground, ★★★★ for Sonoma's Lost Coast

FASCINATING HISTORY comes alive at Fort Ross, established in 1812 by members of the Russian-American Company as they steadily moved from Russian through Alaska and down the west coast of North America in search of sea otter pelts.

For the next 30 years, Fort Ross served as a Russian base for hunting sea otters, growing wheat and other crops for Russian settlements in Alaska, and trading with Spanish settlements farther south along the California coast. Named for its connection with Russia (*Rossiia*), Fort Ross marked Russia's southernmost outpost along the California coast.

The Russian-American Company departed in 1841, selling its holdings to American John Sutter, who had established a fort in the Sacramento valley. Fort Ross later became the property of George W. Call, who managed an

8,000-acre ranch and used the cove below Fort Ross to ship lumber, dairy, and other products to points south. In 1906 the state of California acquired the Fort Ross buildings and surrounding area, creating one of the state's very first state parks in the process.

Over the years, the state has extensively restored the Fort Ross buildings, including the oldest surviving original structure, Rotchev House (built in 1836). Today, the restored site provides a striking window into the state's pre–Gold Rush past, as well as access to an exemplary stretch of Northern California coast.

The Hike visits historic Fort Ross and then descends to the nearby tranquility of Sandy Cove, a peaceful and sheltered strand that delights for a short outing. From there, the path travels along the headlands to nearby Reef Campground, where a remote section of coast can be accessed.

Reef Campground is the end of the hike for all but the most intrepid adventurers. Those willing to take on an ankle-busting, wave-threatened coastal landscape with heart-pumping rock scrambles and tidal threats can continue south for six miles on a point-to-point journey along Sonoma's Lost Coast, a remote and challenging journey that exits at Russian Gulch Beach parking area.

Note that hiking Sonoma's Lost Coast is an extremely serious and committing endeavor that can only be completed at low tides. There is no exit anywhere along the route—steep and inaccessible cliffs back the shoreline for the length of the hike. If you become trapped by the tides, you will be stranded in a dangerous, wave-swept area. The majority of the route involves travel over boulders and loose rocks, with little easy-going sand. The reward is a landscape seldom visited by people, where the region's abundant wildlife will be shocked to see you come around the bend.

To Reach the Trailhead Follow Hwy. 1 to Fort Ross State Historic Park, 11 miles north of Jenner. An $8 day-use fee is charged. For those attempting Sonoma's Lost Coast, the Russian Gulch Beach parking area is 8.0 miles south

of the turnoff for Fort Ross. A car shuttle is required to return to your starting point.

Description From the parking lot (0.0/140'), head first to the excellent park visitor center to pay your day-use fee and enjoy quality displays about the site's history. Head out the rear of the visitor center to find the paved path that leads to the fort, passing under extensive Monterey cypress and crossing a small creek. You quickly reach the fort (0.2/130'), where you can wander around to your historic heart's content.

From the fort, follow the wide dirt path down toward Sandy Cove. As you descend, you can see the stairs on the far side of the beach that mark your continuing route to Reef Campground. You descend toward the alder-lined drainage of Fort Ross Creek, where a signed trail heads left to visit the site of the Russian Cemetery, a minor historical side-trip.

You quickly reach Sandy Cove (0.5/00'), where a gravelly beach provides a pleasant place to rest and explore. Prominent outcrops of greywacke, a type of sandstone common throughout California's coastal areas, forms much of the surrounding bluffs.

Continuing, ascend the opposite staircase (marked REEF) to the blufftop, which offers a nice view of Sandy Cove and the fort. The trail heads south, passing abundant lupine, irises, and sea daisies. The gully that contains Reef Campground becomes visible as the trail curves around, and soon you descend a singletrack path to reach the lower end of the campground. Turn right to follow the campground road to its end, where a narrow trail leads down to a rocky beach (1.1/00') that can be accessed with some mild scrambling. Enjoy the wild scenery here and then retrace your steps.

Sonoma's Lost Coast

Remember: *Sonoma's Lost Coast should be attempted only during low tide.* Mid- to high tides make certain sections impassable and dangerous. Large waves and swells increase the risk, even at lower tides—if the surf is running high, don't try it. (Mileage for this section is listed separately from the main trip.)

Description For those intrepid hikers considering this trip, the first mile provides a reality check of what lies ahead. From the beach by Reef Campground (0.0/00'), begin by rock-hopping continuously over boulders, cobbles, kelp, and driftwood—the typical conditions underfoot for the majority of the adventure—and quickly round a first rocky point (0.3/00'). Soon thereafter follows a second point (0.7/00'), which requires a heart-pumping scramble near the waves and over some substantial boulders, including a narrow slot between the cliff and an overhanging rock. If this section gives you pause or concern, turn back—similarly challenging sections await ahead in multiple locations.

Continuing your ankle-breaking journey, you next reach the mouth of Mill Gulch (1.2/00'), where a pretty cascade forms a small pool, a pleasant rest stop. Continuing, you pass intermittent streams trickling down the slopes and next reach diminutive Timber Creek (1.9/00'). Beyond lies a long black sand beach, backed by sheer and towering cliffs. Waves routinely wash to the cliff base. Depending on wave conditions, the next half mile can be one of the most unnerving and exposed sections of the route.

Past the beach, you pass a potential (but steep and difficult) escape hatch to Hwy. 1 above (3.0/00'), followed by a stretch of nasty angular cobblestones, and then reach a wide sandy beach, the longest and nicest of the hike. You return to the rocks along a narrow section (3.9/00'), where the ocean encroaches closely even on a moderate tide. The coast then curves around to reveal two large incisor-like rocks thrusting upward from the shore like giant canines (4.5/00').

After surmounting this obstacle, you now see the hike's final hurdle—a narrow cleft pinned between the cliffs and a large, distinctive dome-shaped rock. A steep scramble up this chute and down the other side brings you to rockier beach (4.9/00'), where a large sea lion colony often inhabits the offshore rocks.

A short sandy beach then curves around to a final close-hemmed section, where the waves come close again against the cliffs even at midtide. Shortly beyond, the topography

The historic buildings of Fort Ross

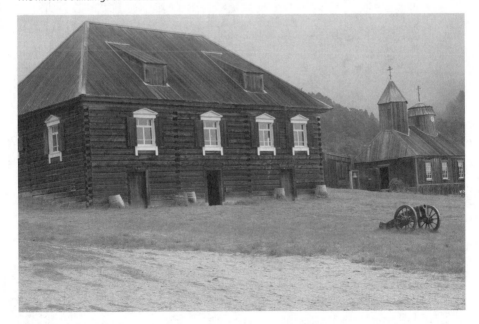

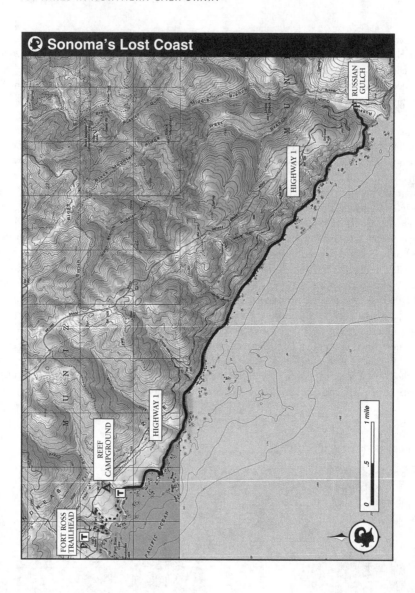

Sonoma's Lost Coast

makes further coastal progress clearly impossible (5.5/00'). At this point, an obvious use trail steeply climbs the slopes to a grassy divide (5.6/130'), where you can savor exceptional views north of your completed route and south to Bodega Head (Trip 39).

After a continued steep climb, the path forks; continue straight to follow the singletrack trail as it winds along the bluffs with views of the ocean below. You curve left above a small creek and then descend into an area intermittently thick with poison oak.

After a final section of dense foliage, you emerge in the parking lot for Russian Gulch Beach (6.0/20'). Take a deep breath—you made it!

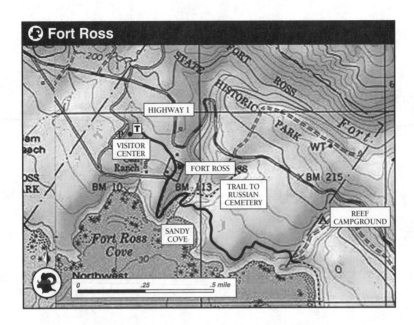

Nearest Visitor Center Fort Ross State Historic Park Visitor Center, 707-847-3286, adjacent to the main parking area, is open Friday–Monday 10 a.m.–4:30 p.m. September–June, with extended hours in July and August.

Nearest Campground The park's Reef Campground is open seasonally (April–October) and offers 21 sites on a first-come, first-served basis ($35).

Additional Information www.parks.ca.gov, fortross.org

The rugged terrain of Sonoma's Lost Coast is not for the faint of heart.

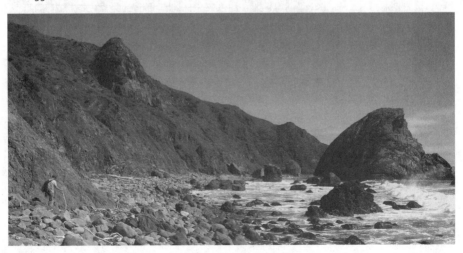

HIKE 41 Manchester Beach ○ 🚶 👫

Highlights	A little-visited strand of sand and the San Andreas Fault
Distance	4.0 miles round-trip
Total Elevation Gain/Loss	Negligible
Hiking Time	1–2 hours
Recommended Map	USGS 7.5-min. *Point Arena*
Best Times	Year-round
Agency	Manchester State Park
Difficulty	★★

JUST NORTH OF POINT ARENA is a miles-long beach that receives minimal use, yet offers a delightful coastside experience of beachcombing. A bonus visit to the San Andreas Fault increases the appeal. Manchester Beach is much less visited than other coastal destinations on Hwy. 1 and offers an exceptional opportunity to beat the crowds, though you should also be prepared for minimal maintenance and facilities; the cash-strapped state park system has largely neglected it in recent years.

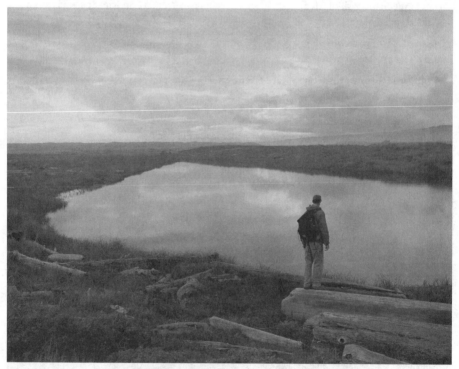

Massive driftwood and ephemeral lagoons punctuate the terrain of Manchester Beach.

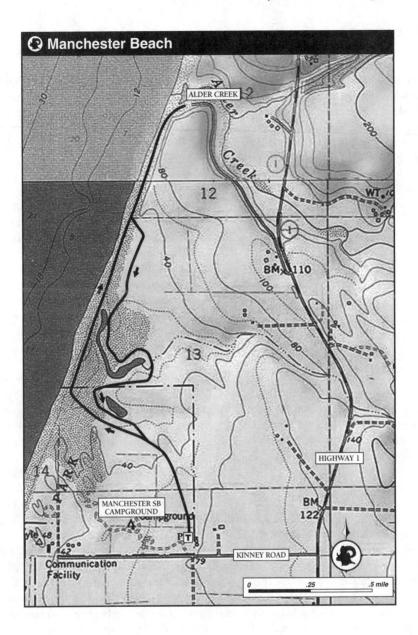

The Hike is a loop that first heads to the beach and travels north along the sand to Alder Creek, where the San Andreas Fault slices from land to ocean and steelhead and salmon spawn in winter. The hike then returns among the inland dunes, where several backcountry (environmental) campsites offer opportunities for an overnight visit. Dogs are not allowed. Note that the beach may be closed in the spring to protect piping plovers during their nesting season.

To Reach the Trailhead Take Hwy. 1 north past Point Arena to Kinney Rd., 6 miles north of Point Arena Lighthouse Rd. and 0.7 mile north of the general store in the small town of Crispin. Proceed down Kinney Rd. for 0.4 mile, passing a large KOA campground on the right, and then turn right onto a short unpaved section of road signed for WALK-IN ENVI-RONMENTAL CAMPSITES. A large, circular parking area marks the trailhead, where water is available.

Description From the trailhead (0.0/70'), strike out on the wide trail, which quickly heads into coastal scrub populated with coffeeberry, bracken fern, and abundant lupine. You quickly encounter a sign about the area's endangered mountain beavers.

Considered the world's most primitive living rodent, mountain beavers can be found in locations throughout the Pacific Northwest. In this area, a genetically distinct subspecies, the Point Arena mountain beaver (*Aplodontia rufa nigra*), can be found only within a 24-square-mile area; Manchester State Park is near the center of its limited range. Stout and compact, mountain beavers reach about 1 foot in length and weigh 2–4 pounds. They are mostly unrelated to true beavers (*Castor* spp.).

Mountain beavers spend most of their time in underground burrow systems, emerging only to forage on vegetation. You'll see the surface traces of their tunnels throughout this hike. They are easily collapsed by errant steps; please help protect this endangered species by watching for—and avoiding—their tunnels.

Continuing, you quickly reach open views of the coastal landscape ahead. Point Arena Lighthouse is visible to the southwest, while a striking wave-cut terrace can be seen to the north. This distinctive topographic feature is common along the coast here, formed by wave action and then uplifted above sea level by the area's active tectonic forces.

The trail narrows to packed dirt and winds toward the dunes, soon reaching a lagoon rife with birdlife and frog song (0.4/10'). From here, proceed toward the beach; a series of paths provides multiple access points. Take care to avoid trampling the extensive dune grass, which helps hold the dunes in place.

Large driftwood, much of it redwood logs, appears among the diminishing dunes as you approach the beach. Head north along the sand, enjoying the tranquil beach experience and crashing surf. In the spring and fall, keep an eye on the ocean for the spouts of migrating humpback whales.

As you proceed north, the adjacent bluffs steepen and you pass below an abandoned house on the blufftops above (1.6/0'). Soon you reach the mouth of Alder Creek (1.9/0'), which is often hemmed in by sand during the low-water months of summer.

To locate the San Andreas Fault, look closely at the coastal bluffs on the south side of the creek and identify where the gray-green rocks in the cliffs transition to loose, brown-gray sediment. This sediment marks the location of the fault, which has ground up the surrounding rocks into loose debris. It also marks the fault's northernmost location on land; north of here it remains entirely beneath the ocean until it ends at the Mendocino Triple Junction offshore from Cape Mendocino (Hike 48).

From here, retrace your steps along the beach below the abandoned house and then proceed inland at the first break in the dunes after the bluffs diminish. This deposits you on an old grassy road (2.4/20'), where you turn right to quickly reach a backcountry campsite in the lee of a dune. A picnic table, fire ring, and boarded-up outhouse greet you at the site.

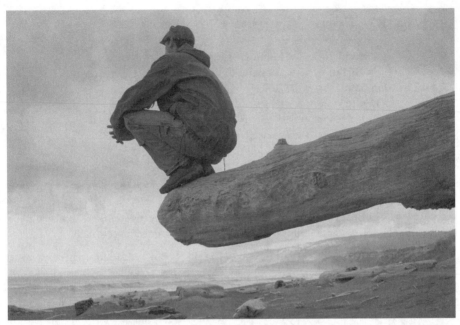

A hiker contemplates the region's tectonic and oceanic power.

Continuing south, the path next curves inland to pass a second decrepit outhouse and then winds past a thick grove of Monterey cypress. Several campsites can be found on the far side of the grove (3.1/20'), where a large, cavelike clearing offers ample tent room in an otherworldly setting.

Past the grove, your route turns to the south, away from the wide and obvious path, and toward the nearby inland lagoon. The trail becomes indistinct at this point, obscured by past coastal flooding and a lack of maintenance. (You may find old trail signs scattered on the ground amid the grass and debris.) Proceed along and around the beachside edge of the lagoon, which varies in shape and extent depending on the year, and make your way back to the large lagoon from the beginning of the hike. From here, return the way you came (4.0/70').

Nearest Visitor Center There is no visitor center in the park. For general information, call the park office at 707-882-2463 or the Mendocino District office at 707-937-5804.

Backpacking Information Overnight camping is permitted at the environmental campsites only ($15 per night; self-register at the trailhead). Water is unavailable at or near the sites—bring sufficient supplies with you.

Nearest Campground Just past the trailhead, the spartan Manchester State Park Campground (41 sites, $25) is a study in contrast with the bustling, amenities-rich KOA campground just up the road. All of the sites are first come, first served; space is almost always available.

Additional Information www.parks.ca.gov

HIKE 42 Fern Canyon ↗ 🚶

Highlight	The lushness of a small coastal river canyon
Distance	5.0 miles round-trip
Total Elevation Gain/Loss	200'/200'
Hiking Time	2–3 hours
Recommended Maps	USGS 7.5-min. *Mendocino* and *Mathison Peak*
Best Times	Year-round
Agency	Van Damme State Park
Difficulty	★

WITH ITS GURGLING ALLEY of green in a verdant canyon, Van Damme State Park provides an easy sampling of the lush ecosystem found just inland from the coast. The highlight is Fern Canyon, a small gorge 400 feet deep that shelters Little River and a lush, regenerating redwood forest. A diminutive coastal river barely 5 miles long, Little River provides critical habitat for coho salmon, steelhead, and a variety of other wildlife. Logged during the late 19th century, the forest has since rebounded to impressive dimensions with only gigantic decaying stumps to remind hikers of the past.

Logging began here on October 15, 1864, in response to the heavy demand for lumber in the burgeoning city of San Francisco. By 1865, more than three dozen schooners were hauling wood from Little River to San Francisco; activity continued unabated for the next 30 years. The redwoods were cut by burly men perched on wide planks known as "springboards," placed approximately 6 feet above the base of a tree, which allowed loggers to fell a tree at a narrower, more easily hewn point. Once cut, logs were floated downriver to be stored and milled near the river mouth. Bull teams, wagons, and a tramway moved trees from the more difficult locations, and skid roads were constructed to access ever farther up-canyon. By 1893 all profitable timber had been cut and the mills closed for good. The Jackson History Trail explores past milling operations in the park with the help of an excellent interpretive brochure, available at the visitor center or entrance station.

The Hike follows wide and level Fern Canyon Scenic Trail along Little River, an easy hike that can be extended significantly by adding the 3.5-mile Pygmy Forest loop at the hike's up-canyon terminus. The sun seldom shines in narrow Fern Canyon, making it cool and damp year-round with winter months colder and wetter than the rest. Fog does not detract from this hike—if anything, it enhances the experience—making it an excellent option for fogbound summer days. The very popular trail does not offer solitude, particularly during summer months. Water is available at the trailhead.

To Reach the Trailhead Drive 3 miles south of Mendocino on Hwy. 1 to the park entrance. Follow the park road to its end behind the campground. An $8 day-use fee is charged.

Description From the trailhead, go through the gate and get an interpretive brochure. It explains the life cycle of the coho salmon with the help of metal fish markers spaced periodically along the hike. As you begin down the wide paved path, note the lush growth around you. Moss, fern, horsetail, huckleberry, stinging nettle, poison oak, thimbleberry, and the seasonal displays of tiger lilies, columbine, and irises cover the ground and cut banks. Tanoaks and Douglas-firs join second-growth redwoods to form the dense canopy overhead.

The trail follows a road constructed during the 1880s to provide up-canyon logging access,

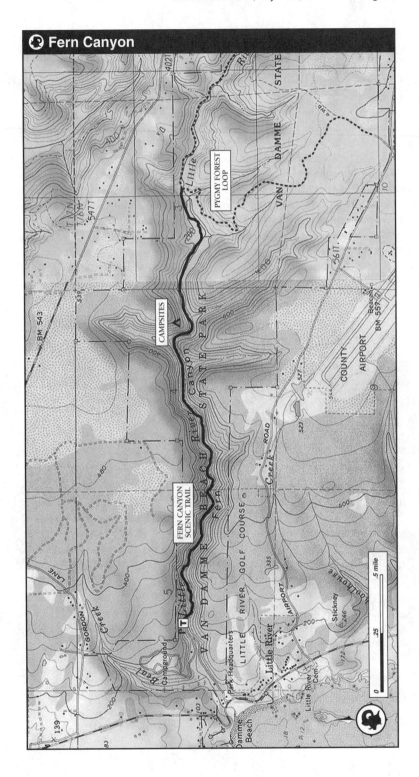

Fern Canyon

which was improved by the Civilian Conservation Corps during the 1930s with the construction of several bridges. As you pass Fish 3, large redwood stumps begin to appear by the trail—look for springboard notches near the tops. Scan the river as you proceed and you may be lucky enough to spot a Pacific giant salamander. Largest of all terrestrial salamanders, they achieve lengths of up to 12 inches and can be identified by their mottled, purplish-brown backs and pale-yellow underbellies. Living in moist places where they can breathe through their skins, they consume everything from insects to fish to frogs to snakes to other salamanders, lunging to grab their prey with sharp, bladelike teeth.

Once cut, a redwood tree immediately sprouts a series of genetically identical saplings from its root system, in time forming a roughly concentric circle of mature trees around the stump known as a "fairy ring." Several good examples of this basal sprouting can be spotted as you continue up-canyon—check around Fish 9. After passing 10 environmental campsites, the trail soon reaches the end of the Fern Canyon Scenic Trail in a large clearing.

Those wishing to continue their hike to the Pygmy Forest can begin the 3.5-mile loop here. Begin on the trail section to the left, a single-track that delves deeper into the canyon. The return stretch is along the wide fire road to your right. Unless you're passionate about ecology, the Pygmy Forest is not as exciting as it sounds. If you don't wish to go farther, return the way you came.

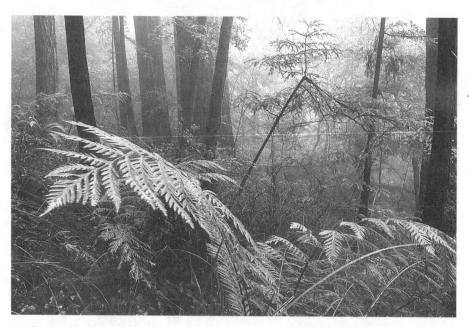

Van Damme's fern-topia is a pteridologist's delight.

Nearest Visitor Center Van Damme State Park Visitor Center, 707-937-4016, is open Wednesday–Sunday 10 a.m.–4 p.m. April–October, and weekends only rest of the year. Also try the district headquarters at 707-937-5804.

Backpacking Information Backcountry camping is allowed only at the 10 small but pleasant environmental campsites ($10–$15, depending on season) tucked along Little River 1.75 miles from the trailhead.

Nearest Campground Van Damme State Park Campground has 74 sites ($35). Reservations are imperative April–September, when tourists and abalone divers routinely fill the campground; visit **reserveamerica.com** or call 800-444-7275.

Additional Information **www.parks.ca.gov**

The North Coast and Klamath Mountains

STRETCHING FROM the Lost Coast north to the Oregon border and east to Mount Shasta, this region includes the hard-to-access strip of coastline north of Hwy. 1, the magnificent old-growth redwood forests along Hwy. 101, and the convoluted ranges of the Klamath Mountains. The coastal topography is usually rocky and often dominated by sheer cliffs. Inland, the Klamath Mountains compose a variety of smaller ranges incised by deep river canyons.

Elevations rarely exceed 8,000 feet. The Trinity Alps and Marble Mountains are two of the more notable subranges.

Annual precipitation, high throughout the entire region, creates thick forests that blanket all but the tallest ridges and peaks. Snow occurs down to roughly 3,000 feet in the winter, and fog envelops the coast during the summer. Highlights include remote locations, luxuriant forests, and some of California's choicest wilderness.

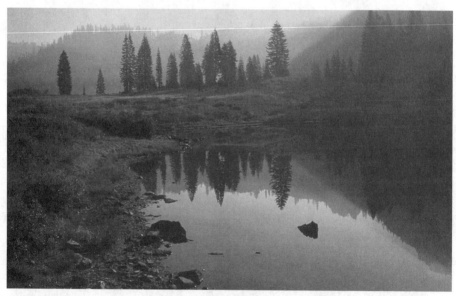

Marble Mountain moment: a reflection in Sky High Lakes Basin (see Hike 55, page 197)

HIKE 43   Humboldt Redwoods ☵

Highlight	A vast forest of redwoods enormous
Distance	7.0 miles round-trip
Total Elevation Gain/Loss	500'/500'
Hiking Time	4–5 hours
Recommended Maps	*Humboldt Redwoods State Park Map,* USGS 7.5-min. *Villa Creek* and *Burro Mountain*
Best Times	Spring–fall
Agency	Humboldt Redwoods State Park
Difficulty	★★★

THE LARGEST CONTIGUOUS old-growth redwood forest on Earth is protected within Humboldt Redwoods State Park. Beyond amazement at individual trees, you experience an entire ecosystem that humbles all other redwood adventures in this book.

Named after the Prussian scientific explorer Alexander von Humboldt, the park began in 1921 with the purchase of 2,000 acres by the Save-the-Redwoods League on the South Fork Eel River. With completion of a railroad linking Humboldt County to the Bay Area in 1914 and construction of the Redwood Hwy. in 1922, increasing tourism and logging activity magnified pressures on the diminishing old-growth redwood forests. In 1927, California created a statewide system of parks and passed a bond measure to provide matching funds for the acquisition of state park lands. The Save-the-Redwoods League immediately began soliciting private donations and, in 1930, J. D. Rockefeller contributed a remarkable gift of $2 million to purchase 10,000 acres along Bull Creek owned by the Pacific Lumber Company. His generosity and farsightedness now protects this unrivaled redwood forest.

Humboldt Redwoods State Park today comprises 53,000 acres, of which 17,000 nurture old-growth redwood forest. Most of the Avenue of the Giants winds through the eastern section of the park and the entire Bull Creek watershed is now protected in its western portion. Efforts to restore park watersheds damaged by past logging are ongoing.

The Hike loops around the lower section of Bull Creek on Bull Creek Trail and winds through a continuous forest of gargantuan old-growth redwood trees. Note that you must cross Bull Creek twice to complete the loop. A seasonal footbridge offers easy crossing from early May until late September. You'll need to ford the creek at other times, however, which can become difficult to dangerous during the rainy months of fall, winter, and spring.

To Reach the Trailhead Take Hwy. 101 to Dyerville, turn east on Mattole Rd. (signed for Rockefeller Forest), and proceed 1.4 miles to the trailhead turnoff on the left. A short but steep drop on a one-lane dirt road leads you to a roundabout with ample parking.

Description At the trailhead (0.0/140'), humongous redwoods rise all around you, including several particularly stupendous specimens— the first in a nearly endless parade of redwoods enormous. Begin your journey on Rockefeller Loop Trail, which almost immediately reaches a junction. Your return route enters from the right, but you bear left to remain on Rockefeller Loop Trail as it travels adjacent to the nearby South Fork Eel River.

Colossal trees are everywhere around you. And yet they are almost all redwoods, with few of the other tree species that commonly intermix elsewhere. Why? Substantial flooding can occur on Bull Creek, driven by heavy winter rains and the surrounding steep topography. Massive amounts of sediment are deposited

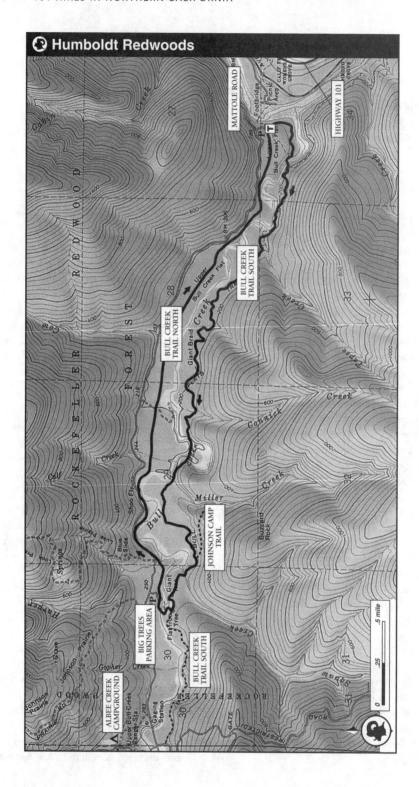

Humboldt Redwoods

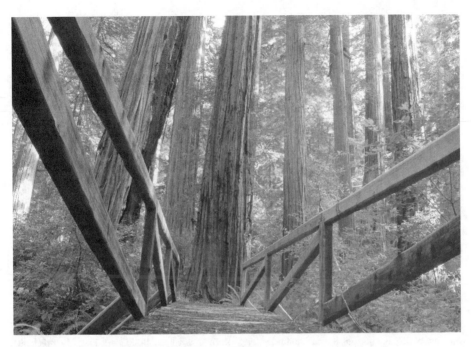

Stupendously large old-growth redwoods predominate along Bull Creek.

along the valley bottom during major flood events, which buries the base of trees beneath many inches (sometimes feet) of sand, dirt, and debris. This smothers and kills the root systems of most tree species. Redwoods, however, have the unique ability to sprout new roots from the base of their buried trunks, which allows them to adapt to, and survive, such events.

Redwoods are not immune to other consequences of flooding, however. As floodwaters erode riverbanks, they slowly undercut the trees above, eventually felling them. Several trees here lean precariously near the water. Others have already toppled to the ground, their enormous root balls now rising nearly 20 feet off the ground.

Continuing, you pass through an enormous cut in a fallen tree and then reach a junction (0.2/140'). Well-trod Rockefeller Loop Trail continues straight, but you bear left here and drop to Bull Creek near its confluence with the Eel River. Cross the seasonal footbridge, climb a few steps cut into a mudbank, and then rise

steeply to reach an unposted junction. Bear left here to curve around toward the Eel River and reach another unposted junction. River Trail continues left here, but your route turns right to begin an uphill traverse.

You curve back around into the Bull Creek drainage, its waters now far below. Huckleberry bushes and sword ferns fill the understory, and a few massive old-growth Douglas-firs can be spotted in places—their crustier, rougher bark easily distinguished from the surrounding redwoods.

You next reach a signed junction for Bull Creek Trail (0.5/190'). Proceed straight and up on singletrack Bull Creek Trail as it cruises gently along the slopes. The triple leaves of white trillium sprout around you. Intermittent views of the flats below look across large expanses of old-growth.

The size and number of mega-trees steadily increase as you slowly climb and then descend to return to the valley bottom. You next pass beneath the monstrous root ball of a fallen tree, cross a bridge over crystalline Tepee Creek (1.0/190'), and then wind along the edge of substantial flats populated by a dense collection of massive old-growth.

The trail crosses a bridge over Connick Creek (2.3/410') and curves down to Bull Creek itself, where it makes a big turn by a gravel bar. The trail briefly transitions to grassier singletrack as it passes through a small meadow. Returning to ancient forest, you cross the Miller Creek bridge (2.8/330') and pass a fallen tunnel tree large enough to walk through upright.

Widening, the trail takes a circuitous route through a section of many fallen giants and then reaches the junction with Johnson Camp Trail (3.3/420'). Go straight on Johnson Camp Trail, which soon crosses a substantial bridge over Squaw Creek near its confluence with Bull Creek.

Bear right at the next junction (3.6/300') to quickly reach the Giant Tree—a champion specimen. Though not the tallest redwood, its massive bulk has long put it as a contender for largest redwood by mass. The continuing route emerges by the flowing creek, where a wide gravel and dirt path leads down to the seasonal bridge. Cross (or ford) the creek to quickly reach the Big Trees parking area on the far side.

Your route back to the trailhead is on Bull Creek Trail North, which strikes out from the far side of the lot. The trail stays briefly near the creek, where large old growth looms among thicker understory trees. After crossing the bridge over Harper Creek (3.9/330'), the trail cruises near Bull Creek and leads to the Blue Slide Picnic Area (5.0/430'), where picnic tables can be found in an open meadow.

The continuing route stays near the creek before heading briefly to the park road, which it follows for approximately 0.2 mile. The posted trail soon bears off the pavement to the right and winds between the road and creek, reentering phenomenal old-growth as the trail curves back toward Bull Creek.

The trail runs near the creek on a flood plain populated by young trees, then curves intermittently between younger and older terrains to eventually return along the creek. You then cross substantial Cow Creek (5.4/400') on another solid wooden bridge and enjoy a long stretch of continuous and massive old-growth in an area known as Upper Bull Creek Flat. The creek remains nearby, and you eventually return to it via a nice stone walkway and small staircase.

Ascending briefly, you then resume your tour of the old-growth flats, which ultimately returns you back to Rockefeller Loop Trail (6.9/140'). Go left to return to the parking lot (7.0/140').

Nearest Visitor Center Humboldt Redwoods State Park Visitor Center, 707-946-2263, is 4 miles south of the Mattole Rd. turnoff along the Avenue of the Giants. It's open daily 9 a.m.–5 p.m. April–September, and daily 10 a.m.–4 p.m. the rest of the year.

Nearest Campgrounds Albee Creek Campground (40 sites, $35; open mid-May–September) is 3.5 miles west of the trailhead on Mattole Rd. Burlington Campground (57 sites, $35; open year-round) is near the visitor center on the Avenue of the Giants. Reservations are recommended during the summer; visit **reserveamerica.com** or call 800-444-7275.

Additional Information humboldtredwoods.org

HIKE 44 North Yolla Bolly Mountain ☉ 🚶

Highlight	Remote adventuring in the northern Coast Range
Distance	11.2 miles round-trip, 8.6 miles out-and-back to North Yolla Bolly Mountain
Total Elevation Gain/Loss	3,100'/3,100'
Hiking Time	6–10 hours
Recommended Maps	*A Guide to the Yolla Bolly Wilderness* by the US Forest Service, USGS 7.5-min. *North Yolla Bolly Mountains*
Best Times	May–October
Agency	Yolla Bolly Wilderness, Shasta-Trinity National Forest
Difficulty	★★★★★

NORTH YOLLA BOLLY MOUNTAIN rises 7,863 feet atop the rough and remote terrain of the northern Coast Range, a summit with dramatic views of a vast wilderness seldom visited by hikers. Located in the northeast portion of 151,000-acre Yolla Bolly Wilderness, the journey to the peak highlights some of the majesty—and challenges—of this little-visited region. It's a hidden gem for hikers who really want to get away from it all, but you must be willing to take the challenge of rough roads and faint-to-nonexistent trails to experience it.

Located west of the northern Sacramento Valley, where the northern Coast Range mashes against the Klamath Mountains, the terrain of Yolla Bolly Wilderness rises above 7,000 feet, higher than just about anywhere else in the Coast Range. Its northerly location and higher elevations result in ample precipitation that nourishes a robust forest of mighty trees, punctuated by bare ridgelines rising high above it all.

This is not granite country. As is common throughout the Coast Range, it is instead a diverse assemblage of sedimentary and metamorphic rocks that have been crushed against the continent and driven skyward by tectonic forces. The wilderness gets its name from the Wintun Indian language; *Yo-la* translates as "snow-covered" and *Boli* meant "high peak."

The Hike ascends North Yolla Bolly Mountain from Rat Trap Gap trailhead, which can be accessed only via a twisting, unpaved, and rough 18-mile access road. The journey first ascends to reach a long ridgeline that extends west from North Yolla Bolly Mountain, then travels directly along the ridgeline's open grasslands to the rocky mountain peak. An out-and-back trip to the summit is more straightforward than the continuing loop, which requires a challenging off-trail descent from the summit to Pettijohn Trail. From there, the hike returns via Yolla Bolly Lake Trail, which visits small, exciting, and scenic North Yolla Bolly Lake along the way.

Water is scarce; a pair of springs provides reliable sources on the initial ascent to the ridgeline and North Yolla Bolly Lake awaits on the far side of the loop, but otherwise the landscape is generally dry.

The wilderness is usually a good early-season option, though snow can linger here deep into April or even May, depending on the season. Call ahead for current conditions.

To Reach the Trailhead Take Hwy. 36 west from Red Bluff for 37 miles, turn left on unpaved Tedoc Rd. (FS 45), and proceed a slow and exciting 17.5 miles to the trailhead. The lower section of the road is most challenging, ascending steeply for 6 miles over open terrain; water ruts in this section may make passage difficult for low-clearance vehicles. The final 12 miles are less challenging, but still rough. Expect the drive from Hwy. 36 to take 60–90 minutes, depending on conditions and vehicle.

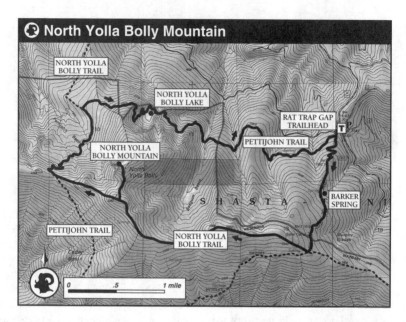

The trailhead is located at the junction of FS 45 and FS 35 and features an established camping area and dilapidated outhouse. No water is available at the trailhead. Note that it is no longer possible to drive between Stuart Gap and Rat Trap Gap on FS 35; a slide has permanently closed the road a mile west of Rat Trap Gap.

Description From the trailhead (0.0/5,950'), strike out past a beat-down trail register and up the wide, obvious trail. Large red firs, Douglas-firs, and ponderosa pines thrust from the surrounding slopes around you. You immediately reach a trail junction, where your return route on Yolla Bolly Lake Trail enters from the right.

Bear left to head toward Barker Camp and enjoy the appearance of substantial sugar pines in the forest mosaic. You ascend steadily on a dusty singletrack trail, making several switchbacks as you climb. The trail eases after 400 feet of climbing and then rises slowly to reach a green gully that marks the hike's first spring (0.9/6,600'). Though more of a seep than a gusher, the spring does provide reliable water; you may need a filter to obtain it. (Approaching Barker Spring offers a better source.)

The trail winds above the top of the spring and continues its steady traverse to reach the flowing spring by the pleasant oasis of Barker Camp (1.4/6,980'), which features a grassy meadow and good potential campsites. The continuing trail levels as it approaches the broad ridgetop, crosses into the wilderness, and then curves around to attain the ridge crest (1.6/7,060'). Here a small cairn marks the junction with unsigned North Yolla Bolly Mountain Trail. Turn right to follow this thin path as it takes a direct line up the broad ridge, initially rising through dense young firs and then returning to more mature forest.

Upon reaching the ridge's first meadow (1.8/7,200'), you enjoy your first grand views to the southeast, including the high summit of 8,098-foot South Yolla Bolly Mountain, the highest peak in the wilderness. At this point, the trail starts to become increasingly faint in the grasslands as it makes a mostly level traverse below the ridgeline. At times, it disappears entirely, though the route finding is straightforward. You pass some striking metamorphic boulders, reenter dense young woods, and then drop slightly to pass below a bare hump on the ridge.

You regain the broad ridge on the far side, where your continuing ridgeline route is apparent ahead. The indistinct trail follows the ridge as it curves to the right, then disappears entirely as the route turns to the northwest and ascends directly along the ridgeline. Views northwest open up for the first time and reveal the rocky high point at the end of the ridge ahead of you (North Yolla Bolly Mountain still hides out of sight). Beyond it, you can spot the abandoned fire lookout tower on Black Rock Mountain.

The pleasure of easy ridgeline walking is enhanced by expanding views west toward the upper watersheds of the Eel and Mad Rivers, which flow west toward the ocean. At the end of the ridge, the exposed terrain transitions to a rock and tree garden just below the rocky high point (3.9/7,800'). You can quickly ascend to the top, where you'll discover a collection of hardy foxtail pines, easily recognized by the long and distinctive needle structures that give this species its name.

Nearby North Yolla Bolly Mountain is now visible for the first time, on the far side of a saddle to the north. To tag the summit, relocate the trail in the saddle between the first rocky summit and a second just beyond, and then drop steeply down lupine-covered slopes into a stand of red fir. Upon reaching the saddle (4.1/7,620'),

the trail vaporizes once again and it's a choose-your-own-route to the top, where an easy walk-up to the summit (4.3/7,863') leads you to an amazing view, as well as a summit register in a heavy metal cylinder.

Admire the world in 360-degree glory. Look east across the Sacramento Valley; on clear days you can pick out Lassen Peak 80 miles away. To the north is Black Rock Mountain and its lookout tower. Peering west, you can see across the Eel and Mad River drainages nearly to the ocean. To the south, peaks and ridges roll to the horizon in almost endless succession.

Now a crucial choice awaits hikers attempting to complete the loop. Per the US Forest Service (USFS) map of the wilderness, North Yolla Bolly Trail continues from the saddle immediately north of the summit and drops steeply down the western flanks of the mountain before traversing west to join Pettijohn Trail. At the time of research, however, I was unable to locate the upper portion of this trail, which was indiscernible. Those with strong navigational skills may consider following this

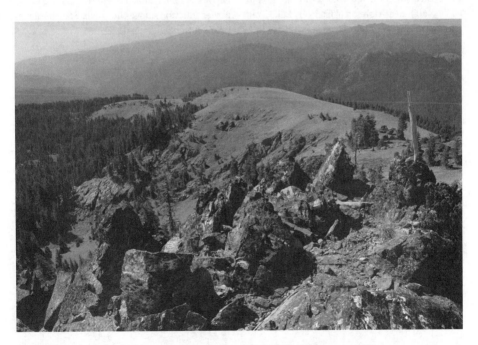

The rugged, remote, and seldom-visited landscape of Yolla Bolly Wilderness awaits.

route nonetheless—and may be able to locate the trail farther down—but the terrain is steep and forested in many places, reducing visibility and increasing the difficulty.

Alternatively, you can retrace your steps across the saddle to the main ridgeline (4.7/ 7,800') and make a descending 0.6-mile off-trail traverse down the southern flanks of the ridge to reach Pettijohn Trail (5.3/7,160'), which crosses the main ridge in the next saddle to the west. Though steep and ankle torquing at times, this option provides the advantage of open slopes and clear views of the route ahead, which makes route finding straightforward.

Upon reaching the saddle and Pettijohn Trail—however you went—enjoy the view of imposing North Yolla Bolly Mountain and then savor the well-worn trail as it heads down the shady north side of the ridge. A series of steep traverses and nearly a dozen switchbacks lead to a pair of seasonal flowing water sources—some of the very upper sources of the Trinity River watershed.

Ponderosa pines reappear on the descent to the posted junction for Yolla Bolly Lake Trail (6.7/6,460'). Bear right on Yolla Bolly Lake Trail and make a sustained and steady climb to a rocky crest with views into the rugged valley of North Yolla Bolly Lake (7.4/6,900'). A series of nine switchbacks leads you to an established campsite by the lakeshore (8.1/6,520'), though the best site is in the boulders by the lake's inlet. It's a scenic spot, punctuated by huge red firs and views of the surrounding cliffs.

The trail winds around the lake and past large boulders to cross the outlet, then immediately resumes its traverse along the steep slopes. Rising and then dropping steeply, you next curve past a barge-shaped megaboulder and meander through a garden of giant rocks. The airy traverse offers intermittent views east—watch for Lassen Peak in the distance—as it undulates into the rugged drainage of Beegum Basin, which is highlighted by sheer granite-esque slabs.

The trail curves around the drainage, crosses a crystalline creek and another smaller source, then reenters dense, shady fir woods. A cruising traverse leads you into the next drainage, where the route descends gently among large and mature Douglas-firs, a few trickling springs, and another flowing creek lush with ferns and gooseberries. A final gentle descent returns you to the earlier junction above the trailhead, where you turn left to head home (11.2/5,950').

Nearest Visitor Center Yolla Bolly Ranger Station 530-352-4211, 9.6 miles west of the Tedoc Rd. turnoff on Hwy. 36., is open Monday–Friday 8 a.m.–4:30 p.m. year-round.

Backpacking Information No wilderness permit is needed, though a valid fire permit is required. Overnight options with water are limited to Barker Springs and North Yolla Bolly Lake.

Nearest Campground Basin Gulch Campground (13 sites, no water) is just west of Yolla Bolly Ranger Station. To reach it, follow Hwy. 36 west of the ranger station for 0.3 mile, turn left on Stuart Gap Road, and proceed 1 mile.

Additional Information www.fs.usda.gov/stnf

HIKE 45 Lost Coast Trail 🚶

Highlights	Daunting coastal cliffs and remote beaches
Distance	16.7 miles one-way
Total Elevation Gain/Loss	3,800'/3,800'
Hiking Time	16–24 hours (2–3 days)
Recommended Maps	*California's Lost Coast* by Wilderness Press; USGS 7.5-min. *Hales Grove, Mistake Point,* and *Bear Harbor*
Best Times	Spring and fall
Agency	Sinkyone Wilderness State Park
Difficulty	★★★★

THE LOST COAST can hardly be considered undiscovered. Ranching, logging, railroads, mills, and seaports have all left their mark on the land. But it is remote, too rugged for Hwy. 1, keeping all but the adventurous away.

The Lost Coast stretches from the Eel River Delta near Ferndale south to Hwy. 1, a distance of more than 70 miles. Offshore is the Mendocino Triple Junction, the point where three tectonic plates meet. North of the junction, the Juan de Fuca Plate dives beneath the Pacific Northwest, triggering the volcanoes of the Cascade Range. South, the San Andreas Fault reaches its offshore terminus, knitting the landscape with a host of faults. All this tectonic mayhem combines to cause dramatic uplift, creating cliffs that tower more than 1,000 feet above the crashing sea. The dark cliffs weather to form unusual black-sand beaches, accessible only where small creeks have carved deep gullies between the bluffs. Sinkyone Wilderness State Park encompasses the southernmost section of the Lost Coast, an area of 7,367 acres that protects more than 22 miles of shoreline.

Wildlife thrives in the park today. A herd of Roosevelt elk, reintroduced from Prairie Creek Redwoods State Park, wanders the coastal bluffs. Black bears and mountain lions prowl inland. Whales and seals can be spotted offshore. Raptors of all varieties soar above. And a few stands of old-growth redwood still remain.

The Hike follows Lost Coast Trail between Orchard Camp and Usal Camp—a strenuous

trek best done in three days. Though this hike travels along the coast, there is virtually no level walking: The trail constantly encounters sheer creek canyons, descending quickly and ascending steeply hundreds of feet at a time. The two ends of Lost Coast Trail lie far apart by road—2–3 hours' driving time—and two vehicles are required for transportation to and from the trailheads.

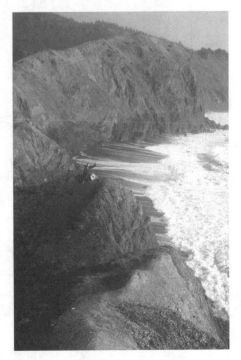

Hooray for California!

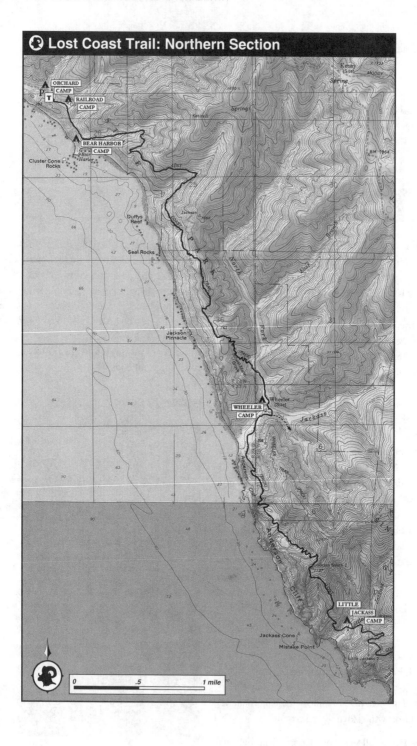

⊙ Lost Coast Trail: Northern Section

A shuttle service is often available from local operators—contact the park or the Bureau of Land Management's King Range Visitor Center, 707-986-5400, open year-round Monday–Friday, 8 a.m.–4:30 p.m., for current information and rates.

While the hike can be done in either direction, this description runs from north to south. Those wishing to day hike from the north trailhead should turn around at Wheeler Camp, making a round-trip of 9.4 miles with an elevation gain/loss of roughly 1,000 feet. Those interested in day-hiking from the south should climb 1,000 feet to the top of the first bluff beyond Usal Beach, a 6-mile round-trip with superlative views of the ocean and coast.

Timing is key. Fog blankets the region from June through mid-September, obscuring views and chilling the air for days on end. Heavy storms usually strike by late October and can inundate the coast with torrential rainfall well into April. From late April through May, storms are less frequent, fog is only occasional, and the lush, green terrain explodes with wildflowers. In late September and October, fog tapers off and weather is most ideal. Avoid holidays and weekends and crowds will be light. Those planning a winter visit should call ahead to verify access: Flooding and slides can close the roads for weeks at a time. Backcountry camping is allowed only at the three designated trail camps (see box page 165). While no water is available at the trailhead, you can find it in abundance along the trail.

To Reach the North Trailhead: Take the Hwy. 101 exit for Redway and Shelter Cove. From Redway, take Briceland Thorn Rd. 18 miles west toward Shelter Cove to Chemise Mountain Rd.—turn left (south). The road rapidly turns to dirt, reaching a four-way junction in 7 miles—turn right onto the least significant road. The descent from here is steep, narrow, and not passable for trailers or RVs. While four-wheel-drive vehicles will have an easier time, low-clearance cars can make a slow descent. The Needle Rock Visitor Center is 3.5 miles from the junction. Here, day-hikers pay a day-use fee per vehicle and backpackers pay their trail-camp fees. The trailhead at Orchard Camp is an additional 2.7 miles south at the road's end. After the first big rains of the season, the road is closed beyond the visitor center, making it necessary to walk this final stretch.

To Reach the South Trailhead: Take Mendocino County (Usal) Rd. 431 north from Hwy. 1. Along Hwy. 1, the easily missed turnoff is located at milepost 90.88, 15 miles west of Hwy. 101 and approximately 3 miles north of Rockport. The one-lane dirt road is impassable for trailers and RVs but easily handled by all other vehicles. In 6 miles you reach the area's first campsites, in a large grassy field. Trailhead parking is 0.3 mile farther on the left, immediately before a small bridge. From here, it's a short walk to the posted trailhead at the road's end. Note that theft has been reported at the Usal Beach trailhead; do not leave valuables in your vehicle.

Description Soon after leaving the trailhead at Orchard Camp (0.0/40'), the trail is joined by a spur trail from Railroad Camp. Then, it winds down to the coastal vista at Bear Harbor (0.4/0'), a rugged coastal access point used in the late 1800s for loading lumber. Nothing remains of prior development but pleasant campsites tucked away from the ocean. Next comes a general introduction to the Lost Coast Trail experience of repeated ascent and descent. Climbing a steep and narrow stream gully, the trail passes through luscious greenery. Large sword ferns splay everywhere, moss covers the thick trunks of alder and California bay, the large leaves of blue elderberry line the stream bank, and every possible nook and cranny bursts with life. You have time to enjoy all this because the trail is remarkably steep. After you attain the ridge, the trail traverses around Duffy's Gulch and through the first grove of old-growth redwoods before gently climbing along the blufftop. Views into the sheer gulch of Jackass Creek open up where the trail makes its steep descent to Wheeler Camp (4.7/10'), passing through another old-growth redwood grove just before the first campsites.

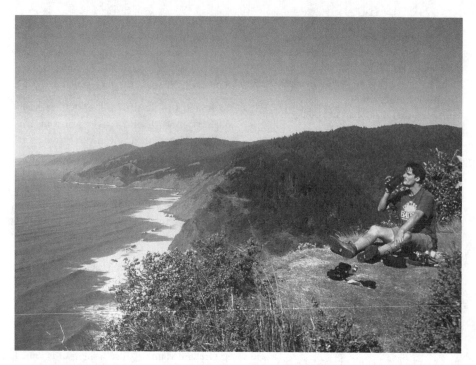

Above the Lost Coast

Wheeler Camp was the location of a wood-processing facility from 1951 until 1960, run by the Wolf Creek Timber Company. The small company town with store, bunkhouse, and school was deliberately burned for liability reasons in 1969. Remnants of the mill include knee-high periscope-like tubes protruding from the ground, which were used to test the underground flow of toxic diesel fuel that leaked from the facility. While no fuel is known to have reached Jackass Creek, to be safe obtain your water upstream from the site. If it's raining or windy, the campsites nearest the redwood grove are nicest. If it's sunny and clear, continue along the trail to uphill sites south of the beach.

On your way to the beach, a trail diverges left as you enter the more open meadow—continue straight, winding along the edge of the beach before climbing steeply to almost 1,100 feet. Keep an eye out for the small trees lining the top of the cliff. Bonsai-sized by exposure to the elements, these trees can be as old as those in the surrounding forest, with remarkably stout

trunks hidden beneath their twisted foliage. Shelter Cove can be spotted north from near the clifftop, before the trail plummets down through dense tanoak forest to Little Jackass Creek Camp (9.2/20'). Sites are fewer than at Wheeler Camp, and farther from the wonderfully secluded beach.

The trail continues inland opposite the creek, quickly entering the Sally Bell Grove, an old-growth redwood stand named for a Sinkyone woman who fled here after a brutal attack on her village at Needle Rock in May 1864 by Lieutenant William Frazier and the Battalion of Mountaineers. Passing many substantial redwoods, the trail makes a very steep ascent to 800 feet before immediately dropping to Anderson Gulch Camp (11.7/250'). Here, the campsites are small and hidden among the trees. You pass the best sites shortly after crossing the creek.

Another brief up-and-down brings you to Dark Gulch (12.3/350'), where the final and most arduous section of the hike begins.

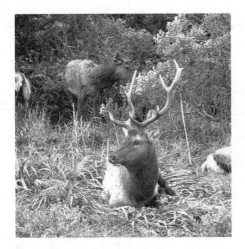

A prolonged stretch of climbing brings you to—at over 1,100 feet—the highest point on this hike, almost directly above the ocean. The thick forest of tanoaks, bigleaf maples, and redwoods opens into fields of low-lying coyote brush and blackberry tangles. South, the trail can be seen winding along the bare ridgetop. Ocean views are exceptional, Usal Beach is visible, and a keen eye can identify Hwy. 1, 7 miles south of here, twisting along the coast before turning inland. It's a gradual descent from here to Usal Beach, ending with several steep switchbacks that deposit you near some nice campsites.

Roosevelt elk roam the Lost Coast.

Nearest Visitor Center The volunteer-staffed Needle Rock Visitor Center is open intermittently depending on staff availability. Park headquarters (also open intermittently, 707-986-7711) is on Briceland Rd. in Whitethorn.

Backpacking Information Backcountry camping is allowed only at the 3 designated trail camps—Wheeler, Little Jackass, and Anderson Gulch. A fee of $5 per night is charged for the trail camps, payable outside the Needle Rock Visitor Center or at the Usal Camp fee station. There is no trail quota.

Nearest Campground There are 18 walk-in campsites scattered around the Needle Rock area, including those in Bear Harbor.

Additional Information www.parks.ca.gov

HIKE 46 Big Flat

Highlights	Endless beach, soaring cliffs, and an idyllic seaside meadow
Distance	17.0 miles round-trip
Total Elevation Gain/Loss	50'/50'
Hiking Time	9–12 hours
Recommended Maps	*King Range National Conservation Area* by the Bureau of Land Management (BLM); *California's Lost Coast* by Wilderness Press; USGS 7.5-min. *Shelter Cove, Shubrick Peak,* and *Honeydew*
Best Times	Spring and fall
Agency	King Range Wilderness and National Conservation Area
Difficulty	★★★

THE KING RANGE LURCHES thousands of feet above from the sea, creating precipitous cliffs that back directly against black-sand beaches. Small streams carve deep ravines through the coastal bluffs, providing water and oceanside campsites for beach-walking hikers. Mountain summits lord over it all. The top of King Peak (4,088'), the highest in the range, is less than 3 miles from the shore. The 42,585-acre King Range Wilderness and surrounding King Range National Conservation Area protects this rugged coastline of the northern Lost Coast, one of the most desolate stretches of sand in America.

The Hike travels along the beach to Big Flat, a rare coastside expanse of level ground awash in profuse spring wildflowers. This is not a hike for the unprepared. The loose and sloping beach is fatiguing underfoot. Strong northwest winds are common, especially in the summer, and there is little to shelter you from its onslaught. A 4.5-mile section of beach (between Gitchell Creek and Big Flat) is passable only at low tide—and is life-threatening at other times. Tide tables are posted at the trailhead; take note of when they occur. Strong storms occur regularly from November through March and can turn the hike's many stream crossings into dangerous torrents. Water is available at the trailhead.

To Reach the Trailhead Take the Hwy. 101 exit for Redway and Shelter Cove. From Redway, take Briceland Thorn Rd. toward Shelter

Cove. In 13.2 miles you'll pass the Bureau of Land Management King Range Office on the left. Continue for another 7.1 miles to Beach Rd. and turn right toward Black Sands Beach, reaching the Black Sands Beach Trailhead and parking area in 0.9 mile.

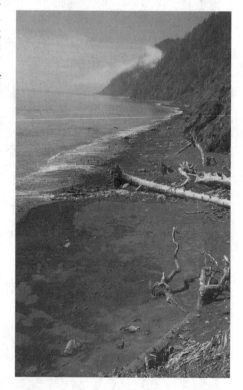

Get lost.

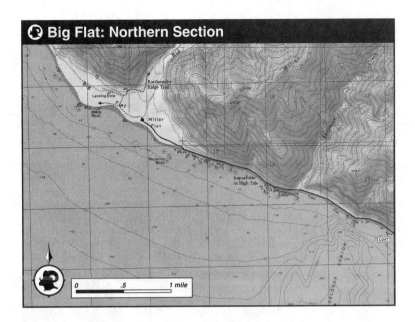

Big Flat: Northern Section

Description A view north from the blufftop parking area (0.0/40') reveals your approaching hike. The broad clearing of Big Flat is discernible in the distance along the shore. Inland, Horse Mountain rises as the first prominent ridgeline, followed next in the distance by Saddle Mountain. The small pyramid of 4,088-foot King Peak peeks out beyond Saddle Mountain, crowning the top of Miller Ridge.

Follow the sidewalk down to the beach. Loosely consolidated layers of dark-colored sand (greywacke) and mud (shale) compose much of the mountains here, eroding to form the beach's distinctive black sand and cobbles. Heading north, you soon pass Telegraph Creek on the right (0.2/0'), followed by a rivulet emerging from below the Kaluna Cliffs. The beach narrows at this point and a giant house-sized boulder bulges from the shore. As you approach Horse Mountain Creek (1.6/0'), you encounter an elaborate driftwood shelter, the first of many to come.

You pass Horse Mountain Trail (1.8/0') just beyond Horse Mountain Creek and wander next to some low terraces. The beach narrows and offshore rocks appear as you approach Gitchell Creek (3.7/0'), which tumbles out of a 30-foot-wide gash in otherwise featureless cliffs. A huge driftwood shelter has been constructed nearby.

The next 4.5 miles of beach are impassable for several hours on either side of high tide (longer if there is significant swell). Time your passage appropriately and don't risk getting caught—there is no escape up the vertical cliffs. Past Gitchell Creek, the beach steepens and hems against sheer outcrops. Huge debris piles lie jumbled at the mouths of steep ravines. Big Flat briefly disappears from sight as you curve around a horseshoe of coastline and pass a pretty stream emerging from a lush alder grove overhead.

You next reach Buck Creek (5.2/0'), which pours into the surf by a wild wall of contorted rock. Numerous campsites (or rest stops) perch just inland from the shore, many with ocean views. The Buck Creek Trail heads uphill from here on its way toward Saddle Mountain, visible in the back of the valley. Past Buck Creek, the beach narrows and boulder fields extend into the tidal zone. Watch for seals hauled out on the rocks. You pass several dainty cascades, then a more significant creek that cuts a razor-thin slice in the cliff face. Next is Shipman Creek

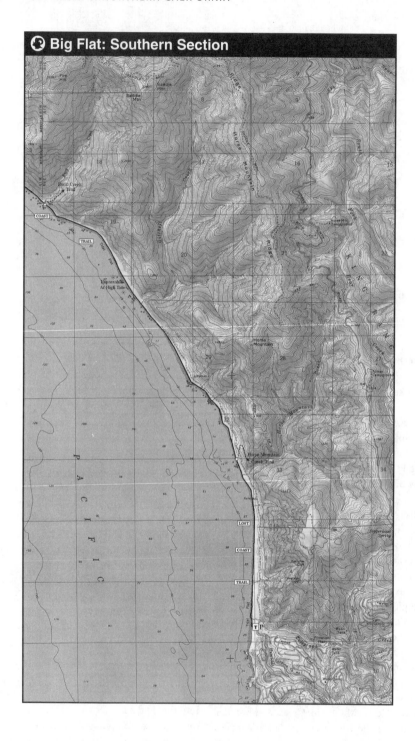

Big Flat: Southern Section

(6.6/0'), a substantial stream that emerges from a broader valley.

Beyond Shipman Creek the beach becomes rockier and strewn with cobblestones, creating the toughest walking conditions yet. Just prior to reaching Big Flat, the cliffs shorten abruptly. There is no obvious path leading off the beach, but you should take your first available opportunity to scramble onto the easy-walking terrain above.

You emerge onto the broad outwash plain of Big Flat (8.2/20'), an open grassland interspersed with boulder piles, stunted Douglas-firs, and profuse wildflowers. Burnt trees lance the surrounding slopes, mute evidence of a 2003 wildfire that scorched much of the western King Range. The trail cruises near the coastline, passing several driftwood shelters, and reaches your final stop at Big Flat Creek (8.5/20'). Retrace your steps to the trailhead.

Nearest Visitor Center BLM King Range Office, 707-986-5400, is 13 miles west of Redway on the way to Shelter Cove. It's open Monday–Friday 8 a.m.–4:30 p.m. year-round.

Backpacking Information Campsites are abundant at Big Flat and around the many creek mouths along the way. A backcountry permit is required, available at the trailhead or from the BLM King Range Office. Campfires are allowed except when a fire closure is in effect (typically late June–late October). Bear canisters are mandatory and can be rented at the BLM King Range Office for $5 per trip with a credit card deposit (violators are subject to a $180 fine), or at the Shelter Cove General Store, 707-986-7733. Camping is prohibited between the parking area and Telegraph Creek 0.2 mile north.

Note that a wilderness-permit quota system is likely to go into effect in 2015 or 2016, which will include the ability to reserve permits online. Contact the King Range office for the latest information.

Nearest Campground Shelter Cove Campground (103 sites, $35) is a private campground next to the airstrip in the center of town.

Additional Information blm.gov/ca/arcata

HIKE 47 King Peak ◯ 🚶 🐐

Highlight	The highest summit in the King Range
Distance	5.1 miles
Total Elevation Gain/Loss	1,950'/1,950'
Hiking Time	3–4 hours
Recommended Maps	*King Range National Conservation Area* by the Bureau of Land Management (BLM); *California's Lost Coast* by Wilderness Press; USGS 7.5-min. *Honeydew*
Best Times	Spring and fall
Agency	King Range Wilderness and National Conservation Area
Difficulty	★★★

WHERE CALIFORNIA bulges farthest west on the northern Lost Coast, powerful tectonic forces have crushed the King Range skyward. Touched by man and then forgotten, the mountains compose a remote topography jammed against the Pacific edge. Less than 3 miles from the sea, 4,088-foot King Peak rises as the highest summit in the range, a heart-pounding destination with difficult access and superlative 360-degree views across the entire rumpled region.

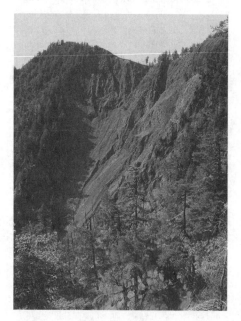

Severe terrain in the King Range

Twenty-five miles northwest of King Peak, Cape Mendocino marks the westernmost point in the Lower 48. Due west from the cape, less than 10 miles from shore, three tectonic plates meet at the Mendocino Triple Junction. Land north lies along an active subduction zone where the tiny Juan de Fuca Plate dives beneath the North American continent in an underwater trench almost 2 miles deep. South, the San Andreas Fault careens offshore, slicing the land in a myriad of related faults. As the triple junction slowly migrates north, combined tectonic forces produce the most seismically active spot in the entire earthquake-prone state. The mountains are pushed upward at an astounding rate and major earthquakes are a frequent occurrence—a 1992 earthquake lifted the entire King Range up 3–5 feet!

The Hike approaches King Peak from the northeast via King Range Rd., a rough and unpaved access road that necessitates a high-clearance vehicle for safe passage. The hike zigzags upward on Lightning Trail and completes a small loop near the summit to pass through pleasant Maple Camp, where a year-round stream and overnight camping area are available. Winter rains can be intense and summer sun can be searing on the often shadeless slopes. These two factors make spring and fall the best times for a visit. No water is available at the trailhead; your only reliable source on this hike is at Maple Camp.

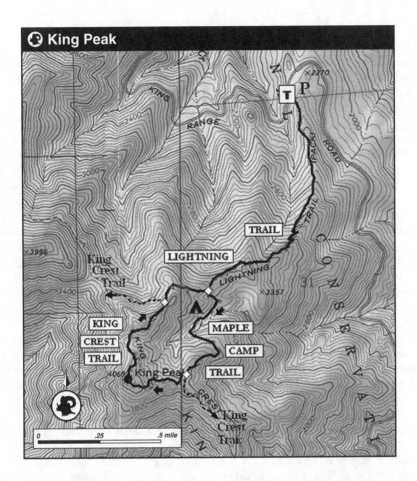

King Peak

To Reach the Trailhead Take the Hwy. 101 exit for Redway and Shelter Cove. From Redway, take Briceland Thorn Rd. toward Shelter Cove. In 13.2 miles, you'll pass the Bureau of Land Management's King Range Office on the left. Continue another 4.8 miles to King Peak Rd., at the top of a divide. Turn right and follow unpaved King Peak Rd. north, reaching Saddle Mountain Rd. on the left in 6.3 miles. Continue straight on increasingly rough King Peak Rd. for 3 miles to King Range Rd. Turn left and follow King Range Rd. 6.6 miles to the trailhead at the road's end, passing Saddle Mountain Rd. on the left 2.3 miles from the King Peak Rd. junction.

Description From the trailhead (0.0/2,220'), strike out on Lightning Trail in the shade of fluttering tanoaks, peeling madrones, and droopy Douglas-firs. As you climb, the broad trail winds past several substantial Douglas-firs, whose blackened trunks provide mute evidence of the 2003 wildfire that burned extensive portions of the western King Range, including much of the area visited by this hike.

Soon you encounter the trail's first switchbacks. Get used to them—you'll encounter 31 over the next 1.7 miles. You enter a burned area populated by dead madrones and young manzanita, then slowly rise close to the ridgeline beneath the shade of twisting canyon live oaks. The zigzags soon resume. Below and to the right, a seasonal creek may become audible; your best access point is just before the end of this section of switchbacks. The steep singletrack trail rises steadily, traverses upslope, and soon encounters its first views northwest, which reveal the terrain of the lower Mattole watershed and Cape Mendocino area.

Then the switchbacks really begin. You rapidly gain 550 feet via 20 switchbacks, interspersed with short traverses. Large, fire-scarred Douglas-firs provide company as you climb. After a final switchback, the trail makes a long gradual traverse to reach the posted junction for Maple Camp (1.7/3,450').

Turn left and follow the trail toward camp. Views quickly appear to the southeast, water becomes audible below, and the rocky path winds downward to meet a laughing brook in a stand of large, unblemished Douglas-firs. A brief rise brings you to Maple Camp (2.0/3,400'), where a half dozen tent sites dot the slopes like rocky nests. Bay trees and a few bigleaf maples shade the creek.

Continuing past camp, the trail runs briefly along the creekbed, crosses the brook, makes a few switchbacks, and then traverses left to enter a sun-scoured world of burnt madrone and manzanita. Views open up to the northeast, then southeast, as you ascend the loose and rocky path through scrub. Glimpses of nearby King Peak appear shortly before you reach King Crest Trail (2.4/3,820').

To the summit! Bear right and head north through the gravelly moonscape on a steady, rising traverse. A few scraggly canyon live oaks provide limited shade as you go. The route attains the ridgeline about halfway up and makes a few final S-turns just below the summit (2.8/4,088'). A three-sided cement shelter nestles just below the top.

The view is tremendous: a 360-degree sweep. The King Range marches away to the north and south, its spine traced by King Crest Trail. The Big Flat Creek watershed pours into the ocean to the west; Shubrick Peak guards its northern flanks. Farther north, the Mattole River flows in the midst of rumpled topography; a keen eye can spot its riverbed. The deep drainage of Shipman Creek is next to the south, separated from Big Flat by Miller Ridge. The Buck Creek watershed is just beyond, separated from Shipman Creek by Fire Hill. In the southern distance, you can make out the Kaluna Cliffs near Shelter Cove and the coastline of Sinkyone Wilderness (Hike 46) on the farthest horizon. More than 10 ridges recede into the eastern distance and the high bumps of the Trinity Alps (Hike 54) dimple the northeast horizon.

Begin your return journey by following King Crest Trail north from the summit, running down the ridgeline through open manzanita and other low-lying chaparral. The trail drops slowly, offers one last view west, and then makes a brief traversing climb. Resuming the descent, the trail switchbacks eight times, enters shady oak woods, and reaches Lightning Trail (3.3/3,720'). Turn right and head down Lightning Trail, enjoying another bout of switchbacks that deposits you at the earlier junction for Maple Camp (3.7/3,450'). Retrace your steps to the trailhead (5.4/2,220').

Nearest Visitor Center BLM King Range Office, 707-986-5400, is 13 miles west of Redway on the way to Shelter Cove. It's open Monday–Friday 8 a.m.–4:30 p.m. year-round.

Backpacking Information Maple Camp is the best option and provides the hike's only reliable water source; a 3-sided cement shelter just below the summit of King Peak is another (dry) option. A backcountry permit is required, available at the trailhead or from the BLM King Range Office. Campfires are allowed except when a fire closure is in effect (typically late June through late October). Bear canisters are mandatory and can be rented at the BLM King Range Office for $5 per trip with a credit card deposit (violators are subject to a $180 fine), or at the Shelter Cove General Store, 707-986-7733. Note that a wilderness-permit quota system is likely to go into effect in 2015 or 2016, which will include the ability to reserve permits online. Contact the King Range office for the latest information.

Nearest Campgrounds Tolkan Campground (9 sites with water, $8) is on King Peak Rd., 3.5 miles north of Briceland Thorn Rd. Horse Mountain Campground (9 sites without water, $5) is 3 miles farther.

Additional Information blm.gov/ca/arcata

HIKE 48 Punta Gorda Lighthouse 🥾 🧍 🐕

Highlight	A remote, abandoned lighthouse
Distance	6.4 miles round-trip
Total Elevation Gain/Loss	100'/100'
Hiking Time	3–4 hours
Recommended Maps	*King Range National Conservation Area* by the Bureau of Land Management (BLM), *California's Lost Coast* by Wilderness Press, USGS 7.5-min. *Petrolia*
Best Times	Spring and fall
Agency	King Range Wilderness and National Conservation Area
Difficulty	★★

ELEVEN MILES north of the Mattole River mouth, Cape Mendocino marks the westernmost point in the lower 48 states. Due west from the cape, less than 10 miles from shore, three tectonic plates meet at the Mendocino Triple Junction. Land north lies along an active subduction zone where the tiny Juan de Fuca Plate dives beneath the North American continent in an underwater trench almost 2 miles deep. South, the San Andreas Fault careens offshore, slicing the land in myriad related faults. As the triple junction slowly migrates north, combined tectonic forces produce the most seismically active spot in the entire earthquake-prone state. The mountains are pushed upward at an astounding rate and major earthquakes are a frequent occurrence—a 1992 earthquake lifted the entire King Range up 3–5 feet!

Twenty-one miles south of Cape Mendocino is Punta Gorda, another bulge in the coastline

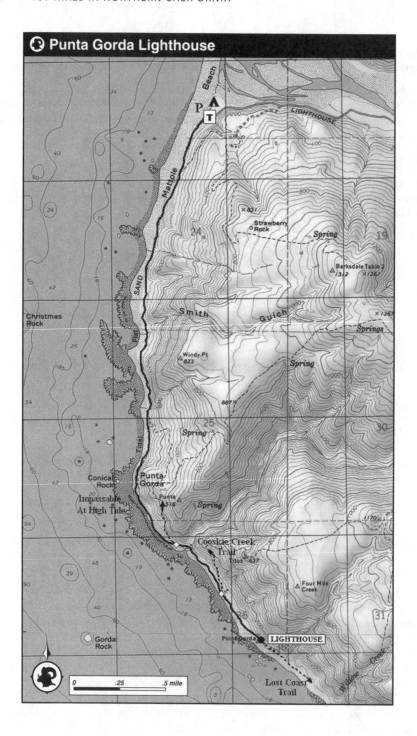

Punta Gorda Lighthouse

sheltering remote Punta Gorda Lighthouse. Staffed for only 40 years, the lighthouse was shut down in 1951. The whole region bears traces of a 19th-century boom that busted, leaving the landscape empty and forgotten by today's world. The first oil well in California was drilled near Petrolia in 1865, and ranching and logging quickly pruned the sweeping hills and ridges. Today, the mouth of the Mattole River marks the northern limit of the King Range National Conservation Area, 60,000 acres of land protected south along the coast and inland through the heart of the King Range; 42,585 acres were set aside as designated wilderness in 2006. The seaside mountain topography catches a lot of rain, making this area the wettest in the entire state. While the mouth of the Mattole River receives an average of 50 inches per year, the surrounding ridges have recorded in excess of 200 inches—nearly 17 feet—during wet years.

The Hike follows the coastline south from Mattole River to Punta Gorda, a sandy walk that ends at the lighthouse turret. Just south of sheltering Cape Mendocino, the coastline here is reputed to have regular fog-free days during the summer months, a rarity on the North Coast. Spring and fall are the best times to come; avoid winter when storms swelling Fourmile Creek are likely to obstruct the hike. The region around Punta Gorda can be treacherous at high tides—tide tables are usually posted at the trailhead and your hike should coincide with low tide. People are few out here, and supplies are limited and very expensive. Water is available at the trailhead.

To Reach the Trailhead You have to drive a lot of twisting roads. The easiest approach is via Ferndale, 5 miles west of Hwy. 101 on Hwy. 211—the turnoff from 101 is located at Fernbridge. In Ferndale, turn right off Main St. onto Ocean Rd., and then turn immediately left at Fifth St. to head south toward Petrolia, 30 miles away. One mile south of Petrolia, turn

right on Lighthouse Rd. and follow it 5 miles to the campground and day-use parking lot at the road's end. It is also possible to get here by taking sinuous Mattole Rd. west from Humboldt Redwoods State Park to the town of Honeydew, 25 miles (60–90 minutes) from Hwy. 101. Cross the Mattole River and continue west (downstream) on Mattole Rd. for 15 miles to reach Lighthouse Rd.

Description From the trailhead, go through the gate by the information sign and head south through the dunes to quickly reach a fenced-off shell midden once used by the Mattole Indians. Interpretive signs explain its potential archaeological significance and provide an excellent diagram of the tectonic forces at work in the region. Looking north, the striking point of Cape Mendocino can be seen jutting into the ocean beyond the nearby Mattole River drainage.

As you head south, follow either a trail often found running below the base of the steep bluffs or the sandy beach. Note the slopes covered with coyote brush, cow parsnip, lupine, yarrow, and mint, but beware the extensive poison oak. Wildlife is rich in the offshore waters, and you may see harbor seals eyeing you from inside the breakers. As you slowly round Punta Gorda to reach Fourmile Creek, the lighthouse appears down the coast, dwarfed in scale by the landscape.

Private property is located near the mouth of Fourmile Creek (2.5/0')—please respect the owner's rights and privacy. Crossing the creek—which can be challenging to dangerous during high water—and continuing south, you soon reach the lighthouse, where informative placards detail the site's history. The tower itself is sometimes open and accessible from the inside via a very tight stairway ladder; it makes a great spot for lunching and relaxing. While the Lost Coast Trail continues 21 miles south along the beaches to Shelter Cove, you avoid that long, sandy walk by returning the way you came.

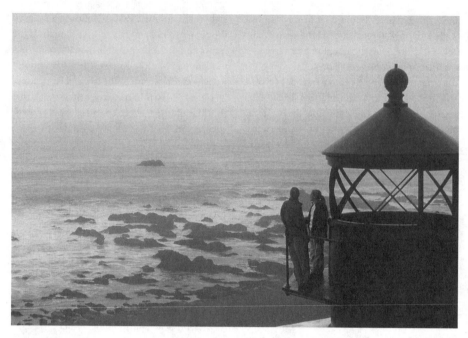

Punta Gorda Lighthouse

Nearest Visitor Center There are no visitor centers remotely close to this hike. The best source of information is the BLM King Range Office, 707-986-5400, 13 miles (30–45 minutes) west of Redway on the way to Shelter Cove. It's open Monday–Friday 8 a.m.–4:30 p.m. year-round. The BLM also has an office in Arcata at the north end of town, 707-825-2300, open Monday–Friday 7:45 a.m.–4:30 p.m.

Backpacking Information Beach camping is permitted along this hike and at points farther south along the coast. A backcountry permit is required, available at the trailhead or from the BLM King Range Office. Campfires are allowed except when a fire closure is in effect (typically late June–late October). Bear canisters are required and can be rented for a nominal fee at the Petrolia General Store (cash only, including deposit) or the BLM King Range Office (violators are subject to a $180 fine). Proper human-waste disposal is critical along the beaches—bury it at least 6 inches deep in the sand of the intertidal zone. Backcountry camping is prohibited within 500 feet of the campground.

Note that a wilderness-permit quota system is likely to go into effect in 2015 or 2016, which will include the ability to reserve permits online. Contact the King Range office for the latest information.

Nearest Campground Mattole Beach Campground (9 sites with water, $8) is located at the trailhead.

Additional Information blm.gov/ca/arcata

HIKE 49 Prairie Creek Redwoods Q

Highlight	Vast and primeval old-growth redwood forest
Distance	6.2 miles round-trip
Total Elevation Gain/Loss	800'/800'
Hiking Time	3–5 hours
Recommended Maps	*Redwood National and State Parks: North* by Redwood Hikes Press, USGS 7.5-min. *Fern Canyon*
Best Times	Spring–fall
Agency	Prairie Creek Redwoods National and State Parks
Difficulty	★★★

DISCOVER CALIFORNIA at its most primeval, where vast old-growth forest tucks tight against a wild shore roamed by Roosevelt elk. Protected in the early 1900s, Prairie Creek Redwoods State Park contains some of the finest examples of old-growth forest anywhere, a diverse world of prehistoric proportions where stupendous redwoods are joined by massive specimens of Sitka spruce and Douglas-fir.

The Hike begins from the north end of Gold Bluffs Beach, a remote strand that can only be accessed by a seasonal dirt road. After traipsing beneath the dripping walls of Fern Canyon, the journey heads inland to complete a magnificent loop through untouched old-growth forest and returning to the shore by Gold Bluffs Beach campground. From there, a mile-long walk along the sand (or easy-walking dirt road) returns you to the trailhead. Morning fog is common in summer, though it often burns off by afternoon.

To Reach the Trailhead Take Hwy. 101 three miles north of Orick and turn left on Davison Road, signed for Gold Bluffs Beach. In 0.3 mile, the pavement ends by Elk Meadow Day Use Area (watch for the namesake animals). Continue down the dirt road, which is easily passable for low-clearance vehicles; trailers are prohibited. In 3.4 miles you reach the entrance station (staffed daily April–September, 8 a.m.–8 p.m.), where you'll need to pay the day-use fee ($8, cash only). Overnight visitors can also register here for Gold Bluffs Beach campground.

The road emerges by the beach a short distance ahead, runs alongside steep bluffs, and passes the campground turnoff 1.9 miles past the entrance station. Just beyond the campground, the road passes through a gate and immediately reaches the Miner's Ridge Day Use parking area, an alternative starting point if you prefer to start, rather than end, with the coastal/beach section (or if the coming ford in the road is impassable).

The road next crosses a substantial creek—potentially hazardous or impassable in high water—and proceeds for 1.0 mile on a much rougher road to reach the Fern Canyon trailhead and parking area. Note that the road to Gold Bluffs Beach is open year-round, but may close due to flooding during the rainy season.

Description From the trailhead (0.0/10'), strike out along the wide and sometimes muddy path by alders and young Sitka spruce. Lush ferns grow in the tree branches, testament to the area's regular supply of moisture. You quickly reach the entrance to Fern Canyon (0.1/10'), where you rock-hop across Home Creek.

Now curving inland, you soon encounter the 40-foot cliffs that rise on either side of the narrow canyon. Vertical gardens of moss and ferns highlight the route along the gravelly canyon bottom; the avid pteridologist can identify seven different fern species on the walls here, including five-finger, deer, lady, and large sword ferns. You navigate a maze of fallen trees to work your way up the canyon, which begins to open up past a very large fallen Sitka spruce.

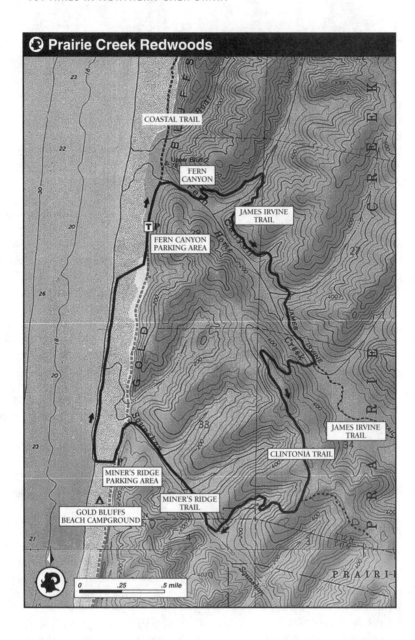

Your continuing trail appears on the left, signed for Loop Trail (0.3/70'), though you can also explore Home Creek a short distance farther before continuing.

Loop Trail climbs a small set of stairs and then steepens quickly as it ascends more than 50 steps, switchbacks left, and is joined by a stout fence that protects you from tumbling into the creek far below. You now enter an emerald world of tall and mossy Sitka spruce—note the trees' distinctive flaky, puzzle-piece bark—and reach the junction with James Irvine Trail (0.5/180').

Follow James Irvine Trail, which soon leads to the first of many signed memorial groves, dedicated to the supporters who helped protect this area. Redwoods begin to appear intermittently as the trail levels; the creek remains audible far below.

After crossing a stout bridge over a deep gully, you next reach the junction Friendship Ridge Trail (0.8/190'), which heads left. Remain instead on James Irvine Trail, which curves around to cross a bridge over a flowing creek that pours through a small fern-draped chute more than 30 feet beneath you.

The trees now begin to increase markedly in size as you make a steep rising traverse that eventually levels out to contour high above Home Creek. The forest becomes a more even mix of Sitka spruce and redwoods as the trail weaves along the slopes. You cross another gully—a slot barely four feet wide yet more than 30 feet deep—and pass a posted spur trail to Cozzens Grove (a short, overgrown, and challenging side trip). You cross another bridge and climb again among unending redwood trees. Douglas-firs intermittently appear, while the presence of Sitka spruce diminishes to only a few in the stream below.

The route runs close to the now quiet headwaters of Home Creek, then crosses the stream for the first time on a stout bridge evocative of a miniature Golden Gate Bridge. Continuing, you climb among increasingly large redwoods and reach the junction with Clintonia Trail (2.0/330').

Bear right to follow Clintonia Trail as it rises slowly, passes abundant trillium in the understory, and traverses steep, fern-carpeted slopes. The path makes a slow U-turn to surmount the lush ridge, home to some particularly large redwoods.

The trail widens and leads next to a bench that admires a gigantic crazy-topped redwood easily 12 feet in diameter. Continuing, you pass a posted junction for several named groves—a thin spur trail offers a short side trip—and then quickly reach Miner's Ridge Trail (3.0/470').

Turn right on Miner's Ridge Trail to begin your return toward the beach. The level trail immediately passes a giant stump cave on the right and then some large redwoods, including one titan with a full-blown tree growing from a burl on its side.

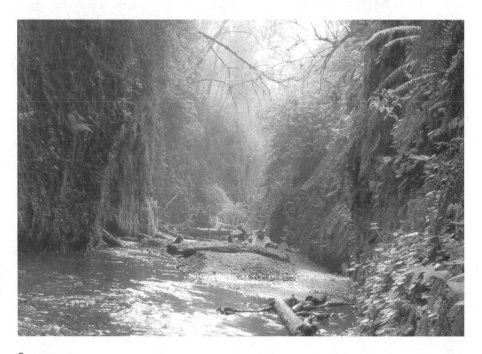

Fern canyon

The path winds above a deepening drainage to your right, descends a few stairs, and then begins a more earnest drop. The switchbacking trail is visible below as you follow it downward and back around the gully. The descent quickens. Redwoods diminish as the forest thickens and transitions to a collection of younger, even-aged Sitka spruce. Tall and old mossy alders rise overhead as you curve right to start following audible Squashan Creek below, cross a series of five small bridges and one larger bridge, and then pass through head-high wood rose bushes.

The trail crosses one final large bridge and encounters the far end of an unpaved service road, which you follow as it runs flat and level through second-growth Sitka spruce forest. You pass Miner's Ridge Trail Camp (closed), which has a decaying outhouse and two small water towers.

The road crosses Squashan Creek and then reaches Gold Bluffs Beach Road by a gate, a short distance north of the day-use parking lot (5.0/10'). From here, make your way to the beach (or walk north on the road) and proceed north.

The beach is a sandy expanse of dunes backed by low bluffs. It was named for the early discoveries of the precious metal along the beach here, though gold was not present in sufficient quantities to make it a worthwhile endeavor over the long term. Tons of crab debris and monstrous mussel shells instead speckle the sand today.

As you head north, watch for the Roosevelt elk who roam these dunes; a small herd of roughly 50 animals calls this area home. Their tracks and droppings are usually evident even when the animals are not—they often bed down in the tall dune grass, which can make them hard to spot. During mating season—roughly six weeks from late August through early October—you may hear the bellowing calls of bull elk as they challenge each other for mating rights. *Approaching elk is both hazardous and illegal; observe them safely from a distance. If they are altering their behavior because of your presence, you are too close.*

The walking is generally easy, particularly in the wet sand near the water line. You eventually reach the outflow from Home Creek, which currently forms a curving waterway and lagoon that separates you from the road if you cross its mouth. Head inland instead along the south side of the waterway to reach the road, then proceed the short remaining distance to the Fern Canyon parking area (6.2/10').

Nearest Visitor Center Prairie Creek Redwoods State Park Visitor Center, 707-488-2039, is on Drury Pkwy. along the eastern edge of the park. To reach it, follow Hwy. 101 north for 2.2 miles past the Gold Bluffs Beach turnoff and take the signed exit for Drury Pkwy. Turn left and proceed 1.2 miles to reach the visitor center on the left. Open daily, 9 a.m.–5 p.m. in summer and Thursday–Monday 9 a.m.–4 p.m. in the off-season.

Nearest Campgrounds Gold Bluffs Beach Campground (26 sites, $35) is available on a first-come, first-served basis from mid-April until late September. It typically fills by late morning during the busy summer months; show up early at the Gold Bluffs Beach entrance station or visitor center to secure a spot. Elk Prairie Campground (75 sites, $35) is just past the visitor center on Drury Parkway. Reservations are recommended in summer; call 800-444-7275 or visit **www.parks.ca.gov**. For camping updates, including availability, call 707-488-2171.

Additional Information www.parks.ca.gov

HIKE 50 Klamath River Mouth ✎ 🏃

Highlight	Gigantic driftwood in a powerful place
Distance	1–2 miles round-trip
Total Elevation Gain/Loss	Negligible
Hiking Time	1–2 hours
Recommended Map	USGS 7.5-min. *Requa*
Best Times	April–October
Agency	Redwood National Park
Difficulty	★

IT IS A WORLD like no other, an enormous sandy spit regularly swept clean by the fury of the ocean. Driftwood litters it, enormous stumps are buried within it, a mighty river flows behind it, and the Pacific breaks upon it.

The Hike explores the length of the broad sandbar formed at the Klamath River mouth, an easy hike that places you deep within nature's domain. *This can be a dangerous place—especially near the mouth itself—where strong surf and high tides can completely wash across the spit and sweep the unsuspecting into the Klamath River and out to sea. Do not venture onto the sandbar if you see water washing across it, and keep children close at hand.* While the hike can be done year-round, torrential winter rains are worth avoiding. The mouth of the Klamath is included within Redwood National Park, but this is not an official or posted trail. Crowds will be minimal. No water is available at the trailhead.

To Reach the Trailhead Take Hwy. 101 a half mile south of its Klamath River crossing, turn west onto Klamath Beach Road, and proceed 3.3 miles to a day-use area near the river level. Park in the pulloff along the road and proceed to the gate along the roadside.

Description From the gate, proceed down the grassy road and past some scrappy alders pruned by the wind and salty air here. You next pass a collection of Yurok ceremonial structures—please respect this facility and remain on the path—and soon drop onto the sand near a large molar-shaped sea stack.

From here, enjoy exploring the sandbar and its collection of massive driftwood. The spit is roughly 0.5 mile long—the exact location of the river mouth shifts over time—and the washed-up remains of many a gigantic redwood tree can be found along its length. Flint Rock Head (175') can be seen protruding from the jagged coast a mile south.

Surpassed in size only by the Sacramento, the Klamath River is the second largest river in California, draining 15,500 square miles as it winds 263 miles from its headwaters in the Cascades of southern Oregon. Supporting the state's largest run of salmon and steelhead, it also provides habitat for a great diversity of life in the estuary tucked behind its mouth. Starry flounder, Pacific lamprey, American shad, and striped bass are but a few of the species that swim in the nearby waters. The wetlands just inland also attract numerous shorebirds, including godwits, willets, pintails, buffleheads, and green-winged teals. Harbor seals and sea lions can often be seen on the offshore rocks north of the river or frolicking in the surrounding waters. Osprey and spotted owls nest in the surrounding forest, and bald eagles are occasionally sighted here as well.

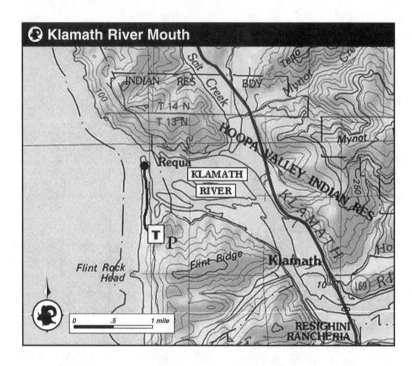

Nearest Visitor Centers Redwood National Park Headquarters and Visitor Center, 707-465-7306, is in Crescent City at 2nd and K Sts. Also try Kuchel Visitor Center, 707-465-7765, to the south in Orick. Both facilities are open daily 9 a.m.–5 p.m. in summer and 9 a.m.–4 p.m. during the off-season.

Nearest Campground Flint Ridge Walk-In Campground (8 sites without water, free) is 1.5 miles south of the trailhead on unpaved Coastal Drive. Accessing these delightful sites requires a quarter-mile walk uphill.

Additional Information nps.gov/redw

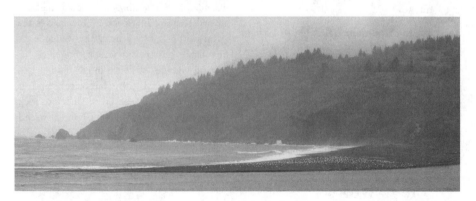

The Klamath River meets the sea

HIKE 51 Damnation Creek ↗

Highlights	Extraordinary old-growth forest and remote coastal access
Distance	4.2 miles round-trip
Total Elevation Gain/Loss	1,200'/1,200'
Hiking Time	3–4 hours
Recommended Maps	*Redwood National and State Parks: North* by Redwood Hikes Press, USGS 7.5-min. *Sister Rocks* and *Childs Hill*
Best Times	April–October
Agency	Del Norte Coast Redwoods State Park
Difficulty	★★

DAMNATION CREEK flows a scant 2 miles to the sea, yet slices a gorge more than 1,000 feet deep and preserves an isolated, undisturbed old-growth forest within its sheltered walls. Its mouth provides the only coastal access point for 3 miles in either direction, a remote and rugged slice of the North Coast.

Damnation Creek lies within Del Norte Coast Redwoods State Park, one of three state parks founded during the 1920s and included today within the Redwood National and State Parks system. There are currently 856 known plant species within the parks and 202 native wildlife residents, including the threatened marbled murrelet and northern spotted owl. The parks are collectively designated a World Heritage Site and International Biosphere Preserve, testament to their unique and irreplaceable qualities. Damnation Creek is a choice example.

The Hike is a quick descent into the Damnation Creek drainage on more than 20 gentle switchbacks, passing through an awe-inspiring forest to reach a rocky and isolated beach. While fog can obscure the far-reaching coastal views, it enhances the primeval tranquility of the forest and should not dissuade you from this hike. Fog is heaviest during the summer months, with spring and fall providing the most consistent sunshine. The trail is open year-round, but torrential winter rains are best not trifled with. Expect cool conditions at all times and bring a warm sweater. Crowds are relatively light, but you are seldom entirely alone. No water is available at the trailhead.

To Reach the Trailhead Take Hwy. 101 north of the Klamath River bridge for 12 miles to milepost 16.0, and park in the dirt lot on the west side of the highway. The turnout is easily missed, so keep your eyes open. Approaching from the north, the trailhead is 3 miles south of the Mill Creek Campground turnoff.

Description From the trailhead, the wide, root-studded path rises briefly to its highest point (1,100'); it passes through a thick ground cover of redwood sorrel and wild ginger while, overhead, enormous redwoods tower above spindly rhododendron trees. After cresting the divide the trail gradually descends, soon reaching the wide dirt road of the Coastal Trail, a former Hwy. 101 roadbed. Cross the road and continue down the posted steep, strenuous trail. As you begin the long switchbacking descent, Douglas-firs become increasingly common; they are easily identified by their rough, unfurrowed bark, so distinct from that of redwoods. Fire scars are abundant in the trees along the trail, and several exciting caverns can be found within their ponderous trunks.

Sitka spruce are a special highlight of this hike and begin to appear about halfway down the gorge. You can identify them by the flaky scales on their trunks and their small feathery cones. Growing in a narrow 1,800-mile-long coastal belt extending from Northern California to Alaska, these majestic trees can achieve heights in excess of 300 feet, and have long been prized for their golden wood. Pound for pound stronger than steel, this spruce has been used

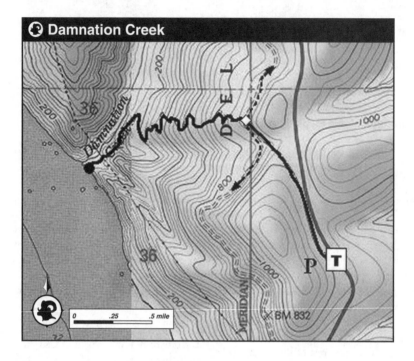

Damnation Creek

to build boats, airplanes, and the soundboards of concert harps, grand pianos, and violins. The victims of heavy logging, few old-growth stands remain—the trees around you are some of the largest left in California.

Thimbleberry and salmonberry twine thickly among the brush as the trail approaches the bottom. The thin trickle of Damnation Creek is heard for the first time where the trees, unable to withstand the salt-laden sea air, suddenly thin. You encounter the ocean at a small promontory, and the adventurous can explore along the coast for some distance both north and south. Then, back up you go.

Nearest Visitor Centers Redwood National Park Headquarters and Visitor Center, 707-465-7306, is in Crescent City at 2nd and K Sts. Also try Kuchel Visitor Center, 707-465-7765, to the south in Orick. Both facilities are open daily 9 a.m.–5 p.m. in summer and 9 a.m.–4 p.m. during the off-season.

Nearest Campgrounds Mill Creek Campground (145 sites, $35), 3 miles north of the trailhead, is open May–September only. Year-round campgrounds can be found in Prairie Creek and Jedediah Smith Redwoods State Parks.

Additional Information nps.gov/redw

HIKE 52 Boy Scout Tree Trail ⬈

Highlight	Mighty, lush old-growth forest
Distance	5.6 miles round-trip
Total Elevation Gain/Loss	750'/750'
Hiking Time	3–4 hours
Recommended Maps	*Redwood National and State Parks: North* by Redwood Hikes Press, USGS 7.5-min. *Hiouchi*
Best Times	April–October
Agency	Jedediah Smith Redwoods State Park
Difficulty	★★

NORTH AMERICA'S temperate rain forest extends from northwest California to Alaska in a narrow coastal strip where rainfall is significant year-round and snow is infrequent. The coastal redwood forest range extends north from Big Sur to a few miles past the Oregon border and exists in a narrow belt. Jedediah Smith Redwoods State Park is one of the few places where you can experience the rare juxtaposition of these two impressive worlds.

Even by the region's rainy standards, the area here is exceptionally wet, receiving more than 100 inches of rain annually—second only to the high ridges along the Lost Coast and King Range (Hikes 45–48). All this moisture feeds a jungle of massive ferns and an understory considerably more lush than any other location in this book.

Flowing through the park is the Smith River, the only major undammed river system left in California. Roughly 300 miles of it are designated as part of the National Wild and Scenic River System—more than on any other river in the country—and its waters support healthy runs of salmon and steelhead throughout the winter months. In 1990 Congress created the Smith River National Recreation Area upstream from the state park to preserve land in the Smith River watershed, helping to protect the long-term health of this pristine corner of California.

The state park is named for Jedediah Smith, who between 1822 and 1830 became the first Anglo-American to reach California from the east, the first to cross the Sierra Nevada, the

first to travel the length of the state, and, in 1828, the first to reach the Pacific Ocean overland through northwest California, camping near the future state park. During his travels he was mauled by a grizzly bear and almost lost an ear, nearly died in the Colorado River when 10 of his 19 men perished, and survived an Indian attack farther up the coast in 1828 that killed 16 of his 20-man party.

The Hike follows the length of Boy Scout Tree Trail as it travels through continuous old-growth forest to splashing Fern Falls near the park's western border. You will likely see other hikers on this spectacular and popular trail, especially during the summer months. Winter rains can be torrential and can close the access road—call ahead if you are contemplating a visit at this time. Regardless of the season, you can expect cool and damp conditions year-round.

To Reach the Trailhead The drive to the trailhead alone is worth the effort, an exceptional journey along narrow and unpaved Howland Hill Road as it passes through miles of old-growth forest between Hwy. 199 and Crescent City. The trailhead can be accessed from either the north or west; approaching from the north provides superior old-growth driving. Howland Hill Rd. is easily passable for low-clearance vehicles; trailers and RVs are not permitted.

To access the trailhead from the north, take Hwy. 199 east from Hwy. 101 for 7.4 miles to South Fork Rd. The turnoff is 2.4 miles past

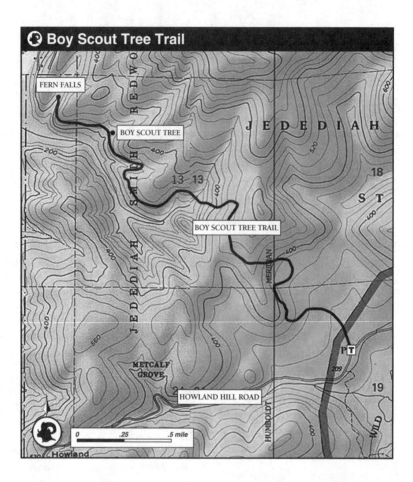

⊘ Boy Scout Tree Trail

the state park entrance, just beyond the Myrtle Creek crossing. Turn right on South Fork Rd. and quickly right again on unpaved Howland Hill Rd./Douglas Park Dr. In 1.2 miles, you enter the state park and the road turns to dirt. From here, continue 3.3 miles to reach the trailhead on the right. Watch for the small parking area and trailhead; it is poorly signed.

To access the trailhead from the west, take Hwy. 101 just south of Crescent City center and head east on Elk Valley Rd. Proceed 1.1 miles and turn right to follow Howland Hill Rd. for 3.6 miles to the trailhead. Note that the pavement ends 1.5 miles past Elk Valley Rd.; 0.3 mile past this point you reach a fork in the road, where you bear left toward Stout Grove to reach the trailhead 1.8 miles past the fork.

Description At the trailhead (0.0/200'), you can admire more than 20 old-growth redwoods in the surrounding woods, while also taking note of the mossy western hemlock that leans over the road near the parking area. Readily identified by its small lacy needles, western hemlock is common throughout the temperate rain forest and has needles that closely resemble those of mountain hemlock—very short and continuously wrapping the ends of its drooping branches. Western hemlocks often grow on fallen trees, or nurse logs, which provide a place for seeds to germinate above the thick and mossy forest floor. Elevated above the understory below, the trees gradually grow roots through the log and into the ground. As the log rots away, the trees are left standing in a line with their roots exposed above the surface—a distinctive sight.

Strike out on the wide and root-laced trail, where you can quickly spot a nurse log supporting young western hemlocks. A few massive Douglas-firs join the gargantuan redwoods as you walk through a world of wet, green walls of understory ferns and foliage. As you proceed, keep an eye on the understory for salal, oxalis, western azalea, rhododendron, trillium, huckleberry, salmonberry, numerous spring wildflowers, and the nine species of ferns found within the park.

You cross a small creek on a bridge by a fallen log sprouting with azaleas, then make a slow steady rise on the well-trod path. Extensive redwoods surround you; several easily exceed 10 feet in diameter. The path winds uphill on gentle slopes, levels out, and then curves right. Western hemlocks fill the understory and midstory of the forest here, and substantial huckleberry bushes—some more than 10 feet tall—grow out of snags and root balls.

Dozens and dozens of redwoods fill the forest in all directions as you continue, ducking under a fallen log along the way that nurses a 20-foot-tall western hemlock. Rhododendrons abruptly appear in the forest, here more akin to small trees than shrubs. You make a slow traversing rise and crest an almost imperceptible divide (1.0/450'). Fern colonies extend high above on the craggy bark of Douglas-firs.

The trail then starts its descent into the Jordan Creek drainage, which flows west to Crescent City rather than north to the Smith River. The creek becomes audible as you drop among a thickening understory punctuated by extensive hemlocks. A steep, curving switchback leads right with the aid of some worn wooden steps, and then a steep, muddy, and rooty drop leads you to the creek, which you cross on a bridge (1.6/220').

After a short rise, you resume the muddy and occasionally rocky descent and soon a flight of stairs puts you at the crossing of a small creek. Large redwoods still populate the

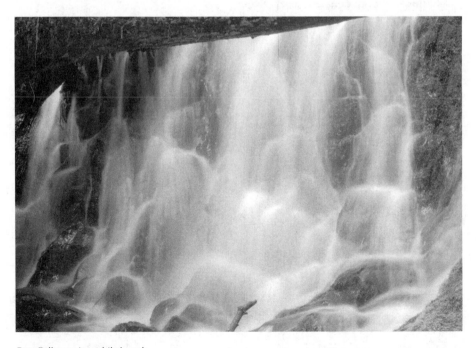

Fern Falls awaits at hike's end.

jungly mix here, and the first Sitka spruce of the hike can be spotted as you proceed. The trail abruptly narrows as it curves around a steeper slope and into a small gully, where several old-growth Sitka spruce can be found in moss-coated glory.

The trail makes two tight switchbacks, crosses over a tributary, and then cruises downward along the creek gully. You soon encounter an unsigned but obvious spur trail on the right (2.5/240'), which climbs briefly but steeply to reach the Boy Scout Tree. A megaspecimen more than 20 feet in diameter, it was formed by the fusion of two separate trees and makes for a worthwhile side trip.

Continuing, you drop down toward the creek bottom and cross a bridge over another feeder stream. The forest abruptly transitions to one dominated by old-growth Sitka spruce and its distinctive puzzle-piece bark, then returns to redwoods as the trail winds along the slopes. Fern Falls awaits at trail's end (2.8/180'), a lovely cascade sheeting over a 20-foot drop. Return the way you came.

Nearest Visitor Centers Hiouchi Information Center, 707-458-3294, is 0.2 mile west of the park entrance on Hwy. 199. It's open daily 9 a.m.–5 p.m. May–September and closed in the off-season. Redwood National Park Headquarters and Visitor Center, 707-465-7335, in Crescent City at 2nd and K Sts., is open daily 9 a.m.–5 p.m. in summer and 9 a.m.–4 p.m. during the off-season.

Nearest Campgrounds The state park campground (90 sites, $35) lies almost entirely within impressive old-growth forest and is open year-round. Reservations are essential in summer; visit **reserveamerica.com** or call 800-444-7275. Otherwise, try the national forest campgrounds east of Gasquet on Hwy. 199.

Additional Information www.parks.ca.gov

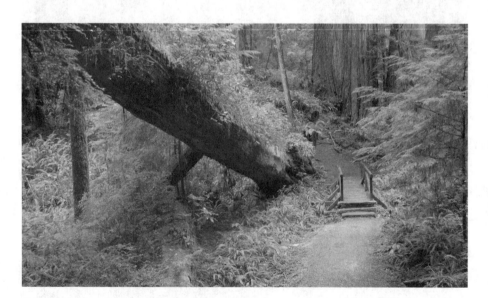

Remarkably lush vegetation fills the forest along Boy Scout Tree Trail.

HIKE 53 Hogan Lake ⚐ 🧍 🐐

Highlight	A rugged pocket of granite wilderness
Distance	6.0 miles round-trip to Hogan Lake, 7.6 miles round-trip to Big Blue Lake
Total Elevation Gain/Loss	1,800'/1,800' to Hogan Lake, 2,700'/2,700' to Big Blue Lake
Hiking Time	5–8 hours
Recommended Maps	*Marble Mountain and Russian Wilderness Map & Guide* by the US Forest Service, USGS 7.5-min. *Eaton Peak*
Best Times	June–September
Agency	Russian Wilderness, Klamath National Forest
Difficulty	★★★

A JAGGED BURST of granite rises skyward in the heart of the Salmon Mountains. Lakes pock the rocky landscape in serene settings. Big Blue Lake—one of the largest and highest in the wilderness—awaits in a steep off-trail setting beneath rugged mountain flanks. Along the way, at trail's end, is scenic Hogan Lake.

The Salmon Mountains are one of the many small ranges included within the greater Klamath Mountains geographic province, an area stretching from near the Pacific coast to just west of Mount Shasta, which includes most of northwest California. The region preserves an ecological story begun millions of years ago when California was composed of low-lying hills and had little topography. A more tropical climate produced abundant rainfall, providing habitat for lush forest. As the tower mountain ranges started to rise 15 million years ago, the climate began to change. Rainfall diminished, temperatures cooled, deserts formed, and higher-elevation regions became intermittently smothered by glaciers. All but eliminated in the Sierra Nevada, this ancient forest was largely preserved in the Klamath Mountains.

The Klamath Mountains' northerly location and proximity to the sea has kept rainfall abundant. Their lower elevation prevented extensive ice sheets from forming during past ice ages. Their situation at the crossroads of the Cascade Range, Sierra Nevada, and Coast Ranges allows an unusual intermingling of species. As a result, a remarkable ecological diversity is preserved

within the Klamath Mountains—and Russian Wilderness has the greatest diversity of all.

More than 450 plant species exist within the small 12,000-acre wilderness, and 17 different species of conifers have been identified within a 1-square-mile plot around the Russian Peak–Little Duck Lake area: Jeffrey, ponderosa, lodgepole, foxtail, western white, sugar, and whitebark pine; white, Shasta red, and subalpine fir; Douglas-fir; Engelmann and Brewer spruce; incense cedar; mountain hemlock; western yew; and prostrate juniper.

The Hike begins from the Taylor Lake trailhead at the northern end of the wilderness and quickly reaches popular Taylor Lake. From there, it rises over the lake's western ridge and then makes a steady descent on the far side to reach tranquil Hogan Lake. To reach Big Blue Lake, a steep but straightforward route climbs the steep granite flanks that hem the far side of Hogan Lake. Taylor has multiple heavy-use campsites. Hogan Lake is much less traveled than Taylor Lake, but still receives moderate use. Several good campsites can be found around Hogan Lake; Big Blue Lake has a handful of sites carved out of a steep and rocky landscape—scenic but very exposed. No water is available at the trailhead.

To Reach the Trailhead Take Hwy. 3 west of I-5 to the town of Etna. Approaching from the north, follow the signs toward the Etna Business District at a prominent junction where Hwy. 3

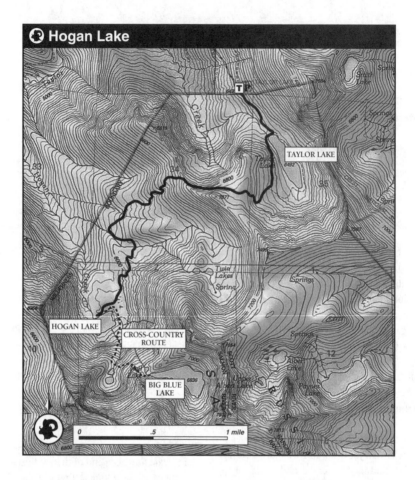

Hogan Lake

curves left. Proceed 0.6 mile to Main St., turn right, pass through the movie-set town center, and continue for 9.8 miles on Sawyer Bar Rd. to Etna Summit; the road narrows and becomes increasingly sinuous as it proceeds. Pause to admire the spectacular view from Etna Summit, which sweeps from the jagged peaks of the Russian Wilderness to the deep headwaters of the Salmon River, before continuing the final 0.3 mile to the Taylor Lake turnoff (FS 41N18) on the left. Proceed 2.2 miles to the trailhead parking area over an initially rough—but low-clearance-passable—road that shifts from dirt back to pavement at its midpoint.

Description From the trailhead (0.0/6,440'), strike out on the wide sandy trail to immediately pass between two incense cedars sporting their distinctive furrowed and fibrous bark. Enjoy views of the steep granite rise across the valley as the trail winds beneath shady white fir, passes a long plank bench, and quickly reaches the tiny outlet creek from Taylor Lake, which nourishes patches of lush wildflowers. Just beyond is the junction for Hogan Lake (0.3/6,500').

To visit Taylor Lake continue straight a short distance ahead. To head to Hogan Lake, bear right at the junction to immediately drop down and cross a steep gully. You now walk along the edge of an old stone dam that hems in Taylor Lake. The lush environment here nourishes dogwoods, leopard lilies, and columbine. Past the dam, the trail curves to briefly run along the west side of Taylor Lake on a rocky but nicely maintained trail.

You begin a traversing climb on sunny and often exposed slopes. Several switchbacks aid in your ascent, which provides expanding views of the surrounding granite slopes. The path eases as it attains the ridge crest (1.1/6,920'), where restricted views north open up to reveal Etna Pass and the mountainous southeast portion of Marble Mountain Wilderness.

Now traversing downward, you pass red fir and hemlock trees in a diverse forest mosaic. The trail reaches its first switchback of the descent, where a short detour brings you to an excellent view of Hogan Lake basin below. From here, the trail soon begins a series of switchbacks that drop you past some nice large trees, including several Douglas-fir and sugar pines. The trail becomes rockier as it approaches the bottom, then crosses a pair of small meadows where it briefly becomes indistinct. Beyond, you climb briefly before dropping once again via a pair of switchbacks to a delightful meadow framed by a backdrop of towering granite peaks.

Cross the meadow and proceed the short, level distance to reach a well-established campsite by Hogan Lake's north shore (3.0/5,950').

If you're continuing to Big Blue Lake, look at the steep rocky slopes across the lake to identify the route. Big Blue Lake awaits over the top of the slopes to the left. To the right is a smaller lower basin, where several shallow ponds can be found.

The off-trail route first climbs diagonally, from left to right, over mostly open granite toward the smaller lake basin on the right, then cuts back left to traverse toward Big Blue Lake. Small cairns mark much of the route. To follow it, head left (clockwise) around the lake, where a clear use path leads you to the start of the ascent.

You climb up mostly open terrain and cross the outlet from the lower basin early on—approximately 100 feet above Hogan Lake. The route then follows a granite ramp upward toward the lower basin—a pleasant destination with a pleasant campsite. To skip this stop and

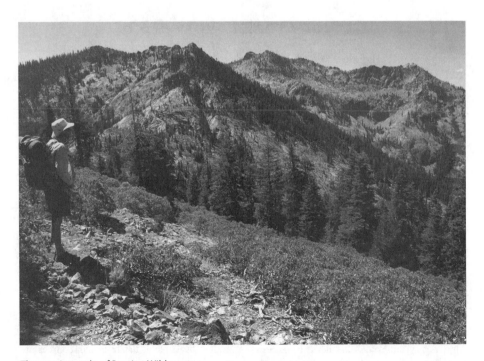

The granite peaks of Russian Wilderness

head directly to Big Blue Lake, you cut left prior to reaching the lower basin to recross the outlet creek in an alder thicket at around 6,500 feet. From here, traverse upward toward Big Blue Lake and then turn more directly upslope on either side of the outlet creek to reach the lakeshore (3.8/6,840').

Surrounded by rocky terrain that slopes deeply into the water, the cerulean waters of Big Blue Lake plunge deeper—96 feet— than any other lake in the wilderness. Enjoy this wild spot, take a dip in its refreshing waters, and then return the way you came (7.6/6,440').

Nearest Visitor Center Scott River Ranger Station, 530-468-5351, on Hwy. 3 in Fort Jones by the intersection with Scott River Rd., is open Monday–Friday 8 a.m.–4:30 p.m.

Backpacking Information No wilderness permit is required, though a valid campfire permit is needed.

Nearest Campgrounds Idlewild Campground (11 sites with water, $10), is located in the headwaters of the Salmon River, 10 steep miles beyond Etna Summit on Sawyer Bar Rd. Scott Mountain Campground (7 sites without water, free) is located at Scott Mountain Summit on Hwy. 3, 20 miles south of Etna.

Additional Information www.fs.usda.gov/klamath

HIKE 54 Canyon Creek Lakes 🡕 🚶 🐕

Highlight	A serrated granite divide above lush wilderness
Distance	15.0 miles round-trip
Total Elevation Gain/Loss	3,000'/3,000'
Hiking Time	12–14 hours
Recommended Map	USGS 7.5-min. *Mount Hilton*
Best Times	Late June–October
Agency	Trinity Alps Wilderness, Shasta-Trinity National Forest
Difficulty	★★★★

A LAND of deep canyons and jagged granite ridges, the Trinity Alps are the greatest alpine highlight of the Klamath Mountains. Impossibly alluring, they crown the thick forest of the region, a vibrant playground of lakes, rivers, and wildlife.

The Hike follows Canyon Creek Trail to Lower Canyon Creek Lake in the heart of the Trinity Alps, a very long day hike that can easily be turned into a two- or three-day adventure. The

Klamath Mountains receive heavy precipitation and, despite the relatively low elevation of this hike, snow can linger on the trail into June. Crowds funnel into this small area in unfortunate numbers during July and August, making September and even early October the best times to visit. Fishing is possible in the lakes, but Canyon Creek is too small for angling. While no water is available at the trailhead, sources are plentiful along the way.

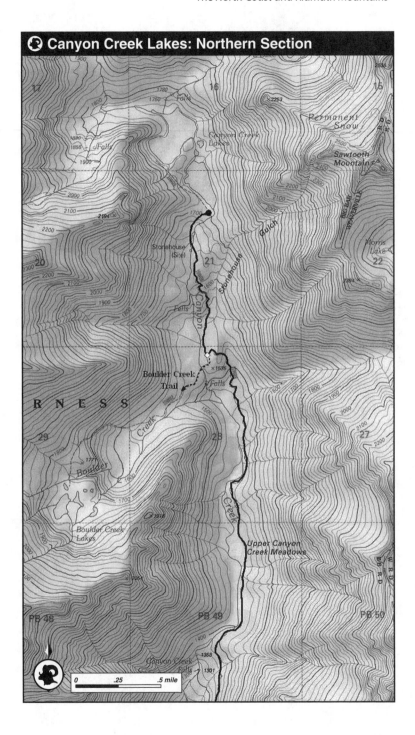

⊙ Canyon Creek Lakes: Northern Section

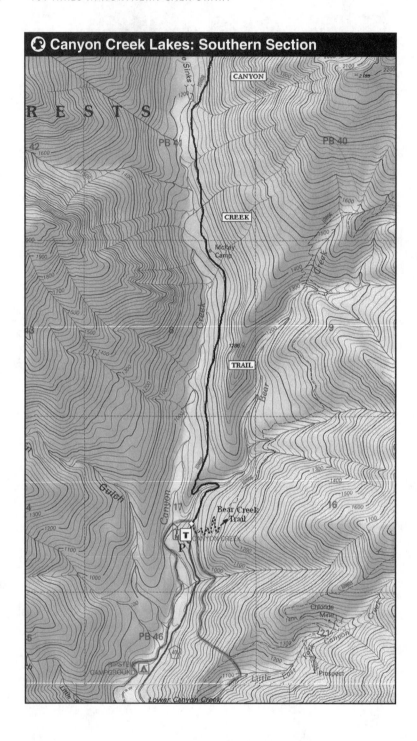

Canyon Creek Lakes: Southern Section

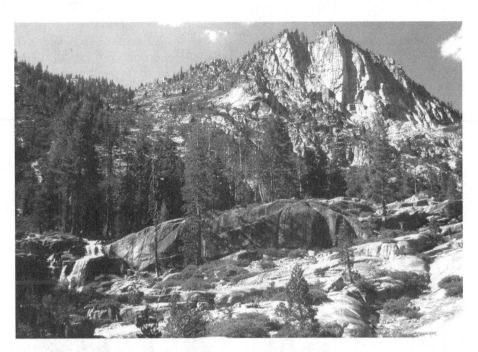

The granite landscape of the central Trinity Alps

To Reach the Trailhead Take Hwy. 299 to Junction City, 8.5 miles west of the intersection of Hwys. 3 and 299 in Weaverville and 6.5 miles east of East Fork Rd. and the turnoff for Helena. Turn north on Canyon Creek Rd. (Hwy. 401)— the turnoff is directly opposite the Junction City Store—and follow the increasingly narrow paved road 13.5 miles to the large parking lot at the road's end.

Description From the trailhead (0.0/3,150'), both paths leaving the parking lot quickly join to reach a posted junction for Bear Creek Trail—head left on Canyon Creek Trail. Entering the wilderness, the trail passes beneath ponderosa pines, Douglas-firs, incense cedars, madrone, black oaks, bigleaf maples, dogwoods, and alders. Thimbleberry and vine maple thrive in the lush understory. Initially traversing above rushing Bear Creek, you soon descend to cross the transparent stream. A few canyon live oaks can be seen as you climb out of the gully to begin paralleling above Canyon Creek.

While Canyon Creek is often visible below through the trees, access is generally not possible. The pale granite boulders that fill the creekbed are in stark contrast to the dark metamorphic rocks of the opposite peaks, and are representative of the overall regional geology. Occupying all of northwest California, the Klamath Mountains are a complex geologic mosaic formed from a wide variety of metamorphic rocks, which accreted to the continent over the past few hundred million years. Once connected with the northern Sierra Nevada, the mountain range was intruded by magma rising through the crust in enormous subterranean bubbles between 120 and 150 million years ago. Solidifying as granite before reaching the surface, these bubbles became exposed as erosion stripped away the overlying rock. Unlike the heavily intruded central and southern Sierra, the Klamath Mountains contain only isolated pockets of granite—the Trinity Alps are the most spectacular example. The rocks of Canyon Creek have been washed down from the granitic heart of the mountains, but here the trail still winds above a complex metamorphic assemblage. However, you soon cross the geologic divide where soaring peaks of granite become visible up-canyon.

The trail steadily climbs above Canyon Creek, becoming increasingly rocky as it navigates a few intermittent switchbacks before reaching beautiful Canyon Creek Falls (3.8/4,450') and the first easy river access. The falls mark the halfway point for the hike, and the end of the deep V-shaped river gorge of lower Canyon Creek. Above the falls, relatively recent glaciation has carved the valley into a broad U, with a delightfully flat canyon bottom. Vegetation is lush, and California redbud, huckleberry oak, and seasonal wildflowers line the trail. Leaving the vicinity of the creek, the trail switchbacks 200 feet to reach the junction with Boulder Creek Trail (6.0/5,000').

Continuing up-canyon on Canyon Creek Trail, notice the appearance of mountain hemlock and western white pine in the forest mix. As the trail begins to climb again, notice the glacial polish in evidence on nearby rocks. Red fir and aspens appear next. Soon the final push to Lower Canyon Creek Lake begins near another beautiful waterfall, this one only visible through the trees. Becoming rocky and narrow, the trail is marked by numerous small cairns as it climbs 200 feet to a rock-hop across Canyon Creek. The lake is just ahead (7.5/5,606').

With a backdrop of Wedding Cake (8,569') and more distant Thompson Peak (9,002') at the head of the canyon, the lake is scenic. It also harbors numerous specimens of Brewer spruce around the shore. The rarest spruce in the world, Brewer spruce exists only in scattered locations throughout the Klamath Mountains and is easily identified by its distinctive dangling branches. Useless for lumber, and growing in generally remote locations, the tree has been little studied and its origins remain a mystery.

Several adventurous side trips are possible from the lake. Past the lake's northwest corner, more rugged Upper Canyon Creek Lake is accessible via a short brushy scramble. Tiny El Lake perches northeast nearly 800 feet above the upper lake and is reputed to be excellent for fishing. Thompson Peak, the highest summit in the Trinity Alps, cannot be bagged from this approach without technical equipment. Revel in the majesty of these mountains before returning the way you came.

Nearest Visitor Center Weaverville District Ranger Office, 530-623-2121, on Hwy. 299 on Weaverville's west side, is open Monday–Friday 8 a.m.–4:30 p.m.

Backpacking Information A wilderness permit is required and available free either outside the Weaverville District Ranger Office or at the Junction City Forest Service fire station (0.1 mile east of Canyon Creek Rd.). Campsites are abundant in the valley above Canyon Creek Falls, but only a few good sites exist around Lower Canyon Creek Lake; there are none at the upper lake. Black bears are common in the area—hang your food or bring a canister. No quota is currently in effect for this very popular trailhead.

Nearest Campground Ripstein Campground, on Canyon Creek Rd. 0.7 mile before the trailhead, has excellent walk-in sites (10 sites without water, free).

Additional Information www.fs.usda.gov/stnf

HIKE 55 Marble Rim ⤢ 🚶 🐕

Highlights	Serene lakes, mountains of marble
Distance	17.4 miles round-trip
Total Elevation Gain/Loss	2,800'/2,800'
Hiking Time	10–14 hours
Recommended Maps	*Marble Mountain and Russian Wilderness Map & Guide* by the US Forest Service, USGS 7.5-min. *Marble Mountain*
Best Times	Mid-June–October
Agency	Marble Mountain Wilderness, Klamath National Forest
Difficulty	★★★★

DESIGNATED A PRIMITIVE AREA in 1931 and established as one of California's first wilderness areas in 1953, Marble Mountain Wilderness protects nearly a quarter-million acres of pristine California. You might think that the deep lakes, striking mountains, lush forest, abundant wildlife, and isolation would attract droves of hikers. But they don't.

The Hike ascends to the impressive cliffs of Marble Mountains via serene Sky High Lakes Basin, a long day hike best done as an easy overnight trip. Despite the low elevation, snow lingers on the trail well into June and usually returns by the end of October. This is (deservedly) the most popular hike in the wilderness, but crowds will be light relative to other alpine regions of the state. Fishing is possible in the Sky High Lakes. Water is available at the trailhead until late September, and sources are plentiful along the hike.

To Reach the Trailhead Take Scott River Rd. 14.5 miles west from Fort Jones on Hwy. 3 to Indian Scotty Campground and turn left (south) onto Forest Service Rd. 44N45, posted for Lovers Camp. Bear left at the immediate fork and continue on the sinuous, one-lane paved road as it climbs 7.5 miles to a large parking lot at the road's end.

Description From the trailhead (0.0/4,150'), start out on Canyon Creek Trail, passing two established campsites and entering the lush forest. Douglas-firs, tanoaks, and bigleaf maples

are common sights overhead, and trail markers, wild ginger, and ferns line the path. In 0.1 mile, the trail reaches a confusing intersection of unpaved roads—continue on the trail found diagonally across the road. Passing a wilderness boundary sign hammered to a Douglas-fir, you soon reach a posted fork (0.7/4,250') in the level trail. The trail to Red Rock Valley heads left, but you continue right on Canyon Creek Trail toward Marble Valley.

While the hike parallels rushing Canyon Creek for several miles, it remains unseen below you for the duration. Crossing flowing Death Valley Creek, the trail then climbs briefly before dropping to cross Big Rock Fork. The logs that litter the bouldery watercourse provide evidence of the ferocity that winter rains and flood bring to the region's otherwise small streams. Shortly thereafter, the trail abruptly turns upslope and begins climbing steeply uphill. Intermittent switchbacks eventually bring you to the junction for Marble Valley (4.1/5,320'). Marble Valley provides faster and more direct access to the Marble Mountains but entirely misses Sky High Lakes Basin. If you are short on time, bear right and continue uphill to the Marble Valley Cabin (closed to the public) and the Pacific Crest Trail (PCT) junction. Head south on the PCT until you reach the Marble Rim Trail. This marble-strewn route also makes an excellent return trail at the end of the day.

Bearing left toward Sky High Lakes, you climb more gradually and soon pass another

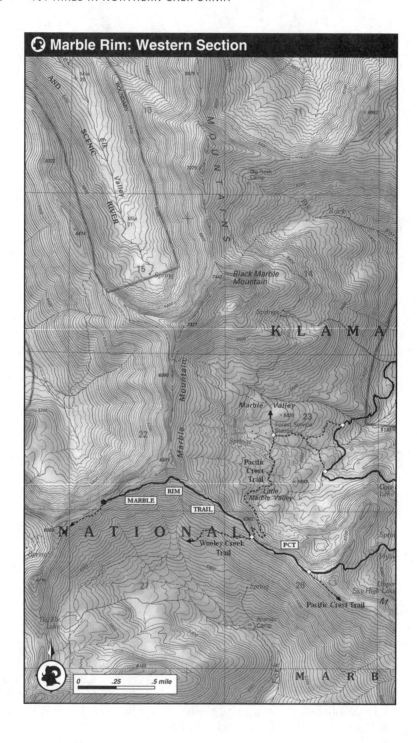

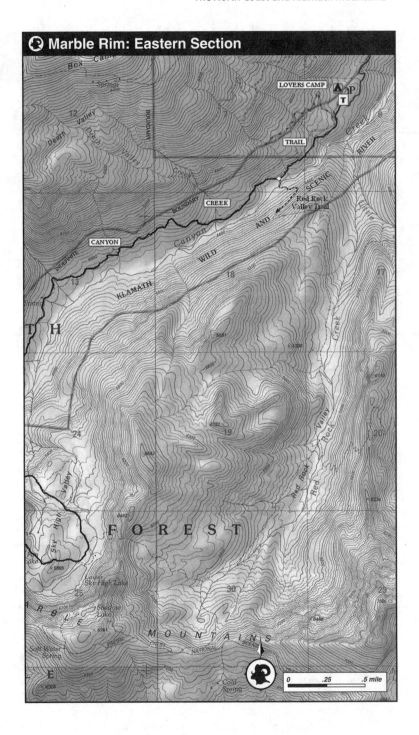

⊙ Marble Rim: Eastern Section

LOVERS CAMP

TRAIL

SCENIC

Red Rock
Valley Trail

CREEK

CANYON

WILD

AND

KLAMATH

FOREST

MOUNTAINS

0   .25   .5 mile

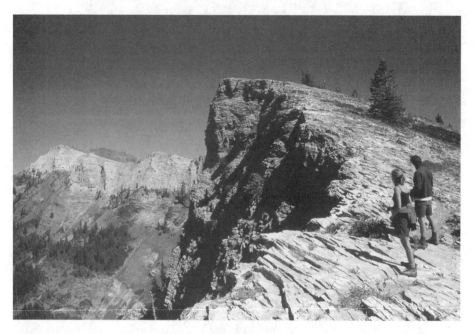

Marble Rim

junction for Marble Valley (4.4/5,500') on the right. Curving east, the trail offers the first views of the Marble Mountains to the west before making a final ascent into Sky High Lakes Basin. After you crest a final rise, diminutive and willow-choked Gate Lake welcomes you to the gently rolling basin.

Carved out by recent glaciation within the past 2 million years, the basin holds several lakes. While use paths crisscross the area, the actual trail leads first to larger Lower Sky High Lake (6.0/5,775') in the basin's southeast corner, before turning west toward tiny Frying Pan Lake, and then climbing out of the basin. The trees are diverse—white fir, red fir, mountain hemlock, western white pine, and large groves of aspen can all be found. In addition, a rare stand of subalpine fir grows here as well. A common tree throughout the Pacific Northwest, subalpine fir's range extends north to the subarctic. But in Northern California it only occurs here and in scattered locations within nearby Russian Wilderness, and both

populations are more than 50 miles distant from the next closest stand in southern Oregon, according to Ronald Lanner in *Conifers of California*. Despite existing at the extreme southern limit of their range, the trees seem to be thriving. Identify them by their narrow spire shape, strongly aromatic crushed needles, and close resemblance to red fir. Within the lakes amphibians thrive: frogs, tadpoles, and the ubiquitous, orange-bellied roughskin newt all entertain along the shorelines. In early October, cattle graze here as well.

Continuing west toward the Marble Mountains, the trail climbs steeply up the slopes and offers superlative views of the entire basin before attaining the divide and reaching a junction with the PCT (7.1/6,400'). From the ridge, the entire drainage of Wooley Creek reveals itself within a horseshoe of peaks dominated west-southwest by granite Medicine Mountain (6,837'). From its headwaters here, Wooley Creek plummets more than 5,000 feet through dense, undisturbed forest to join the Salmon

River 20 miles away. Its entire pristine watershed is protected within the wilderness.

Once on the ridge, turn right and follow the PCT descending gently northwest to a four-way junction (8.6/6,230'), where you continue straight toward Marble Rim. Right leads down into Marble Valley, the possible shortcut or return route mentioned above. Left drops down in just over a mile to Big Elk Lake, visible southwest in an open grassy area. Now climbing again toward the marble slopes, the trail remains below the divide until it reaches the low, treeless notch along Marble Rim (8.7/6,480').

Part of the complex geologic mix of the Klamath Mountains, the Marble Mountains most likely originated more than 200 million years ago from coral reefs surrounding an ancient offshore island or landmass. Over the millennia, the reefs' skeletal remains collected in thick layers that eventually solidified into the sedimentary rock limestone. Smashed into North America, the limestone was transformed to marble and exposed by erosion to form the spectacular cliffs before you. North, Rainy Valley trails away more than a thousand feet below. Southeast are the jagged peaks of the highest mountains in the wilderness, and the Trinity Alps (see previous hike) can often be seen on the distant southern skyline. Return as you came via Sky High Lakes Basin or take the Marble Valley shortcut.

Nearest Visitor Center Scott River Ranger Station, 530-468-5351, on Hwy. 3 in Fort Jones by the intersection with Scott River Rd., is open Monday–Friday 8 a.m.–4:30 p.m.

Backpacking Information No wilderness permit is necessary, but a valid campfire permit is required—get it at any national forest visitor center. Sites are abundant in the Sky High Lakes Basin.

Nearest Campgrounds Free overnight camping is permitted in sites around the trailhead. Otherwise, try Indian Scotty Campground (28 sites, $10), at the Lovers Camp turnoff from Scott River Rd.

Additional Information www.fs.usda.gov/klamath

HIKE 56 Castle Dome ↗

Highlight	Jagged pillars of granite
Distance	5.4 miles round-trip
Total Elevation Gain/Loss	2,300'/2,300'
Hiking Time	3–5 hours
Recommended Map	USGS 7.5-min. *Dunsmuir*
Best Times	April–October
Agency	Castle Crags State Park
Difficulty	★★★★

RAKING THE SKY, a jagged protrusion of granite bursts from the slopes above I-5. Needle-sharp spires, bulbous domes, a mania of fantastical granite blades, Castle Crags is unlike anywhere else in California. Add to this views of Mount Shasta and you have a hike that must be done.

The Hike follows the steep trail to Castle Dome (4,966'), a tall, round peak in the middle of Castle Crags. Unlike trails in nearby high-elevation areas, this hike usually becomes free of snow by April and does not receive snowfall again until November. While summer months are crowded, spring and fall offer increased solitude and views of a snow-mantled Mount Shasta. While no water is available at the trailhead, sources can be found by the visitor center, in the campground, and halfway at Indian Springs.

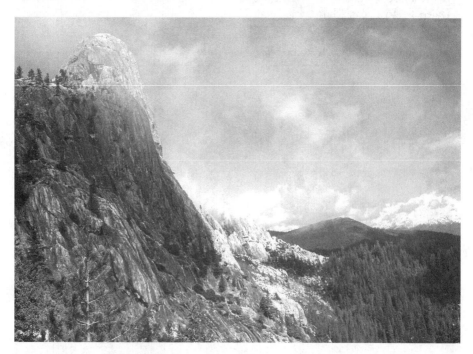

Castle Dome and distant Mount Shasta

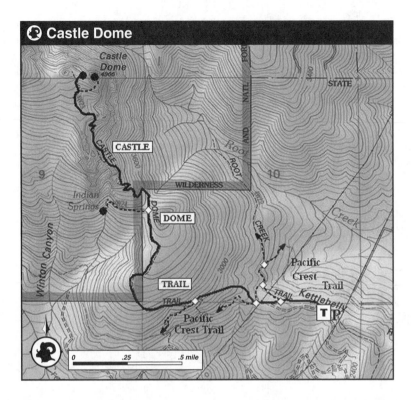

To Reach the Trailhead Take the Castella off-ramp from I-5 and head west, immediately turning right into Castle Crags State Park. Turn right past the entrance station toward Crags Trail and Vista Point and proceed 2 miles, passing the campground before reaching the parking lot at the road's end—RVs and trailers are prohibited on this steep and narrow road. An $8 day-use fee is charged.

Description From the trailhead at the west end of the lot (0.0/2,580'), the level doubletrack trail begins climbing among second-growth Douglas-firs, incense cedars, bigleaf maples, alders, ponderosa pines, black oaks, and poison oak to quickly reach a junction with Root Creek Trail—bear left and continue on Castle Crags Trail. After a few switchbacks, the trail crosses the Pacific Crest Trail beneath some power lines (0.4/2,680') and continues climbing. Canyon live oaks begin to appear and the small Indian Creek drainage is visible below

you to the west, before a gradually rising traverse brings you to the junction with Bob's Hat Trail (0.6/2,910')—continue upward on Castle Crags Trail. Crossing into Castle Crags Wilderness, the rising trail briefly levels out on the eastern slope of Indian Creek, and offers the first tantalizing glimpses of granite crags and the deep east–west drainage of Castle Creek. Formed between 170 and 225 million years ago when the Klamath Mountains and Sierra Nevada were joined as one continuous mountain range, the granite of Castle Crags closely resembles the rock of the eastern Sierra Nevada in both age and composition.

At the posted junction for Indian Springs (1.5/3,560'), a brief and highly recommended side trip leads to a series of lush springs emerging from the hillside and dribbling out of cracks in a mossy 25-foot-high block of granite. Back on the main trail, the route gets rocky and steep, switchbacking rapidly as sugar pine and increasing manzanita line the path. Mount Shasta soon appears for the first time beyond the sheer east face of Castle Dome. The fire lookout on top of Mount Bradley (5,556') is visible between the two.

Weaving through jagged pillars of granite surmountable only by spiderpeople, the trail, occasionally hewn into solid rock, begins to diverge into a maze of use paths near the top. The wider main trail is generally easy to follow; it terminates at a fenced overlook with a view into the deep crevice between Castle Dome and the neighboring crags. The thick ground cover of the upper crags is primarily manzanita and huckleberry oak; the trees are sugar and ponderosa pine. The summit of Castle Dome (2.7/4,966') can be bagged from the south with some precarious scrambling—follow the easiest route up the south face and wrap around to the east. Return the way you came.

Nearest Visitor Center Castle Crags State Park Visitor Center, 530-235-2684, at the park entrance, is open daily May–September and sporadically October–April.

Backpacking Information While not allowed within the state park, backcountry camping is allowed within Castle Crags Wilderness—no wilderness permit is needed. A few possible sites exist around Castle Dome, but there is no water above Indian Springs.

Nearest Campground Castle Crags State Park Campground has 76 sites ($25). Reservations are recommended in the summer; call 800-444-7275 or visit **reserveamerica.com**.

Additional Information **www.parks.ca.gov**

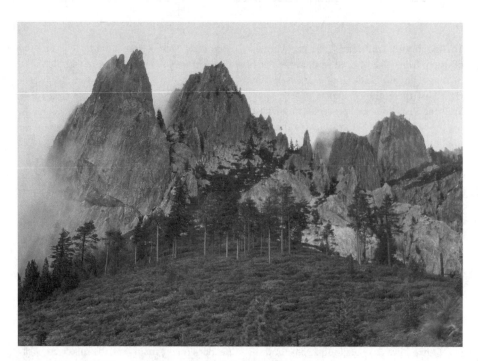

Jagged, thrusting pillars of granite

HIKE 57 Heart Lake 🥾 🐕

Highlight	The quick and easy Shasta-Trinity experience
Distance	1.8 miles round-trip
Total Elevation Gain/Loss	700'/700'
Hiking Time	1–2 hours
Recommended Map	USGS 7.5-min. *Seven Lakes Basin*
Best Times	June–October
Agency	Shasta-Trinity National Forest
Difficulty	★★

JUST NORTH OF Castle Crags Wilderness, tiny Heart Lake perches among boulders and trees high above Castle Lake. The massif of Mount Shasta looms beyond, a great geographic transition easily observed without the physical punishment of other nearby hikes.

The Hike climbs past Castle Lake to reach Heart Lake, an easy hike with easy access that provides a quick sample of the region's geography. Fishing for brook and rainbow trout is popular in deep Castle Lake. Water is available at the trailhead.

Note that a portion of this hike travels over private land that recently changed ownership. While the long-established trail continues to receive regular use, its status may change in the years ahead. Please respect private property and remain on the trail throughout this hike.

To Reach the Trailhead Take the Mount Shasta exit from I-5 and head west, immediately turning left (south) at the stop sign by the fish hatchery. Continue straight on W. A. Barr Rd. for 2.6 miles, bearing left on Castle Lake Rd. at the Y-junction immediately after crossing the outflow from Siskiyou Lake. Castle Lake Rd. twists uphill for 7.5 miles to a large circular paved lot at the road's end.

Description From the trailhead, drop down to Castle Lake (5,436'). Known to the local Shasta-Wintun Indians as "Castle of the Devil," home of the evil spirit Ku-Ku-Pa-Rick, Castle Lake is one of the most extensively studied mountain lakes in all of California. Numerous informative placards highlight the work done here over the past 60 years. The wide trail strikes south along the lake's east shore among white fir and lodgepole pine, passing several heavily used primitive campsites before reaching a posted sign for Little Castle and Heart lakes.

The narrower trail begins to climb, traversing above Castle Lake and becoming increasingly rocky and root-strewn. Red fir begins to appear trailside, tantalizing views begin to appear between the peaks, and you soon crest the low divide above Castle Lake. The junction for Heart Lake is precisely at this divide. Continuing straight on the obvious trail leads to Little Castle Lake in a quick half mile, but the unposted spur to Heart Lake strikes a hard right from the main trail and soon reaches its destination. Western white pines appear here, Mount Eddy (Hike 58) is visible northwest through a notch in the ridge, and Mount Shasta is apparent in its entirety.

Castle Lake is located at the eastern edge of the Klamath Mountains, a geologically complex range whose ancient rocks vary in age from approximately 80 to 300 million years old. You are so close to the edge of this geologic province that you can see beyond it to the young rocks mantling Mount Shasta, rocks formed less than 10,000 years ago. Here in the eastern Klamath Mountains, however, the peaks are composed primarily of the Trinity Complex—the largest exposure of ancient seafloor in all of North America. Yet the rocks around you are granite,

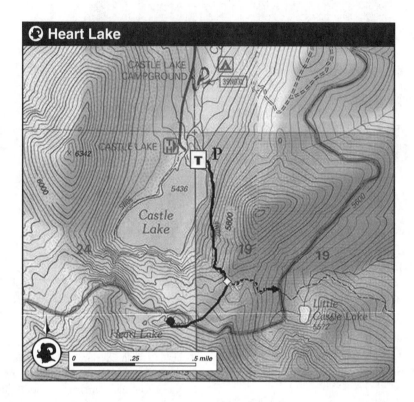

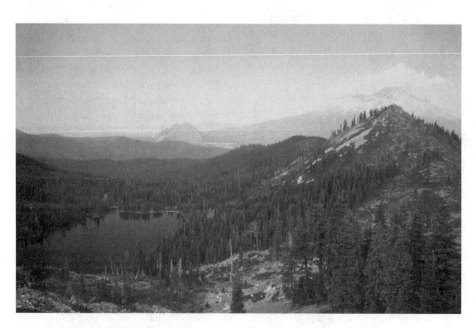

Looking north toward Castle Lake and cloud-capped Mount Shasta

the exposed surface of a small bubble of magma that rose through the older rock between 170 and 225 million years ago and solidified before reaching the surface. Castle Crags (Hike 56), a mere 6 miles south of here, represents the southern edge of this granite outcropping. The darker rocks of the Trinity Complex can be found mixed in with the lighter granite on your return trip. So back you go!

Nearest Visitor Center Mount Shasta Ranger District Office, 530-926-4511, in the town of Mount Shasta at 204 W. Alma St. (parallel to Lake St.), is open daily 8 a.m.–4:30 p.m. Memorial Day–Labor Day, and Monday–Friday only the rest of the year.

Nearest Campground Castle Lake Campground, a half mile north of the lake on Castle Lake Dr. (6 sites without water, free), is always full on weekends. There is a maximum stay of 3 nights.

Additional Information www.fs.usda.gov/stnf

HIKE 58 Mount Eddy 🏂 🚶 🐕

Highlights	Killer views of Mount Shasta and the Klamath Mountains
Distance	10.0 miles round-trip
Total Elevation Gain/Loss	2,100'/2,100'
Hiking Time	5–7 hours
Recommended Maps	USGS 7.5-min. *South China Mountain* and *Mount Eddy*
Best Times	Mid-June–September
Agency	Shasta-Trinity National Forest
Difficulty	★★★★

DWARFED BY ITS towering neighbor, the rocky rise of Mount Eddy may not immediately catch your attention, but, if you want a secluded valley and a summit with sweeping 360-degree views, it should.

The Hike ascends Mount Eddy (9,025') from the west, passing through a broad valley with easy access to Upper Deadfall Lake before steeply climbing to attain the summit. The high elevation of Mount Eddy means that snow can linger well into June and return anytime in October. Crowds are unfortunately thick during the summer months, when as many as 60 cars can be found parked at the trailhead. Fishing is good in Upper Deadfall Lake, and wildflowers are abundant in June and July. No water is available at the trailhead, but it can always be obtained from Deadfall Creek 2.5 miles from the trailhead.

To Reach the Trailhead Take the Edgewood exit from I-5—2 miles north of Weed—and go west. Just past the freeway, turn right and then quickly left in 0.2 mile to stay on Stewart Springs Rd. for 4.2 miles. At the wooden gate marking the entrance to Stewart Springs, turn right onto Forest Service Rd. 17. Proceed 9.5 miles on the paved road to the posted Parks Creek Trailhead on the left, just past the divide. An alternate trailhead can be found 1.4 miles farther down the road, from a gravel lot at a

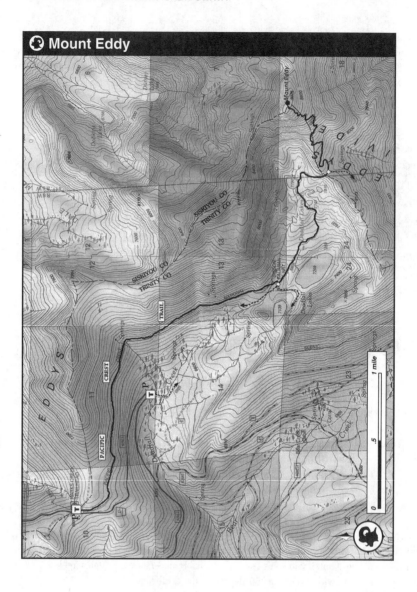

Mount Eddy

sharp U-turn in the road. The trail leading from here follows Deadfall Creek along the valley bottom and avoids some areas of recent logging activity, joining the trail described below in 1.5 miles and adding an extra 750 feet of elevation gain to the hike.

Description From the trailhead (0.0/6,850'), the hike begins on the Pacific Crest Trail (PCT) and briefly parallels the road as it passes among Jeffrey pine, white fir, and western white pine.

It then curves east to begin a long, gradually rising traverse above the valley that soon passes through an area of recent logging activity. As views open up, the glacial origin of the valley is readily apparent in its broad U-shape.

In season, wildflowers abound along the trail—please do not pick them. The reddish-brown rocks here are part of the Trinity Complex, the largest exposure of ancient seafloor found in North America. Accreted to the continent roughly 250 million years ago, these rocks weather to form a nutrient-deficient soil that provides habitat for many rare and unusual plants found only where such rocks are exposed. Let them live.

Reaching the valley floor, you come to a four-way junction (2.6/7,230'). The PCT continues straight and the trail from the alternate trailhead joins from the right, but you turn left toward Mount Eddy, visible due east from here. Lodgepole pines now predominate. In 0.1 mile you reach an unmarked spur trail that splits right to Upper Deadfall Lake—fishing and swimming opportunities abound around the lakeshore.

Back on the main trail, your route quickly steepens where the trail switchbacks to reach several ponds in a small basin, the last source of water for this hike. As the trail continues to climb, an unusual stand of foxtail pine appears among mountain hemlock and western white pine.

Foxtail pine exists in two distinct populations separated by a gap of nearly 300 miles: one in the Klamath Mountains, of which the trees around you are the easternmost representatives and one in the southern Sierra Nevada, found primarily in Sequoia and Kings Canyon National Parks. How such a wide gap developed remains unresolved, but it seems likely that the two populations are remnants of a once extensive forest across California. Closely related to the ancient bristlecone pine (Hike 95), foxtail pines are able to survive in soils inhospitable to most other conifers. They are easily identified by the namesake needle clusters that extend densely along the branches.

Reaching a divide (4.0/8,000'), you come to another junction—turn left and begin the grueling push to the top. The rocky path switchbacks more than a dozen times as it climbs the south ridge and provides increasingly airy views. Approximately halfway to the top, scrubby whitebark pines, the only conifer capable of surviving at such high elevations, have been twisted into krummholz form by the harsh elements. Ever-tightening switchbacks finally deposit you on the summit (5.0/9,025').

An old abandoned fire lookout, blown over during the winter of 1998–99, crowns the summit and provides some shelter from windy conditions. The view is unbelievable: Mount Shasta dominates the landscape east above the thin ribbon of I-5 and the perfect cone of Black Butte (6,325'). To the west, a large stretch of the Trinity River drainage can be identified, and the distant peaks of the Trinity Alps (Hike 54) rake the skyline southwest. Due west are the mountains of Russian Wilderness, and Marble Mountain Wilderness (Hike 55) forms the skyline west-northwest. Return the way you came.

Nearest Visitor Center Mount Shasta Ranger District Office, 530-926-4511, in the town of Mount Shasta at 204 W. Alma St. (parallel to Lake St.), is open daily 8 a.m.–4:30 p.m. Memorial Day–Labor Day, and Monday–Friday only the rest of the year.

Backpacking Information A campfire permit is required. Besides a large campsite by Upper Deadfall Lake, the adventurous can sleep on the often-windy summit of Mount Eddy.

Nearest Campgrounds There are several campgrounds along Hwy. 3, including Scott Mountain Campground (7 sites without water, free), 5 miles north of the junction of Hwy. 3 and Forest Service Rd. 17, and Eagle Creek Campground, 6 miles south of the junction (10 sites, water available; $10). Hwy. 3 can be accessed from the trailhead by driving west on FS 17 for 13 twisty miles.

Additional Information www.fs.usda.gov/stnf

Shasta and the Modoc Plateau

INCLUDING ALL of northeast California from Mount Shasta east to Nevada and Lassen Peak north to Oregon, this region is a starkly unique place. The landscape is entirely volcanic, an extensive plateau averaging around 4,000 feet in elevation and dominated by two active volcanoes—Mount Shasta and Lassen Peak. Cinder cones, defunct volcanoes, lava flows, and the notable Warner Mountains add a distinctive topography to the land.

Annual precipitation is low and summer temperatures are high, creating deserts and dry forests. Snow falls across the plateau in the winter. Highlights include the volcanic wonderlands of Mount Shasta and Lassen Peak, the Warner Mountains, and some of the emptiest corners in the state.

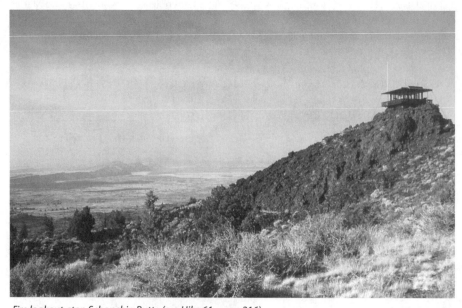

Fire lookout atop Schonchin Butte (see Hike 61, page 216)

HIKE 59 Hidden Valley

Highlights	The mountain. The views.
Distance	6.0 miles round-trip
Total Elevation Gain/Loss	2,300'/2,300'
Hiking Time	4–6 hours
Recommended Maps	*Mount Shasta Wilderness Recreation Map* by Wilderness Press, USGS 7.5-min. *McCloud* and *Mount Shasta*
Best Times	July–October
Agency	Mount Shasta Wilderness, Shasta-Trinity National Forest
Difficulty	★★★★

AN ACTIVE VOLCANO, Mount Shasta towers over the landscape of Northern California and hides a secluded world of rock and snow on its southwest flank. Hidden Valley awaits. Mount Shasta (14,142') is part of the Cascade Range of volcanoes that extends from Northern California to northern Washington State, and includes such notable peaks as Mount St. Helens and Mount Rainier. With a volume of roughly 80 cubic miles, Mount Shasta is substantial—the largest of the Cascade Range—and while its vents have been active for at least 100,000 years, the bulk of the current mountain has been constructed over only the past 10,000 years in a series of at least 13 separate eruptions. Hotlum Cone at the summit has erupted eight times during this period, covering the mountain and surrounding landscape with lava and debris flows. Its most recent eruption occurred in 1786, and there is no doubt that the mountain will flare again—current studies indicate that, on average, eruptions take place once every 250–300 years.

The Hike follows the popular trail to Horse Camp from Bunny Flat before continuing on an open cross-country traverse over loose and rocky slopes to Hidden Valley, a secluded depression offering outstanding views of the mountain. Because Mount Shasta is primarily a mountaineer's playground and Bunny Flat is the principal trailhead for the summit, crowds will be thick during mountain-climbing season (roughly April–July). The period following climbing season is best for hikers as crowds

decrease drastically and the snow preferred by aspiring climbers melts off the trail. No water is available at the trailhead. Horse Camp has a freshwater spring and provides the hike's only water source. Dogs are allowed on this hike but prohibited in the area around Horse Camp.

To Reach the Trailhead Take I-5 to the town of Mount Shasta and proceed east on Lake St. to join Everitt Memorial Hwy. and continue toward the mountain—Bunny Flat Trailhead is 12 miles from town on the north side of the road.

Description At the trailhead (0.0/6,900'), be sure to complete a self-issued day-use permit before striking out on the wide trail. Shasta red fir, manzanita, and lupine surround you as the trail climbs above a broad, dry meadow swept clean by the occasional heavy winter avalanche.

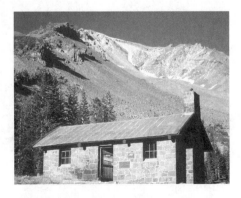

Sierra Club hut at Horse Camp

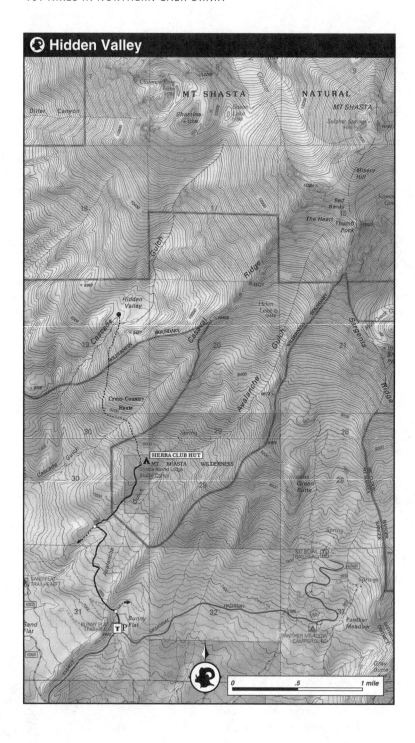

Hidden Valley

Use trails crisscross the area—stay on the main trail and bear left at the next obvious junction.

Winding through open forest, the path curves west toward the edge of Avalanche Gulch, climbing more steeply now along the edge of a lateral moraine carved by recent glaciation. A trail from Sand Flat trailhead joins from the left (1.0/7,330') and you soon cross the wilderness boundary. The steady ascent leaves the shaded forest just before reaching the open vistas of Horse Camp (1.7/7,880'). The Sierra Club hut here is a historic shelter open to everyone for browsing, relaxing, and reflecting. The hut is manned by a seasonal caretaker until early October, and supplies are available here in the event of an emergency. The standard climbing route is visible northwest, winding east around the distinctive Red Banks near the top before reaching unseen Misery Hill and the final push to the summit. Campsites and well-marked trails crisscross the area around Horse Camp, and an excellent outhouse is nearby.

From Horse Camp, the route to Hidden Valley follows a generally distinct trail that has been marked in recent years by wands to minimize hiker impact. Please stay on the marked route—the loose slopes are easily scarred. The rocky route begins beyond the northern campsites and

is clearly discernible as it immediately begins climbing north out of Avalanche Gulch. Lassen Peak (10,457'), the southernmost volcano of the Cascade Range, soon appears southeast beyond the eastern ridge of Avalanche Gulch. Cresting a rise, the trail levels out briefly in a flat bowl (2.0/8,100') where spectacular views west open up. The Eddys rise across the valley, with the high point of Mount Eddy (9,025'; see Hike 58) visible just south of the perfect cone of Black Butte (6,325'). Beyond Mount Eddy, the distant skyline peaks of the Trinity Alps (Hike 54) can be picked out southwest on a clear day.

As the route begins climbing steeply out of the bowl, shrubby and twisted whitebark pines appear among the rocks, shrunken to krummholz form by the powerful elements so high on the mountain. The final trail section is less discernible, where the route scrambles above sheer Cascade Gulch to crest into barren Hidden Valley (3.0/9,220'). Shastina (12,330') dominates to the north, a subsidiary cone formed between 9,300 and 9,700 years ago. The southern edge of Hidden Valley is part of Casaval Ridge, the sharp spine winding northwest toward the main summit, which offers some of the mountain's more technical routes when snow and ice are present. Return the way you came.

Nearest Visitor Center Mount Shasta Ranger District Office, 530-926-4511, in the town of Mount Shasta at 204 W. Alma St. (parallel to Lake St.), is open daily 8 a.m.–4:30 p.m. Memorial Day–Labor Day, and Monday–Friday only the rest of the year.

Backpacking Information A wilderness permit is required and is available free anytime at the trailhead or outside the Mount Shasta Ranger District Office. A donation is requested for camping in the sites around Horse Camp. The only other options are the small sites in Hidden Valley, which don't have water. Be sure to follow the guidelines for the human waste pack-out program if you are camping beyond an outhouse—supplies are available at the trailhead. While you will often find a community fire by the Sierra Club hut, no campfires are allowed elsewhere on the mountain.

Nearest Campgrounds Panther Meadows Walk-In Campground (10 sites without water, free) is 2 miles east of Bunny Flat Trailhead on Everitt Memorial Hwy. Also try McBride Springs Campground (12 sites, $10), on Everitt Memorial Hwy. Both are usually full during the summer, especially on weekends.

Additional Information www.fs.usda.gov/stnf, shastaavalanche.org

HIKE 60 Sheepy Ridge 🥾👨‍👧

Highlight	The land of a million birds
Distance	0.6 mile round-trip
Total Elevation Gain/Loss	180'/180'
Hiking Time	1 hour
Recommended Map	USGS 7.5-min. *Hatfield*
Best Times	Year-round
Agency	Tule Lake National Wildlife Refuge
Difficulty	★

TULE (*TOO-LEE*) LAKE sits in the Klamath Basin, a region of vast wetlands providing habitat for 353 species of birds. Many are migratory, stopping over to rest and refuel before continuing on their journeys. Geese, swans, and ducks of all types pass through, peaking in numbers during March and early November and swelling the number of birds in the Klamath Basin to more than 1 million. Winter is a magical time—Tule Lake freezes over and raptors of all kinds congregate here. From December through February, the Klamath Basin hosts the largest concentration of bald eagles in the contiguous United States—more than 500 can be present in the Basin—and Tule Lake is one of the best spots to observe them. During the summer, resident ducks and other waterbirds raise their young, livening the area with their darling broods. Options for birdwatching include an auto tour, self-guided canoe trails, and reservable photo blinds. The visitor center (see box page 215) has all the details.

The Hike climbs Sheepy Ridge behind the Klamath Basin Wildlife Refuges Visitor Center, an easy hike that is primarily an introduction to adventuring around Tule Lake. It offers broad views of the landscape from an unusual stone hut perched above the sheer cliffs. The exposed trail is scorching during summer months, so sun protection is essential. While snow can cover the trail in the winter, the Tule Lake region is worth visiting year-round for its ever-changing seasonal birdlife. Water is available at the trailhead.

To Reach the Trailhead Take East–West Rd. west from the town of Tulelake on Hwy. 139. In 4.8 miles, turn left on Hill Rd. to reach the visitor center in 0.5 mile. The trail starts in the upper parking lot. Approaching from Lava Beds National Monument, take Hill Rd. 9.3 miles north from the park road—the junction is immediately west of the Lava Beds north entrance station.

Description Pick up an interpretive brochure at the trailhead before you begin. Climb through rabbitbrush and sage, making three switchbacks before traversing over to the stone lookout at the trail's end. Constructed by the Civilian Conservation Corps in 1938, the enclosed hut offers respite from the sun's blistering rays.

Sheepy Ridge was formed as the adjacent land to the east slipped downward along a long, linear fault, forming a north–south ridge that extends more than 10 miles south into Lava Beds National Monument. Looking south down the ridge, notice the several cinder cones east of its terminus. The farthest east is Schonchin Butte (Hike 61). The collapsed form of Medicine Lake Volcano (Hike 63) occupies the distant southern skyline. As you face east, the perfect squares of reclaimed wetland surround Sump 1-A and the northern section of Tule Lake. The hills of Oregon recede into the northern distance.

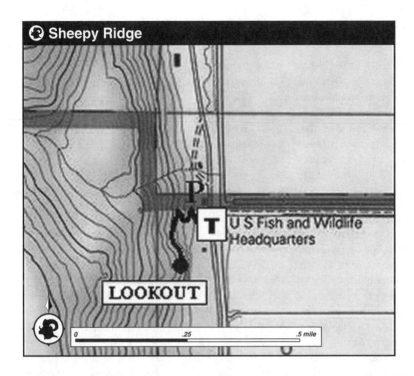

Nearest Visitor Center Klamath Basin National Wildlife Refuges Headquarters and Visitor Center, 530-667-2231, is open 8 a.m.–4:30 p.m. Monday–Friday and 10 a.m.–4 p.m. on weekends and holidays.

Nearest Campground Indian Well Campground (43 sites with water, $10) is in Lava Beds National Monument.

Additional Information fws.gov/refuge/tule_lake

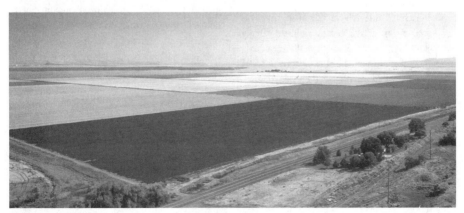

Tule or not Tule?

HIKE 61   Schonchin Butte ✔

Highlight	A sweeping vista of volcanic wasteland
Distance	1.4 miles round-trip
Total Elevation Gain/Loss	500'/500'
Hiking Time	1–2 hours
Recommended Map	USGS 7.5-min. *Schonchin Butte*
Best Times	Year-round
Agency	Lava Beds National Monument
Difficulty	★

LAVA BEDS NATIONAL MONUMENT is a land smothered by recent lava flows, pocked with cinder cones, devoid of all surface water. A world both hostile and fascinating, it's almost entirely visible from the fire lookout atop Schonchin (SKON-chin) Butte (5,253').

This is an active volcanic area. The entire landscape was formed less than 1 million years ago, when lava spilled across the surface and smothered it beneath thick flows of black basalt. Much of the lava originated in Medicine Lake Volcano to the west, but several vents within the monument have been active during the past 10,000 years. The Modoc Plateau is a part of the earth's crust that is undergoing extension, thinning and cracking in places as it is pulled apart. These cracks allow liquid basalt from the earth's interior to well up onto the surface, creating the lava flows and cinder cones seen in the monument today.

Schonchin Butte is a cinder cone that was produced by an active vent sometime during the past 10,000 years. As a new fissure allows magma to rise toward the surface, ground water is overheated, blowing large chunks of rock into a distinct cone shape around the surface opening. Once the actual magma reaches the surface it typically pours out at the base of the cone, flowing with gravity over the land. Schonchin Butte and the Schonchin Lava Flow, which flowed north over the heart of the monument, are textbook examples. This type of eruption is generally small and short-lived, producing a volcano in miniature that rarely erupts again.

The Hike climbs Schonchin Butte via a well-maintained trail to the summit fire lookout, an easy hike with several strategically located rest benches. While the hike is partly shaded, the sun is intense during summer months on the exposed portions of trail. The monument is open year-round and receives light snowfall from November through April. Despite the intense sun, Lava Beds receives most visitors during summer months, making the rest of the year preferable for a hike. No water is available at the trailhead or anywhere along the way.

To Reach the Trailhead Take Hwy. 139 northwest from Hwy. 299—the turnoff is just west of Canby. In 29 miles, turn west onto Hwy. 97. When you reach a fork in 2.7 miles, bear right onto Hwy. 10 and drive 10 miles to the monument border. From here, the visitor center is 4 miles and the turnoff for Schonchin Butte 6.2 miles. (Approaching from the north, the turnoff is 7.3 miles south of the north entrance station.) The unpaved road reaches the trailhead parking area in 1 mile and is easily passable for all vehicles, though RVs and trailers are not recommended due to the tight turnaround. There is a $10 entrance fee, which is valid for seven days.

Description From the trailhead (0.0/4,800'), the wide path traverses up the north flank of the cone. Juniper, sage, rabbitbrush, and mountain mahogany cover the slopes, and the fire lookout is visible above you. After two switchbacks, the trail forks. While both paths

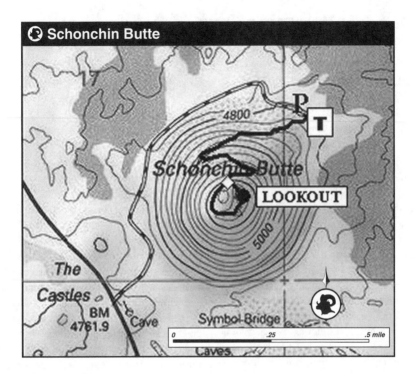

Schonchin Butte

lead to the summit, the left is more direct, but the right traverses around the old cinder crater, providing good views of the lookout's precarious roost. Go for the loop!

A wooden railing rings the lookout and you may have the opportunity to converse with the seasonal worker that staffs this active facility. Placards identify the surrounding landmarks, including Glass Mountain (Hike 63) and Mount Shasta (Hike 59). The fresh-looking, razor-sharp rocks of the Schonchin Lava Flow cover the ground below you to the north, barely colonized by plant life after thousands of years of erosion. Hidden among the cracks at the flow's northern end is Captain Jack's Stronghold, where a small band of Modoc Indians successfully resisted army attack for over six months by using the maze of caves and passageways in the lava flow. Lasting from November 1872 until June 1873, the Modoc War was the last Indian war fought in the United States.

Nearest Visitor Center Lava Beds National Monument Visitor Center, 530-667-8113, is open daily 8 a.m.–6 p.m. in summer and 8:30 a.m.–5 p.m. the rest of the year.

Nearest Campground Indian Well Campground (43 sites with water, $10) is 0.5 mile from the visitor center.

Additional Information nps.gov/labe

HIKE 62 Valentine Cave ⚲👤

Highlight	Spelunking in a lava tube
Distance	0.5 mile round-trip
Total Elevation Gain/Loss	Negligible
Hiking Time	1 hour
Recommended Map	USGS 7.5-min. *Schonchin Butte*
Best Times	Year-round
Agency	Lava Beds National Monument
Difficulty	★

FEEL THE COOL, inky darkness of a cave below a scorching volcanic desert. Lava tubes are formed as the sides and surface of a lava flow solidify, covering with hardened basalt the liquid rock that still courses inside. Once the flow stops, the lava drains away and leaves a hollow tube with several distinctive features inside. Lavicles are formed when liquid rock drips from the ceiling and solidifies. Benches found on the tube walls represent decreasing surface levels brought on by reductions in flow volume. Roof collapse typically exposes the lava tubes, which can wind underground for miles through passages of varying widths.

The Hike is the only one in the book that goes underground, following spacious Valentine Cave

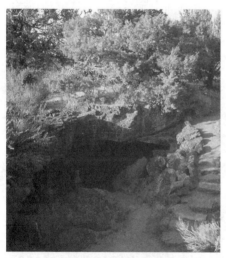

At the entrance to Valentine Cave, cool, inky darkness awaits.

to its terminus well beyond the reach of the sun's rays. It's a good introduction to the 700-plus caves of Lava Beds, most of which are much more challenging to explore. With its cool, constant, year-round temperature, Valentine Cave provides welcome respite from summer heat and winter chill, and is open all year long.

Before heading to the trailhead, you must first check in at the visitor center to receive a pass to enter the cave. The park is working to protect the area's bats from white-nose syndrome, a fatal disease decimating bat populations throughout North America. Cave visitors must complete a short orientation and screening to ensure they are not potentially contaminating the area's caves with the disease-causing fungus.

The hike is short and easy but requires taking important precautions. Sturdy nonslip shoes are essential, and long pants and a warm pullover are recommended. Carry two sources of light with you at all times, but do not use gas or carbide lanterns. The visitor center provides flashlights free of charge during the day and sells inexpensive plastic hard hats, although Valentine Cave has ceilings sufficiently high for you to walk upright. No water is available at the trailhead.

To Reach the Trailhead Take Hwy. 139 northwest from Hwy. 299—the turnoff is just west of Canby. In 29 miles, turn west onto Hwy. 97. When you reach a fork in 2.7 miles, bear right onto Hwy. 10 and drive 10 miles to the monument border. From here, the visitor center is 4 miles. There is a $10 entrance fee, which is valid for seven days. Continue on the

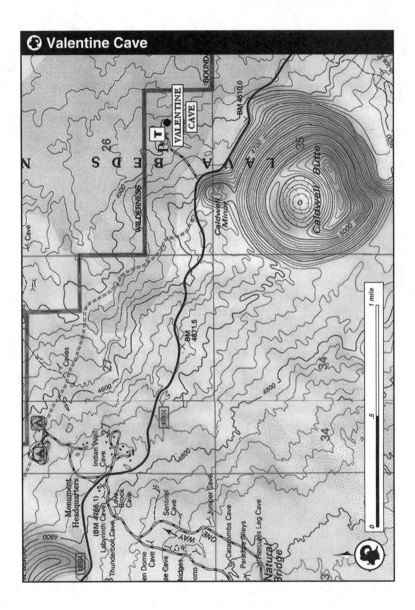

Valentine Cave

park road (Hwy. 10) 1.7 miles southeast of the visitor center and turn left toward Valentine Cave, reaching a substantial parking lot in 0.2 mile. Approaching from the south, the turnoff is 2 miles northwest of the park boundary.

Description A paved trail leads 50 feet to the cave entrance, ringed by junipers and sagebrush. The collapsed blocks preserve solidified *pahoehoe* (puh-HOY-hoy), a ropy type of lava flow formed by basaltic magma. The magma associated with Mount Shasta and the Cascade Range forms blocky, slow-moving flows known as aa (ah-ah). After immediately splitting around a large pillar, the cave resumes its tubelike shape in increasing darkness. Lavicles cover the ceiling and benches. The cave narrows abruptly in the back, terminating in a small crawl space that continues a few feet farther. If the cave is empty of other visitors, turn out your lights to experience utter darkness.

Nearest Visitor Center Lava Beds National Monument Visitor Center, 530-667-8113, is open daily 8 a.m.–6 p.m. in summer and 8:30 a.m.–5 p.m. the rest of the year.

Nearest Campground Indian Well Campground (43 sites with water, $10) is 0.5 mile from the visitor center.

Additional Information nps.gov/labe

HIKE 63 Glass Mountain ↗

Highlight	A recent lava flow laced with volcanic glass
Distance	1.0 mile or less round-trip
Total Elevation Gain/Loss	50'/50'
Hiking Time	1 hour
Recommended Maps	USGS 7.5-min. *Medicine Lake* and *West of Kephart*
Best Times	Mid-June–September
Agency	Modoc National Forest
Difficulty	★

LAVA COOLED SO FAST it turned to glass. Medicine Lake Volcano is larger in mass than nearby Mount Shasta, yet its slopes are so gradual as to be almost unremarkable. It is a shield volcano formed from basaltic lava, an extremely broad mountain very similar to those of the Hawaiian Islands. Measuring 15 miles east–west by 25 miles north–south with a surface area greater than 900 square miles, it is a prominent landmark of the Modoc Plateau.

Unlike the towering stratovolcano of Mount Shasta, Medicine Lake Volcano hardly appears intimidating. This is because the entire top of the mountain collapsed approximately 100,000 years ago in a block 4 miles wide by 6 miles long, forming a large depression, or caldera. Smaller volcanoes welled up along the circular fracture, spilling lava both into the caldera and down the slopes of the mountain.

Glass Mountain, the most recent flow in the Medicine Lake complex, spilled down the volcano's east flanks less than 1,000 years ago. Liquid magma is a soup of chemicals unformed and without structure. Most lava flows are extruded

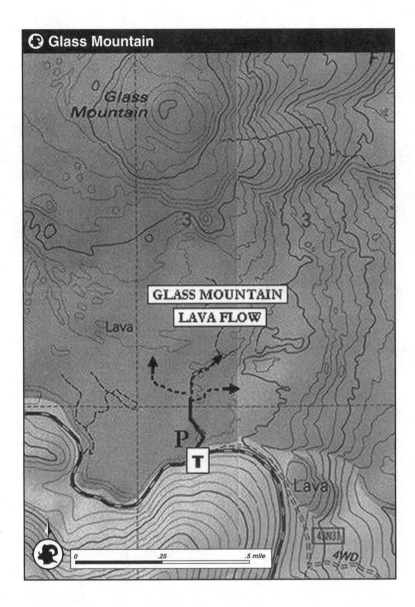

Glass Mountain

slowly enough for the assorted chemicals to gradually cool and form discrete crystals, but occasionally the molten rock cools so quickly that it hardens unchanged, forming black glass, or obsidian. This transformation occurred at Glass Mountain. Americans Indians prized obsidian's sharp edges for knives and arrowheads; at least four different tribes collected here, trading to neighboring tribes more than a hundred miles away.

The Hike is an opportunity to wander around on a recent lava flow and see obsidian in its natural state, though collecting it is prohibited. This is a remote part of California, and odds are that you won't encounter anybody else, regardless of when you come. This hike is at a relatively high elevation for the region—above 7,000 feet—and snow can fly as early as October. No water is available at the trailhead or on the lava flow.

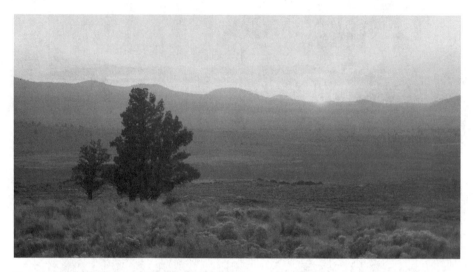

The sun sets behind the remnants of Medicine Lake Volcano.

To Reach the Trailhead A high-clearance vehicle is recommended for the rough access roads, though they are usually passable with care in a low-clearance vehicle. Take Hwy. 97 west from Hwy. 139 for 20 miles to unpaved Forest Service Road 43N99 on the right, the first of three possible turnoffs for Glass Mountain. (Approaching from the west, the turnoff is 4.8 miles east of the junction of Hwys. 49 and 97. Don't be tempted by the GLASS MOUNTAIN signs you see at the first two turnoffs at 1.1 miles and 3.9 miles from the junction.) As you head north on FS 43N99, astonishing views of the flow appear before you reach a small, posted pullout at its base, 3.9 miles from Hwy. 97.

Description From the trailhead (0.0/7,050') head up the obvious path. The lava flow has been worked by heavy machinery, and numerous paths wind this way and that. While none of them really go anywhere, they make for considerably easier walking than over the jagged piles of rock. Obsidian is visible everywhere, glinting in the sunlight, interlaid with enormous amounts of gray pumice. A few scattered lodgepole and western white pines pioneer this moonscape. Mount Hoffman (7,913') is almost due west and Red Shale Butte (7,834') is south, easily identified by the bare red nubbin at its summit. These mountains are two of the smaller volcanoes that welled up along the fracture zone after the mountaintop collapsed. Glass Mountain (7,622') is the bluff visible north, the highest point on the lava flow. Wander as much as you like, but don't lose your bearings in the maze of trails.

Nearest Visitor Center Doublehead Ranger District Office, 530-667-2246, just southeast of the town of Tulelake on Hwy. 139, is open Monday–Friday 8 a.m.–4:30 p.m.

Nearest Campgrounds There are 4 campgrounds around Medicine Lake (72 sites total, $14 per vehicle).

Additional Information www.fs.usda.gov/modoc

HIKE 64   Patterson Lake ⤢ 🚶 🐕

Highlight	The heart of South Warner Wilderness
Distance	10.2 miles round-trip
Total Elevation Gain/Loss	2,900'/2,900'
Hiking Time	8–12 hours
Recommended Maps	*South Warner Wilderness* by the US Forest Service, USGS 7.5-min. *Soup Creek, Eagle Peak,* and *Warren Peak*
Best Times	Mid-June–October
Agency	South Warner Wilderness, Modoc National Forest
Difficulty	★★★★

HERE'S A hike to the heart of a small piece of mountain paradise.

The Hike climbs to Patterson Lake (9,040') through Pine Creek Basin, a strenuous trip that packs in all the wilderness has to offer, from soaring raptors to crystalline creeks, from sweeping panoramic vistas to the largest lake in the wilderness. The hike's second half, climbing out of Pine Creek Basin, is steep, sustained, and shadeless—skin-frying conditions during the summer months. Those looking for a shorter excursion should make the 4.6-mile round-trip to the Pine Creek crossing, a less demanding hike to a wonderful picnic spot. October is the nicest time to visit as aspens turn gold and weather is ideal. Snow can linger well into June along upper sections of the trail. While no water is available at the trailhead, Pine Creek is soon accessible.

To Reach the Trailhead Take Hwy. 64 east from the town of Likely on Hwy. 395. In 9 miles, bear left on Hwy. 5 by a sign for Mill Creek Lodge. Proceed 3 miles to the turnoff for Mill Creek Campground. The paved road turns right but you continue straight on the unpaved but easily traveled gravel road for 1.7 miles to an unposted Y-junction—bear left and continue on Hwy. 5 for 5.3 miles to the posted turnoff for the Pine Creek Trail. Turn right, reaching the parking lot at the road's end in 1.4 miles. Approaching from the north, take Parker Creek Rd. (Hwy. 56) east from Alturas for 14 miles to

where Hwys. 31 and 5 split. Head south on Hwy. 5 for 10.5 miles to the Pine Creek Trail turnoff.

Description An information sign and register mark the start of the trail. From the trailhead (0.0/6,800') the singletrack trail passes through thick white fir where babbling Pine Creek can be heard unseen below you. The firs increase in size and are joined by large ponderosa pines as you cross into the wilderness by an idyllic stream confluence. Fill your water bottles here because the trail next travels away from the creek, seldom approaching it.

Becoming progressively steeper, the trail passes near several, shallow, swampy lakes before reaching the open meadows of Pine Creek Basin (2.3/7,400'). While the trail crosses the creek and reenters the trees, you should continue a short distance ahead to an ideal picnic spot by a small bend in the creek. Of volcanic origin, Warner Mountains' rocks were formed from ash and lava flows extruded on the landscape roughly 30 million years ago. Within the past 2 million years, glaciers carved the upper mountain reaches and formed the broad bowl of Pine Creek Basin.

Back on the main trail, you begin the long, brutal climb to the ridgecrest above. Views become increasingly expansive as the exposed path climbs through sagebrush, mule's ears, and spring-fed patches of corn lilies. A few isolated whitebark pines dot the slopes. Mount Shasta's distinct cone more than 100 miles west becomes visible near the top before you reach

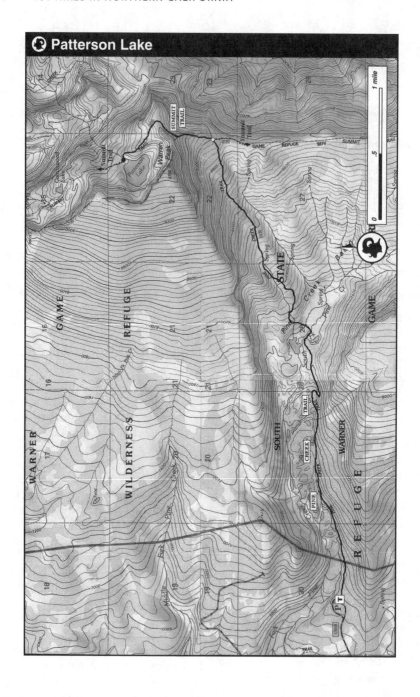

Patterson Lake

the ridge and the junction with the Summit Trail (4.2/9,000').

Views east suddenly open up and the deep basin of Surprise Valley lies below you, brimming with the salt-encrusted trinity of Upper, Middle, and Lower Alkali Lakes. Enclosed by Nevada peaks to the east, the lakes fill depressions in a graben, a valley formed through extension of the earth's crust. Also known as a "pull-apart basin," it occurs when a large block of crust drops along parallel fault lines relative to the adjacent landscape. This is the defining geography of the Basin and Range Province, a distinct geologic region that essentially begins here and continues east to Utah. Surprise Valley is more than 4,000 feet below you on the Summit Trail and, presumably, still dropping. Eagle Peak (9,892'), the highest peak in the Warner Mountains, is visible almost due south.

Turning north, the trail continues to climb before finally cresting a rise and dropping 300 feet to Patterson Lake (5.1/9,040'). Exceedingly deep and green, Patterson Lake was formed 1.8 million years ago through glacial erosion. Backed by the sheer layered cliffs of Warren Peak (9,710'), it boils with rainbow trout and is excellent for fly-fishing. Rest and rejuvenate here before returning the way you came.

Nearest Visitor Centers Warner Mountain Ranger District Office, 530-279-6116, is inconveniently located in Cedarville on the east side of the Warner Mountains and open Monday–Friday 8 a.m.–4:30 p.m. Also try the Modoc National Forest Supervisor's Office, 530-233-5811, on Main St. in Alturas and open Monday–Friday 8 a.m.–5 p.m.

Backpacking Information No wilderness permit is needed, but a valid campfire permit is required. Campsites are located around Patterson Lake and in the Pine Creek Basin.

Nearest Campground Soup Spring Campground is a few miles to the south (8 sites, $12 in summer, free after Labor Day). When approaching from the south, bear right instead of left at the unposted Y-junction and proceed 5.6 miles to the campground turnoff.

Additional Information www.fs.usda.gov/modoc

HIKE 65 Burney Falls ⟳ 🚶

Highlight	A perennial waterfall unlike any other
Distance	1.2 miles
Total Elevation Gain/Loss	200'/200'
Hiking Time	1 hour
Recommended Map	USGS 7.5-min. *Burney Falls*
Best Times	April–November
Agency	McArthur–Burney Falls Memorial State Park
Difficulty	★

PICTURE A VOLCANIC CLIFF 129 feet high. Over its lip, twin waterfalls cascade into an iridescent pool. Springs gush from its face, showering lush vegetation with spray while birds dart through rainbow refractions of light. This is Burney Falls.

The unusual multitiered falls result from two distinct geologic layers stacked on top of each other. The upper layer is the porous Burney Basalt, which allows water to easily percolate to the nonporous formation underneath. Both layers are exposed in the cliff face, where water pours forth in a constant year-round flow. The volume of Burney Creek, spring fed less than a mile above the falls, varies little with season; the entire system gushes a steady 100 million gallons of water a day. The moist corridor below the falls is an ecologic oasis, harboring species not normally seen in the Modoc Plateau. Oregon oak, Douglas-fir, vine maple, flowering currant, and bear clover are at the far limit of their respective ranges, accompanied by the more typical assortment of Jeffrey pine, black oak, and manzanita. The fish of nearby Lake Britton attract osprey and bald eagles, sometimes seen soaring overhead.

The Hike is an easy loop that descends to viewpoints of Burney Falls and explores the ecology of Burney Creek with the help of interpretive placards. The park is open year-round, but snow may cover the trail from Thanksgiving until April. Crowds are extremely heavy from Memorial Day through Labor Day. Fishing is popular (but challenging) in Burney Creek, although strict regulations govern the stretch of water below the falls. Above the falls, standard regulations apply and the fishing is just as good. Water is available at the trailhead.

To Reach the Trailhead Take Hwy. 89 north for 5 miles from the junction of Hwys. 89 and 299 to the park entrance. A day-use fee of $8 per vehicle is charged. Park in the lot across from the visitor center.

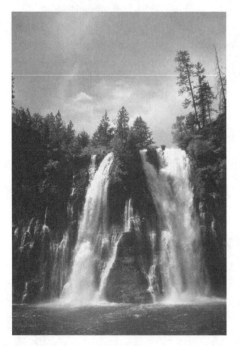

Burney Falls

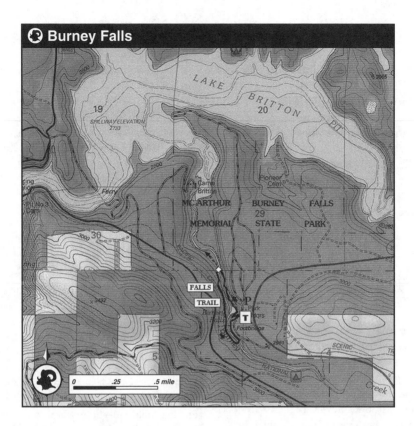

Description From the parking lot, descend to the falls along the wide paved path, enjoying the cool 65°F temperature near the bottom. Continue downstream on the paved trail below large piles of broken Burney basalt. Notice the springs that continually gush from the opposite streambank, indicating surface exposures of the geologic formation below the basalt. Cross the first bridge and continue on the dirt trail that heads an additional 50 yards downstream and splits—go left on the Falls Trail.

Heading uphill away from the creek, the trail quickly reaches the level of the falls. Although unseen, the falls sound louder and more powerful here. Cross the river above the falls on a bridge (memorialized by visitors' chisel marks) to where the trail once again divides. Head left (downstream) to another parking lot where a rock-lined pedestrian path paralleling the road gets you back to the starting point. A half mile upstream from the bridge, the riverbed springs make an interesting side trip.

Nearest Visitor Center The park visitor center, 530-335-2777, is open daily in summer 10 a.m.–4 p.m.

Nearest Campground The state park campground has 104 sites ($35, open year-round) and 24 cabins ($85–$105, open mid-April–mid-October). Reservations are recommended in the summer; call 800-444-7275 or visit **reserveamerica.com.**

Additional Information **www.parks.ca.gov**

HIKE 66 Magee Peak ↗ 🚶 🐴

Highlights	The remote rim of an extinct volcano, plus backcountry lakes
Distance	12.0 miles round-trip
Total Elevation Gain/Loss	3,200'/3,200'
Hiking Time	5–7 hours
Recommended Maps	*Ishi, Thousand Lakes, and Caribou Wildernesses Map & Guide* by the US Forest Service, USGS 7.5-min. *Thousand Lakes Valley*
Best Times	July–September
Agency	Thousand Lakes Wilderness, Lassen National Forest
Difficulty	★★★★

THOUSAND LAKES OFFERS a less traveled wilderness in the Modoc Plateau, complete with alpine lakes and sweeping mountain summits. Here you can contemplate the construction and destruction of a volcano from atop an eroding crater rim.

Spawned from the same volcanic activity that created Lassen Peak, Thousand Lakes Volcano has not been active in historical times. Although it was likely created within the past million years, it has been dormant long enough for a glacier to eat away its northeastern slopes and leave a horseshoe of peaks around the former crater. One of them, Crater Peak (8,683'), is the highest point in Lassen National Forest. Thousand Lakes Wilderness is small, only 16,335 acres, and does not have one thousand lakes—more like a dozen.

The Hike ascends Magee Peak (8,549'), one of the peaks along the volcano's summit rim, passing several lakes along the way. Two of them, Everett and Magee, are roughly midway and make a worthwhile destination for those unprepared for the full ascent. The approach described here from Cypress Trailhead in the northwestern corner of the wilderness receives lighter use than Tamarack Trailhead farther east. While this approach adds about 500 feet of elevation gain, it avoids the popular but less exciting Lake Eiler area. You are more likely to encounter equestrians than hikers on this trail. Fishing is worthwhile throughout the wilderness. No water is available at the trailhead, and

none can be easily obtained for the first 3.5 miles and 1,600 feet of ascent.

To Reach the Trailhead Prepare yourself to cover some dirt roads. Take Hwy. 89 north from the junction of Hwys. 89 and 44 in Old Station for 11.8 miles to the turnoff for Forest Service Rd. 26, 0.3 mile past the Hat Creek Work Center. Approaching from the north, the turnoff is 1.6 miles south of the Hat Creek Fire Station and post office. Reset your odometer at the turnoff and head west on the unpaved road to the first junction (mile 3.6)—bear right to continue on FS 26. Turn left at the next junction (mile 5.3), still continuing on FS 26. At mile 8.3, turn left onto FS 34N60 and follow it to the road's end at mile 11.0. The information sign at the head of the parking area marks the trailhead.

Description From the trailhead (0.0/5,520'), you pass through stands of sugar pine, red and white fir, juniper, and Jeffrey pine before quickly crossing rocky and seasonally dry Eiler Gulch. From here, a steady climb brings you into the wilderness. Shortly after the weathered boundary sign (1.0/6,240') the trail levels out and reaches a junction (1.2/6,330')—go right toward Barrett and Magee Lakes. A left turn would bring you to large but shallow Lake Eiler, a side trip not recommended unless you are desperate for water. Crossing Eiler Gulch, bear right again at two subsequent nearby junctions and stay on the trail (3E04) toward Magee Peak.

The trail switchbacks steeply southwest before leveling out in a forest where western white

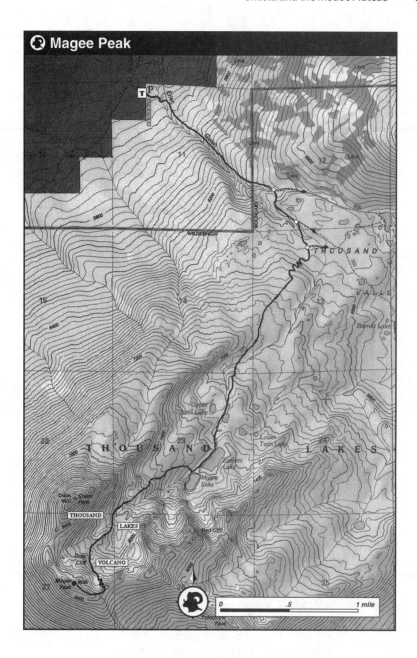

⊘ Magee Peak

and lodgepole pine enter the mix. Mountain hemlock can also be identified near the lakes. After a long, level stretch and a brief climb, you pass dried-up Upper Twin Lake and soon reach Everett Lake (3.6/7,180'). Magee Lake is next, accessed by going left on the unposted spur trail after Everett Lake. Both lakes are pretty and deep—good for relaxing and swimming.

Now climbing again, you enter the heart of the ancient volcano, with Crater Peak towering above to the west. The trees are now almost exclusively mountain hemlock, although a smattering of whitebark pine can also be seen. The views become more expansive as you ascend up-canyon past the prominent red outcrops to the east, climbing nine steep switchbacks on the loose upper slopes to finally reach the summit ridge (5.3/8,400'). Traverse west along the ridge to stand on top of Magee Peak (5.5/8,549').

As you look northeast, the scouring force of the glacier that carved this volcano is obvious. The broad valley formed by the glacier turns east below Freaner Peak (7,485'), a satellite vent of the same volcanic complex. Fredonyer Peak (8,054') is the summit on the ridge extending due east from the crater rim. Lassen Peak (10,457') is an easy landmark to the south, and Chaos Crags (Hike 67) are visible below its northern flanks. The ridge extending west from Lassen Peak ends in Brokeoff Mountain (9,235', Hike 68), the highest remnant of Mount Tehama. This ancient volcano once rose above present-day Lassen Volcanic National Park and was probably contemporary with Thousand Lakes Volcano. Return the way you came.

Nearest Visitor Centers Old Station Information Center, at the junction of Hwys. 89 and 44, is open daily April–December; summer hours are 9:30 a.m.–4 p.m., with reduced hours in the spring and fall. The Hat Creek Ranger District Office, 530-336-5521, is located in Fall River Mills on Hwy. 299 and is open Monday–Friday 8 a.m.–4:30 p.m.

Backpacking Information No wilderness permit is required, but a valid campfire permit is necessary. Both Everett and Magee Lakes have good campsites.

Nearest Campground Honn Campground (6 sites without water, $10) is 2.1 miles south of the turnoff for FS 26 on Hwy. 89.

Additional Information www.fs.usda.gov/lassen

HIKE 67 Chaos Crags ↗

Highlights	An ephemeral frog pond below a 2,000-foot-high jumble of volcanic rock
Distance	4.0 miles round-trip
Total Elevation Gain/Loss	1,050'/1,050'
Hiking Time	2–3 hours
Recommended Maps	*Lassen Volcanic National Park* by Wilderness Press, USGS 7.5-min. *Manzanita Lake*
Best Times	Mid-June–September
Agency	Lassen Volcanic National Park
Difficulty	★★

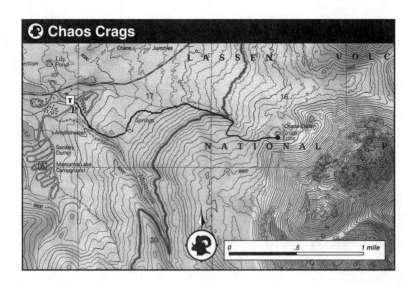

ROUGHLY 1,000 YEARS AGO, lava was extruded from Lassen Peak's northern flank. Too viscous to flow downhill, it piled up as giant domes of solid rock covered in loose rubble—Chaos Crags. A minor explosion about 300 years ago along Chaos Crags' northwestern slope triggered a huge landslide that traveled more than 2 miles to dam Manzanita Creek and form Manzanita Lake. Dubbed the Chaos Jumbles, the chaotic remains of the slide are plainly evident today.

The Hike climbs from the northwest corner of the park to tiny Crags Lake at the base of Chaos Crags. The "lake" is really a small pond fed only by snowmelt, which slowly evaporates over the course of the summer. Although largest in late June, it's never really big enough to be nice for swimming. Depending on conditions, it can be completely dry by August or remain as a tiny puddle throughout the season. Visitation here is relatively light, especially compared with other national parks. No water is available at the trailhead.

To Reach the Trailhead Take Hwy. 89 to the Loomis Museum in the northwest corner of the park, 0.4 mile east of the Manzanita Lake Entrance Station. There is a $10 entrance fee for Lassen Volcanic National Park, valid for seven days. At the east end of the museum parking lot, turn south on the road to Manzanita Lake. The trailhead is almost immediately on the left in 0.1 mile. If there is no space for your vehicle here, park in the museum lot and walk to the trailhead.

Description The path, running within earshot of rushing Manzanita Creek, is initially outlined with large volcanic boulders. Jeffrey pine and white fir comprise this open forest. The trail soon arcs away from the creek into dense trees and shortly passes a lush spring, which feeds a brook lined with alder trees. Sugar pine and red fir begin to appear. A few scattered Douglas-firs can be identified, too, by their distinctive cones around you on the ground. The trail next ascends adjacent to the hummocky moonscape of Chaos Jumbles, occasionally visible through the trees. Chaos Crags increasingly loom east above the treetops, where the trail enters more open terrain carpeted with manzanita scrub. You pass through lodgepole pine a few hundred feet before breaking out into a rough boulder field with epic views of Chaos Crags.

The final stretch to Crags Lake (6,630') is the most challenging, a 100-foot descent through sand and loose rock. Hundreds of tadpoles inhabit the lake, and many mature frogs lurk along the moist shore, hurtling themselves behind nearby rocks at the approach of the curious hiker. Most trees here are sugar pines, although a few white firs and Jeffrey pines can be seen. A small chokecherry sits above the east end of the pond. Also known as Chaos Crater, this basin was created from the blast that triggered the massive landslide of Chaos Jumbles. Above, the pink-scree slopes of Chaos Crags are deceptively high (not recommended for exploration); it's 1,900 feet from the lake to the top of the highest promontory at 8,530 feet.

Nearest Visitor Center Loomis Museum and Visitor Center, 530-595-6140, ext. 5180, is open daily 9 a.m.–5 p.m. mid-June–September, and weekends only Memorial Day–mid-June.

Nearest Campground Manzanita Lake Campground (179 sites, $18) is on the south side of Manzanita Lake.

Additional Information nps.gov/lavo

HIKE 68 Brokeoff Mountain ⬈

Highlights	The eroded lip of an ancient volcano and far-reaching views of contemporary volcanoes
Distance	7.4 miles round-trip
Total Elevation Gain/Loss	2,600'/2,600'
Hiking Time	4–6 hours
Recommended Maps	*Lassen Volcanic National Park* by Wilderness Press, USGS 7.5-min. *Lassen Peak*
Best Times	July–September
Agency	Lassen Volcanic National Park
Difficulty	★★★★

EVERYBODY LIKES to climb Lassen Peak. Instead, you should try Brokeoff Mountain— a less traveled summit with views every bit as exceptional.

Brokeoff Mountain (9,235') is the highest remnant of the former Mount Tehama, a huge stratovolcano, which began erupting 600,000 years ago and grew to be over 11 miles wide at its base. Erosion and structural collapse wasted away the volcano core once major activity stopped 200,000 years ago, leaving only the volcanic slopes. Lassen Peak (10,457') was

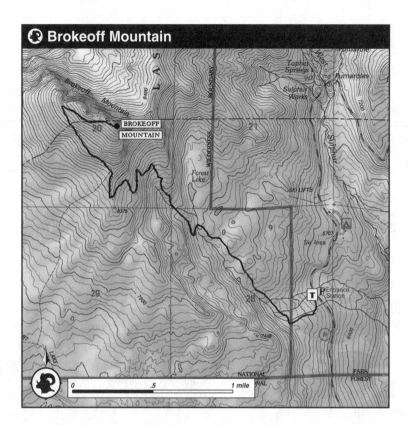

Brokeoff Mountain

formed from more recent eruptions along the eroded eastern flanks of Mount Tehama some 11,000 years ago.

The Hike climbs Brokeoff Mountain from the park road near the south entrance station, a strenuous trip flush with wildflowers in July and early August. Snow can linger a long time in Lassen Volcanic National Park and usually does not disappear on this trail until very late June or early July. While less popular than the Lassen Peak Trail, this hike still receives ample use during the summer. No water is available at the trailhead, but sources are plentiful along the first half of the hike.

To Reach the Trailhead Take Hwy. 89 to the park's southwest edge. The trailhead is 0.4 mile south of the entrance station on the west side of the road. Parking is opposite the trailhead. There is a $10 entrance fee for Lassen Volcanic

National Park, valid for seven days. Those approaching from the south are still required to pay at the entrance station or at the self-registration kiosk at the trailhead.

Description From the trailhead (0.0/6,600'), you immediately start climbing through dense alder thickets. After crossing a small stream, the trail breaks out into a more open forest of red fir, incense cedar, and western white pine. The rocky pyramid of Brokeoff's summit is a beacon already visible northwest above the trees as you continue upward to rejoin the earlier stream. Paralleling the water, the trail crosses a small creek outlet (1.2/7,460') from tiny, unseen Forest Lake, and then starts to climb more rapidly. As you gain elevation, mountain hemlock appear and soon views open up—Lake Almanor is visible southeast, and Forest Lake just below you. Leaving the creek (and your last water source), you traverse below the imposing southeast face of Brokeoff Mountain, making a few switchbacks among dense mats of lupine before cresting the mountain's south ridge (2.4/8,400'). On a steady ascending traverse northwest, you have good views west across the Great Central Valley. All the trees here are mountain hemlock, most bursting with tiny cones. Near the ridgetop, the trail cuts back east, passing below a satellite summit before finally reaching the top (3.7/9,235'). A few scraggly whitebark pines and an anomalous, krummholz Jeffrey pine are growing from the rocky hillside just below the summit.

Grab a seat on the flat summit and admire the view. Looking northeast, Mount Diller (9,087') is the highest peak between you and imposing Lassen Peak. Mount Diller is another remnant of Mount Tehama; the bands exposed below its western ridge are hardened flows that once coursed down the western flanks of the long-gone volcano. North beyond these bands are Chaos Crags (Hike 67) and more distant Thousand Lakes Volcano (Hike 66). Turning east-southeast, Mount Conard (8,204') is the bare, sandy-looking ridgetop across the deep valley of Mill Creek. Some 200,000 years ago, the towering summit of Mount Tehama rose between you and Mount Conard directly above today's Sulphur Works, the parking lot of which is visible more than 2,000 feet below. When you're ready, back down you go!

Nearest Visitor Center The Kohm Yah-mah-nee Visitor Center, 530-595-4480, is located at the southwest entrance of the park off Hwy. 36 on Hwy. 89. It's open daily 9 a.m.–5 p.m. year-round, and closed Mondays and Tuesdays in winter.

Backpacking Information While backpacking is allowed on this hike, the lack of good campsites makes it less appealing than day-hiking. A wilderness permit is required and is available at the visitor center, as well as at the southwest entrance station and the Loomis Museum and Visitor Center, 530-595-6140, ext. 5180. Loomis Visitor Center is open 9 a.m.–5 p.m. daily mid-June–September, and weekends only Memorial Day–mid-June.

Nearest Campgrounds Southwest Campground (20 sites, $14) is a walk-in campground by the southwest entrance station. The Summit Lake campgrounds in the center of the park are the closest drive-in options.

Additional Information nps.gov/lavo

HIKE 69 Devils Kitchen ⤢

Highlight	Geothermal action away from the crowds
Distance	5.0 miles round-trip
Total Elevation Gain/Loss	700'/700'
Hiking Time	2–3 hours
Recommended Maps	*Lassen Volcanic National Park* by Wilderness Press, USGS 7.5-min. *Reading Peak*
Best Times	Mid-June–September
Agency	Lassen Volcanic National Park
Difficulty	★★

CALIFORNIA LIVES, breathing outward in hissing fumaroles and fetid mudpots. While most experience bubbling volcanic activity along the mobbed trail to Bumpass Hell, you should come—away from the crowds—to Devils Kitchen.

Underneath Lassen Volcanic National Park, at least 6 miles deep, is a large body of molten rock. Groundwater encountering it is heated to extraordinary temperatures, sometimes in excess of 500°F. Kept in liquid form by intense pressures found at such depths, the super-heated water rises and flashes to steam near the surface. Boiling pools and billowing fumaroles are the result. Most of the hot water rises vertically to Bumpass Hell, but several substantial lateral flows exist, including the one spewing out at Devils Kitchen.

The Hike is an easy one, following Hot Springs Creek to a substantial area of geothermal activity. It is a quieter section, accessed far from the main park road and receiving light use. A great early summer hike for wildflowers, it generally receives light use in the fall. While no water is available at the trailhead, Hot Springs Creek is accessible early on.

To Reach the Trailhead Take Hwy. 36 to Chester and turn north on Feather River Drive—the turnoff is across from Plumas Bank at the east end of town. In 0.7 mile, bear left at the fork to stay on Feather River Rd. Drive 5.7 miles to another fork. Bear right and follow Warner Valley Road 10.6 miles to the trailhead parking lot, on the left immediately past Warner Valley Campground. The last 3.1 miles are unpaved with steep grades—not recommended for RVs or trailers. A $10 entrance fee is due at the self-pay entrance station just inside the park boundary.

Description At the trailhead (0.0/5,670'), brochures are available for Boiling Springs Lake Nature Trail, a 3-mile interpretive trail to Cold Boiling Lake that parallels this hike for a short distance to Stop 9. Our trail begins on the Pacific Crest Trail (PCT) and immediately heads to Hot Springs Creek, briefly following it before crossing a rusting metal bridge and heading slightly upslope. A hot spring can be seen flowing directly out of the ground at Stop 8, the water almost too hot to touch. This water, along with that from other nearby hot springs, flows into the baths at Drakesbad Guest Ranch, visible across the broad meadow. Unfortunately, the baths are for guests only.

At Stop 9, the trail reaches a four-way junction (0.3/5,730') by a large incense cedar. The Cold Boiling Lake Nature Trail and PCT head left, and straight leads to Drake Lake, but you turn right and head back downslope. You reach another junction immediately prior to recrossing the creek. Turning left here leads to Dream Lake, a nearby shallow pond where beavers can sometimes be spotted, but you continue straight across the alder-choked stream and enter the wide, open meadow. A few paths from the ranch join your trail, now winding along the north side of the meadow. You reenter a dense forest of predominantly white fir (1.1/5,760') and soon reach another junction. An optional return trail splits left to join the trail leading to Drake Lake. A slow and gentle climb ahead toward Devils Kitchen ends by a hitching post atop a small rise, where the sulfuric stench of geothermal activity first assaults your nose.

A 0.5-mile loop trail runs through Devils Kitchen, with informative placards and a stern warning not to go off the trail. Enjoy the fantastic hues of technicolor rock, accompanied by the dull roar of venting fumaroles and the musical bass of bubbling mudpots.

Nearest Visitor Centers The Kohm Yah-mah-nee Visitor Center, 530-595-4480, is located at the southwest entrance of the park, off Hwy. 36 on Hwy. 89. It's open daily 9 a.m.–5 p.m. year-round, and closed Mondays and Tuesdays in winter. Warner Valley Ranger Station, just east of Warner Valley Campground, is open sporadically when park staff are around—try knocking on the door.

Nearest Campground Warner Valley Campground (18 sites, $14) is 0.5 mile east of the trailhead.

Additional Information nps.gov/lavo

HIKE 70 Big Chico Creek

Highlights	Bountiful valley woodlands and a basalt gorge
Distance	3.5 miles round-trip
Total Elevation Gain/Loss	600'/600'
Hiking Time	3–5 hours
Recommended Maps	USGS 7.5-min. *Richardson Springs* and *Paradise West*
Best Times	Spring and fall
Agency	Bidwell Park
Difficulty	★★

BIDWELL PARK provides a living diorama— a glimpse of the bounty and rich diversity of life that once flourished in the Great Central Valley. It's also good for swimming.

In 1905, John and Annie Bidwell donated this land to the city of Chico for the public's use and enjoyment. The third-largest municipal park in the country after New York's Central Park and Portland's Forest Park, it is a beautiful tract along Big Chico Creek, a lush riparian alley winding through dry oak woodlands. Fremont cottonwoods, California bays, willows, Oregon ash, white alders, California box elders, bigleaf maples, and California sycamores line the creek; their trunks are interwoven by the twisting tendrils of wild grapevines. Valley oaks, blue oaks, interior live oaks, canyon live oaks, gray pines, California buckeyes, black walnuts, and Chinese stink trees thrive on the dry slopes away from the creek. Flowers and some trees offer seasonal displays of color, and bird life abounds year-round. In Upper Bidwell Park, sheer canyons carved through erosion-resistant basalt result in wild formations of rock, stripped clean of soil and plant life for long sections.

The Hike winds along Big Chico Creek in Upper Bidwell Park, passing through lush creekside vegetation before threading up through basalt outcroppings to the canyon rim and park road. (A bicycle or vehicle left at Parking Lot P would facilitate an easy return to the trailhead.) While the hike can be done year-round, it is sizzling in the summer months, with daily highs

hovering around 100°F. Fall and spring provide the most ideal temperatures. Sun protection is always worth having. Fishing is prohibited in Big Chico Creek. No water is available at the trailhead. Note that trails are often closed after heavy rains in winter and spring.

To Reach the Trailhead Take Hwy. 99 in Chico to the East 8th St./Hwy. 32 off-ramp, and head east on E. 8th St. for 2 miles to Chico Canyon Rd. Turn left and go 0.6 mile to Centennial Ave. Turn right, and 0.5 mile farther turn right again onto Wildwood Ave., immediately beyond the sign for Upper Bidwell Park. After 1.9 miles of road, with speed bumps by the golf course, you reach a gate, which is open Fridays and Saturdays. If you're here on those days, proceed 0.7 mile past the gate to Parking Lot F on the right. If not, park in nearby Parking Lot E and walk the short distance to the trailhead. The last 0.4 mile is unpaved.

Description From the parking lot (0.0/ 300'), take the widest, most obvious trail down to the creek and begin heading upstream. Throughout this hike, numerous use paths branch this way and that, but the main trail close to the stream is generally obvious. A posted spur trail soon leads down to the Day Camp swimming area, overshadowed by layered basalt—a pancake stack—exposed near the top of the opposite cut bank.

Known as the Lovejoy Basalt, it's a result of volcanic flows 18 million years old that originated somewhere east of present-day Susanville. With no intervening mountains present

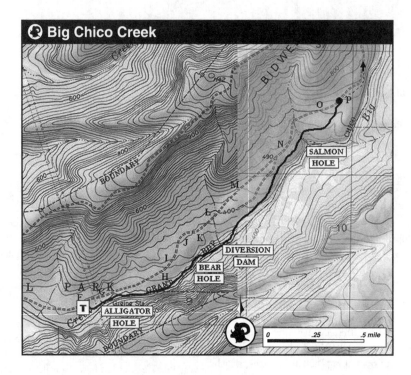

at the time, the flows coursed southwest, nearly reaching the present site of Winters in the middle of the Great Central Valley. Existing rocks in what is now Bidwell Park were coated with a thick layer of erosion-resistant basalt. The underlying rocks compose the Chico Formation, formed approximately 75–100 million years ago just offshore from the continental edge. Sediments washed into the sea were deposited in beds thousands of feet thick, becoming shale and sandstone over time. Where exposed by the down-cutting of Big Chico Creek, this formation provides good soil for the rich plant life around you.

Continuing upstream, you soon reach Bear Hole (0.7/300'), where there's a remarkable change in scenery. Here the creek has not eroded through the Lovejoy Formation and instead flows through surprising basalt formations bare of most vegetation. Numerous signs warn of the swimming hazards in this treacherous section. From here, it is possible to walk along the creek a short distance on the remains of an old cement flume. Passing through a narrow basalt gorge with sheer, 40-foot walls, the flume ends at an old diversion dam. A mildly precarious stairway requires a bit of scrambling to get here. An alternative stretch of trail skirts this section along the canyon rim.

Now at the top of the stairs, follow the shadeless trail along the canyon rim to an overlook of Salmon Hole (1.6/530'), a deep, accessible swimming spot in the gorge below. Beyond this point, the canyon below becomes wider and difficult to access. It is possible to continue to the northern reaches of Upper Bidwell Park, but this hike—having sampled what the park offers—ends where the trail rejoins the park road at Parking Lot P. Return the way you came or via the park road.

Nearest Visitor Center Chico Creek Nature Center, 530-891-4671, is on E. 8th St., 1 mile east of the Hwy. 99 off-ramp, and is open Wednesday–Saturday 11 a.m.–4 p.m.

Nearest Campground Woodson Bridge State Recreation Area (35 sites, $25) is 20 miles northwest of Chico along the banks of the Sacramento River. Take South Ave. 3 miles west of Vina on Hwy. 99.

Additional Information ccnaturecenter.org

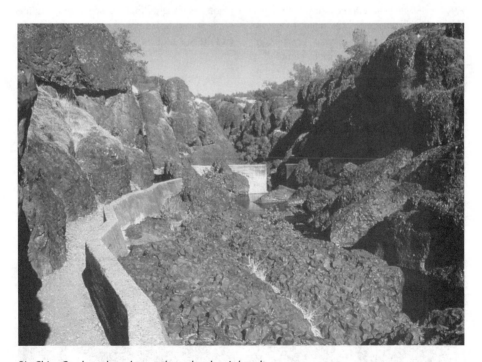

Big Chico Creek pools and pours through volcanic basalt.

The Sierra Nevada

FOR THE PURPOSES of this book, the Sierra Nevada stretches north from southern Sequoia National Park to the edge of the Modoc Plateau near Lake Almanor and includes a few locations east of the range. Ranging in height from more than 14,000 feet at its southern end to barely 7,000 feet at its northern terminus, the range is characterized by jagged peaks, major rivers, and countless alpine lakes. While naked granite composes much of the range, a more complicated geologic mix is prevalent in the northern regions.

Annual precipitation is high and arrives in the form of heavy winter snows that melt throughout the summer, creating a broad forest belt that extends upward to about 10,000 feet. The highest elevations support only bare expanses of rock, snow, and hardy low-lying plants. Highlights include spectacular alpine scenery, unique landforms, deep river canyons, and the magnificent giant sequoia.

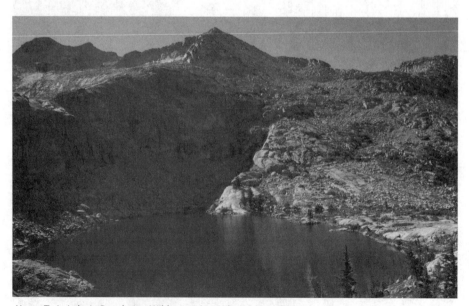

Upper Twin Lake in Desolation Wilderness (see Hike 75, page 252)

HIKE 71   Feather Falls ○

Highlight	The sixth-highest waterfall in the continental United States
Distance	7.4 miles round-trip
Total Elevation Gain/Loss	1,650'/1,650'
Hiking Time	4–5 hours
Recommended Map	USGS 7.5-min. *Brush Creek*
Best Times	April–October
Agency	Plumas National Forest
Difficulty	★★★

ON THE WESTERN FLANKS of the northern Sierra Nevada, Feather Falls Scenic Area protects 15,000 acres of diverse forest and lush scenery. Its highlight is a spectacular overlook of Feather Falls dropping 640 feet down a sheer cliff face. An unusual range of forest diversity provides a secondary bonus; more than 180 species of flowers, 17 species of trees, 20 shrubs, 11 vines, and 10 ferns have all been identified along this hike.

The Hike makes a counterclockwise loop from the trailhead to Feather Falls and back, traveling first along a longer, easier, and more scenic upper trail and returning via a shorter, less-traveled, and steeper lower trail. Note that the bridge over Frey Creek on the lower trail is currently broken but still passable. Poison oak is present on the hike, though not abundant.

To Reach the Trailhead Take Hwy. 162 east from Hwy. 70 in Oroville for 7.3 miles, turn right on Forbestown Rd., and proceed for 6.1 miles to Lumpkin Rd. Turn right on Lumpkin Rd. and follow its winding grade for 10.9 miles to FS 21N35Y. Turn left here and continue 1.7 miles to the large trailhead parking area.

Description From the trailhead (0.0/2,460'), strike out on the wide, smooth trail among young second-growth Douglas-fir, ponderosa pine, and incense cedar. An octacular canyon live oak, its myriad twisting branches lush with gardens of moss, highlights this early section as does another monster live oak with a large fire scar chamber in its trunk.

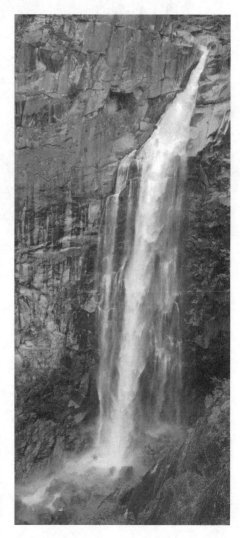

Feather Falls

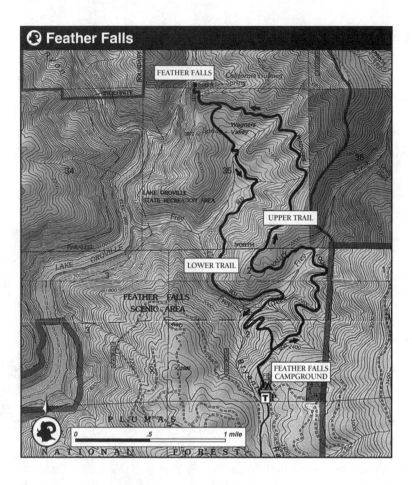

You soon reach a signed fork for the upper and lower trails (0.4/2,380'). Left is the most direct route, but you bear right on the upper trail to curve around a small drainage and pass some large Douglas-firs joined by stout white firs. Joining them in this diverse forest are occasional madrone trees (watch for their peeling bark) and small tanoak and dogwood trees, which are indicative of the increased precipitation this region gets compared to the drier foothills farther south.

You cross the deepest drainage yet on a nice wooden bridge (1.4/2,280') and begin contouring into the Frey Creek drainage. Crossing the creek on a stout three-section bridge (1.5/2,050'), the trail then ascends to reach a bench and excellent view of Bald Rock Dome (2.0/2,260'), a distinctive landmark of the Middle Fork Feather River canyon rising nearly 2,000 feet above the river. Part of the Bald Rock pluton, it's an unusual mass of granite in an otherwise metamorphic landscape.

The continuing trail slowly descends on an easy-cruising section, then rises slightly to reach the far junction of the lower trail (3.6/1,970'). Continuing to the falls, you climb a pair of switchbacks to reach an old concrete section of singletrack trail, which traverses steadily uphill to a fenced overlook of the confluence of Fall River and Middle Fork Feather River far below.

The fence protects you on the left as the path contours toward increasingly visible Feather Falls; then two descending switchbacks lead you to a steep metal staircase. At its end is a decagonal viewing platform perched on a large rock outcrop that overlooks the entirety of Feather Falls (3.9/2,050').

Savor the majesty of this dramatic waterfall, which plummets as a sheeting curtain of thundering water that explodes on the rocks below. To the west, you can peer down the Feather River drainage as it makes its last curves prior to entering Lake Oroville.

After you've reached waterfall saturation, retrace your steps to the earlier junction, and bear right on the lower trail (4.2/1,970') for a faster return to the trailhead. The narrower lower trail descends past a few brief level areas—some of the few potential (but dry) camping spots on this hike—then drops steeply on a mildly overgrown path that eventually levels out in a grove of incense cedar.

Continuing, you traverse steadily downward and make a curving U around a deep drainage. Evidence of recent fire is apparent in the surrounding forest, including dead manzanita bushes and fire-scarred ponderosa pine. You encounter a random bench and then rediscover the old concrete path, which you follow as it briefly drops. The route now ascends steadily into the Frey Creek drainage, passing below some impressive cliffs of granite before reaching a sitting rock with a nice view up-canyon toward Bald Rock Dome.

As you approach Frey Creek, the trail passes its first easy water access by a bench and bouldery moss garden, and then reaches the creek crossing. The wide six-plank bridge here has cracked in the middle and is sagging into the stream, though it remains easily passable. Beyond it, you pass another bench by a massive ponderosa pine and reach the earlier junction with the upper trail (7.0/2,220'). Return the way you came to the trailhead (7.4/2,460').

Nearest Visitor Center Feather River Ranger District Visitor Center, 530-534-6500, is on Mitchell Ave. between 3rd and 5th Aves. in downtown Oroville. It's open Monday–Friday year-round, 8 a.m.–4:30 p.m.

Backpacking Information Backpacking is permitted in the Feather Falls Scenic Area, though the steep slopes and lack of good campsites make this a challenging option. No wilderness permit is needed, though a valid campfire permit is required.

Nearest Campground Five walk-in sites (first come, first served; free) are available at the trailhead and can be accessed via a short walk. Water is available during the summer.

Additional Information www.fs.usda.gov/plumas

HIKE 72 Sierra Buttes 🥾 🧍 🐕

Highlight	A fire lookout with hundred-mile views
Distance	4.6–11.0 miles round-trip
Total Elevation Gain/Loss	1,600'/1,600' to 3,200'/3,200', depending on route
Hiking Time	3–10 hours
Recommended Maps	*Downieville & Lakes Basin Trail Guide* by Sierra Buttes Trail Stewardship, USGS 7.5-min. *Sierra City*
Best Times	July–September
Agency	Tahoe National Forest
Difficulty	★★★★

SIERRA BUTTES SOAR, powerful monoliths of rock burst from the sylvan terrain of the North Fork Yuba River. Atop their highest peak a tower perches—a lookout for wildfire with commanding views.

Part of a complicated geologic puzzle, the rocks of Sierra Buttes were probably formed during the eruptions of ancient undersea volcanoes some 350 million years ago. Accreted to North America more than 200 million years ago, their resistance to erosion has left them exposed as naked mountains today.

The Hike is a long, challenging ascent of Sierra Buttes from Lower Sardine Lake and provides the full Sierra Buttes experience of scenery, lakes, and summit vista. Two alternate access trails—one via the Pacific Crest Trail (PCT), one via Tamarack Lakes—offer shorter routes to the summit. Both these trails miss out on the exceptional views of Sierra Buttes above Sardine Lakes, however. Via the Pacific Crest Trail, the round-trip to the summit is 4.6 miles with an elevation gain/loss of 1,600 feet. Via the Tamarack Lakes, the round-trip is 6.2 miles with an elevation gain/loss of 2,300 feet. With two vehicles or one vehicle and a bicycle, you can begin at Lower Sardine Lake and exit via the PCT, sparing your knees considerable downhill compression. Snow can linger deep into June and the trail is usually not snow-free until July. While the Sardine Lakes are an extremely popular fishing destination with heavy crowds all summer long, only a small percentage of people

are on the trail. Fishing is possible at the Tamarack Lakes and both are planted with fingerling trout. Water is available near the Lower Sardine Lake Trailhead but not at the two alternate trailheads. Sources are scarce along the trail—the Tamarack Lakes near that trailhead are your only sure bet.

To Reach the Trailhead Take Hwy. 49 to Bassetts Station, 5 miles east of Sierra City and 15 miles west of Sattley. Turn north onto Gold Lake Rd., proceed 1.3 miles, and turn left toward Sardine and Packer Lakes. In 0.3 mile the road forks: left leads to the lower trailhead, and right, to the two upper trailheads. Going left, the trailhead is 0.1 mile farther on the right, just before Lower Sardine Lake Campground, and is signed TAMARACK CONNECTION TRAIL 12E08. Going right at the fork, you reach a Y-junction in 2.7 miles by the Packer Lake day-use area—go left and stay on FS 93. The Tamarack Lakes Trailhead is a short 0.2 mile ahead, and the PCT Trailhead a steep and winding 2.1 miles farther.

Description From the Lower Sardine Lake Trailhead (0.0/5,770'), the wide and rocky trail begins climbing through manzanita, Douglas-firs, Jeffrey pines, white firs, and incense cedars. The lookout tower is barely discernible to the naked eye, perched on top of the mountain's highest point. The trail soon climbs a ridge, crossing briefly to the eastern side before returning to begin the fabulous traverse above Sardine Lakes. Dazzling Sierra Buttes overshadow the

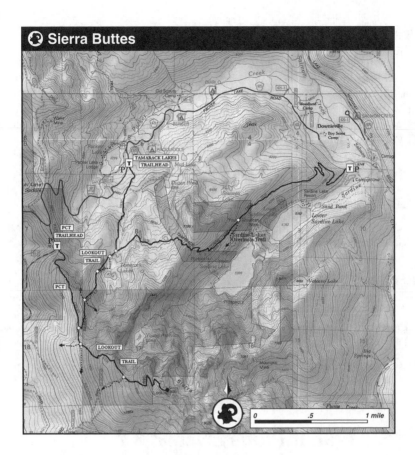

Sierra Buttes

emerald waters of Upper and Lower Sardine Lakes, lending inspiration to your feet as you approach the grueling ridgetop ascent. Along the way, you pass the junction for the Sardine Lakes Overlook Trail (1.7/6,500'). After powering up the steep switchbacks to attain the ridge (2.3/7,050'), you descend briefly and pass two small ponds before reaching the junction with the Lookout Trail (3.2/6,720'). Those approaching from Tamarack Lakes Trailhead join here; you turn left (southwest) on the wide four-wheel-drive road to immediately reach Lower Tamarack Lake. The trail forks just past the lake: left leads down to nicer Upper Tamarack Lake; right is the continuation of the hike. The upper lake is good for some very brisk swimming.

Now on posted Tamarack Connection Trail 12E30, you climb steadily southwest and cross a wide logging road halfway to the ridgetop. The lookout becomes visible southeast between the peaklets before three switchbacks bring you to the ridgetop. The junction with the PCT (4.0/7,350') is located by a large, twisted western white pine. Those approaching from the PCT Trailhead join here, where your trail continues southeast up toward the summit. Winding steeply through large boulders, you stay near or along the ridgecrest and begin the final push to the top. Note your route as it can be difficult to spot on your return, especially when lingering snow obscures the track. The icy, turquoise water of Little America Lake lies below, the lookout sits above, and mountain hemlock grows all around you, climbing the four-wheel-drive access road to the top. Following it up eight switchbacks, you then reach the stairs—as if you weren't tired enough—and 141 steps later you reach the top (5.5/8,591').

The interior of the seasonally staffed lookout is off-limits, but the walkway that surrounds it is open for 360-degree views. The northeast corner of this precarious roost actually juts out into the void beyond the summit cliffs. On a reasonably clear day, Lassen Peak (10,457') is visible more than 70 miles away on the northwest horizon, the peaks of Desolation Wilderness (Hike 75) appear far to the south-southeast, and the Coast Ranges rise beyond Sutter Buttes and the Great Central Valley (a distance of more than 100 miles). Return the way you came or by one of the two alternate routes.

Nearest Visitor Center Yuba River Ranger Station, 530-288-3232, is 7 miles north of North San Juan and 23 miles south of Downieville on Hwy. 49 and is open Monday–Friday 8 a.m.–4:30 p.m.

Backpacking Information A campfire permit is required. The only campsites along this hike are around Tamarack Lakes and receive heavy use.

Nearest Campgrounds Sardine Campground (27 sites, $24), at Lower Sardine Lake, and Packsaddle Campground (12 sites, $24), near Packer Lake, both provide water. More primitive Berger and Diablo Campgrounds (8 and 19 sites, respectively; $20) are on the road to Packer Lake and lack water. Reservations are essential for all campgrounds; visit **recreation.gov** or call 877-444-6777.

Additional Information www.fs.usda.gov/tahoe

HIKE 73 South Yuba River 🥾 🚶 🐐

Highlights	Swimming holes and river access in the Sierra foothills
Distance	8.8 miles round-trip
Total Elevation Gain/Loss	1,800'/1,800', including side trips to the river
Hiking Time	5–6 hours
Recommended Maps	*South Yuba River Recreation Guide* by the US Forest Service, USGS 7.5-min. *North Bloomfield*
Best Times	April–October
Agency	South Yuba Wild and Scenic Recreation Area; Bureau of Land Management, US Forest Service, and California State Parks
Difficulty	★★★

THE SOUTH YUBA RIVER flows through the heart of Gold Country in the foothills of the Sierra Nevada. This region once swarmed with miners and prospectors seeking pay dirt. Today the river flows through a quieter landscape as it cuts through a deep valley in the South Yuba Wild and Scenic Recreation Area. The South Yuba Trail explores a long stretch of it, traversing wooded slopes and dropping intermittently to the riverbanks where high-quality fishing, swimming, lounging, and camping options can all be found.

You can even relive the excitement of the Gold Rush on your hike. The trail travels through

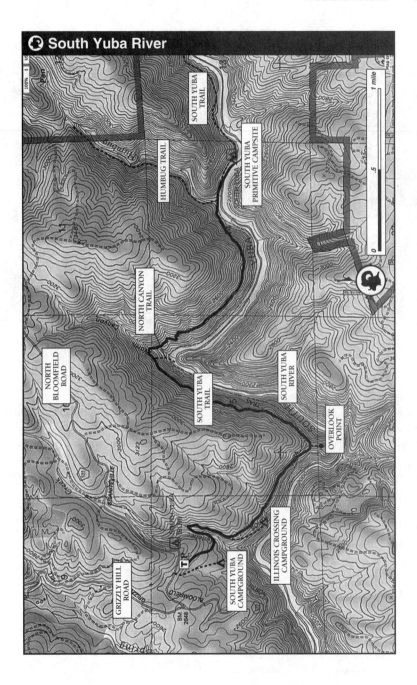

South Yuba River

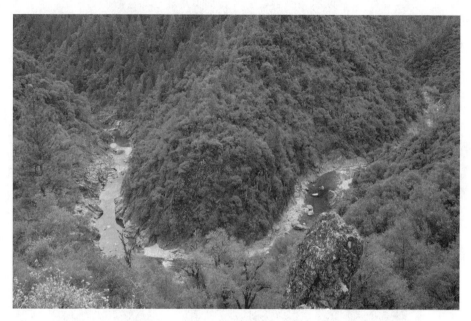

The South Yuba River flows through the Sierra foothills.

a "hands and pans" area, which means that you can legally look for (and keep) gold from the river as long as you use nothing but your hands and a gold pan (no shovels allowed).

The Hike explores the central section of the 15-mile South Yuba Trail on an out-and-back journey to South Yuba Primitive Camp, a designated backcountry camping area near the river. Most of the hike, however, runs high on the slopes above the river; access is possible in only a few locations. The emerald river runs deepest in late spring and early summer and steadily drops as the summer progresses. During dry years, it can diminish substantially by late summer.

The hike's relatively low elevation makes it a viable spring destination; it also means scorching heat is common during the summer months. Poison oak is a common trailside companion on this hike—be watchful.

To Reach the Trailhead Take Hwy. 20/49 a short distance east of Nevada City and then turn left (north) to remain on Hwy. 49. In 0.3 mile, turn right on North Bloomfield Rd.

and proceed 0.6 mile to a T-junction at the top of the ridge; turn right and remain on North Bloomfield Rd. for the next 4.8 miles as it makes an increasingly steep descent over rough pavement to reach the Yuba River. Cross the river and follow the now unpaved—but easily passable—road as it climbs 1.5 miles to reach the junction with Grizzly Hill Road. Bear right to remain on North Bloomfield Rd. for 0.2 mile, and then turn right toward South Yuba Campground. You immediately reach a fork; turn left to reach the trailhead, right to continue to the campground a short distance ahead.

Description From the trailhead (0.0/2,580'), descend the gentle singletrack trail as it winds through a second-growth forest of ponderosa pine, black oak, canyon live oak, Douglas-fir, incense cedar, and an understory of fragrant bear clover. You initially parallel the road to the campground, then gently contour down to curve around the Kennebec Creek drainage, where a short detour upstream leads to a trickling waterfall.

After a brief ascent, you drop to a signed junction (0.8/2,330'). To visit the river, bear right to make a traversing descent 300 feet to Illinois Crossing, where several tenting areas are tucked among the dense woods on the steep slopes above the river. A toll bridge across the river once stood at this site in the 1850s.

Continuing on South Yuba Trail, you cruise through thick forest, passing a few intermittent glimpses of the densely vegetated river canyon. In the 1850s, these same views would have instead revealed an almost completely denuded landscape heavily transformed by mining activity. Manzanita begins to appear on dry and exposed slopes, and poison oak flourishes in abundance.

You next arrive at a posted spur on the right (1.5/2,350') for Overlook Point, which leads quickly to a trio of picnic tables but, alas, no views; surrounding trees block any chance of an overlook these days. From here, South Yuba Trail traverses steadily upward, with continued sporadic views into the canyon below. Though out of sight, the river is clearly audible below.

A slow descent leads you past a view of a distinctive horseshoe bend in the river below, which you can access from the posted junction for North Canyon Spur (2.7/2,360'). This 0.4-mile side trip drops 300 feet via 11 switchbacks to the river below and is one of the nicest destinations on this hike—a very worthwhile detour. A substantial bedrock bench about 20 feet above the river provides access to swimming holes, as well as opportunities for an overnight camp.

Continuing on South Yuba Trail, a pair of switchbacks descends to cross North Creek, and the trail then resumes a rising traverse through dry terrain punctuated by redbud, buckthorn, and manzanita. An ensuing descent then leads you to Humbug Creek Trail (4.1/2,180') on the left; a pair of picnic tables can be found on an open bench about 50 feet upslope.

South Yuba Trail then descends to reach the main trail's first river access—a good opportunity for swimming—and crosses Humbug Creek on a footbridge. A short distance farther, you reach South Yuba Primitive Camp (4.4/2,160'), a shady camping area with two picnic tables, a large fire circle, and convenient river access.

Additional opportunities for exploration await up-canyon on the continuing South Yuba Trail, but this hike returns the way you came back to the trailhead (8.8/2,580').

Nearest Visitor Centers Tahoe National Forest Supervisor's Office, 530-265-4531, is on Coyote St. just north of the Hwy. 20/49 junction. (You pass it on the drive to the trailhead.) It's open Monday–Friday 8 a.m.–4:30 p.m., year-round. Also try the Bureau of Land Management (BLM) Mother Lode Field Office, 916-941-3101, at 5152 Hillsdale Cir. in El Dorado Hills. It's also open Monday–Friday 8 a.m.–4:30 p.m., year-round.

Backpacking Information Overnight camping is permitted throughout this hike, with established sites at Illinois Crossing and South Yuba Primitive Camp. No wilderness permit is needed, but a valid campfire permit is required.

Nearest Campground South Yuba Campground (16 sites with water, $5) is just past the trailhead and open April–mid-October.

Additional Information www.fs.usda.gov/tahoe, tinyurl.com/motherlodefieldoffice

HIKE 74 Rubicon River 🏃 🐕

Highlight	The crystalline Rubicon River
Distance	6.0-plus miles round-trip
Total Elevation Gain/Loss	500'/500'
Hiking Time	1–5 hours
Recommended Maps	USGS 7.5-min. *Bunker Hill* and *Robbs Peak*
Best Times	May–October
Agency	Eldorado National Forest
Difficulty	★★

ORIGINATING IN Desolation Wilderness, the Rubicon River flows through the Sierra foothills on its way to join the Middle Fork American River. Hiking beside this river—clear as glass and emerald green—is a peaceful experience.

The Hike explores a small stretch of the Rubicon River that flows for 10 miles without road access. Traveling the Hunter Trail high along the slopes parallel to the river, the hike provides views into some deep gorges, as well as opportunities to scramble down and explore along the river. There is no end destination for this hike—this description goes 3 miles upstream, but you can continue past this point or turn around earlier without missing any significant sights. The first 1.5 miles are the most dramatic. This low-elevation hike seldom receives snow and is often accessible even in the off-season. Fishing is fair to good, with the water clarity often making for challenging conditions. No potable water is available at the trailhead, but the river is easily accessible.

Note: In the fall of 2014, the King Fire burned 97,000 acres in this area, including almost the entirety of this hike. The trail itself was not damaged, and at press time the US Forest Service expected it to be open in 2015 and beyond; call ahead to check current conditions and access.

To Reach the Trailhead Take Hwy. 49 south from Auburn to the junction with Hwy. 193 in Cool and turn east. Proceed 12.7 miles to the Georgetown stop sign, and turn left on Main St., which becomes FS 1 (also known as Wentworth Springs Rd.) on the other side of town. Follow FS 1 for 20 miles to the junction with FS 2 (11 Pines Rd.) and turn left. The road descends and crosses the Rubicon River in 4.2 miles. Immediately past the bridge, there is a small unmarked dirt road on the right. Park here on the left side of the main road. The trailhead is halfway down the unmarked road, indicated by short wooden posts.

Description From the trailhead (0.0/3,390'), begin your hillside traverse among black oaks, canyon live oaks, ponderosa pines, incense cedars, and Douglas-firs. Fragrant bear clover fills in the understory. The early section also crosses a geologic divide, passing briefly over metamorphic rocks before reaching the more typical granite of the Sierra Nevada. Early on look for schist and other metamorphic rocks in the creekbeds that the path crosses.

Climbing high above the river, the trail peaks at a clearing (1.0/3,710'), which offers views up-canyon and of the opposite slopes rising more than 2,000 feet above the river. It then drops back down; where the trail bottoms out, you pass a spur trail to the river (1.7/3,600'), one of only two good access points. A few small white firs can be spotted as you continue along the more level trail and the canyon slopes become more gradual. Near a significant creek gully where the riverbed is clearly visible, you pass the next river access point. Large, healthy representatives of incense cedars, Douglas-firs,

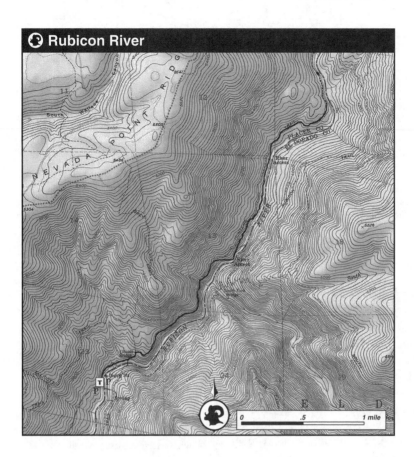

Rubicon River

and ponderosa pines grow along the trail's upper section; it is possible to continue all the way to Hell Hole Reservoir, a 10-mile one-way journey from the trailhead. Turn around whenever you'd like.

Nearest Visitor Center Georgetown Ranger Station, 530-333-4312, 3.2 miles east of the Georgetown stop sign on FS 1, is open daily 8 a.m.–4:30 p.m. May–October, and Monday–Friday only in winter.

Backpacking Information While it is legal to backpack on this hike (valid campfire permit required), finding good campsites can be a challenge. No wilderness permit is required.

Nearest Campgrounds Stumpy Meadows Campground (40 sites, $19; open mid-April–mid-October) is 12 miles east of Georgetown on FS 1. There are a few primitive use sites near the trailhead parking area.

Additional Information www.fs.usda.gov/eldorado

HIKE 75 Island Lake ⬈ 🧍 🐐

Highlight	Alpine lakes in a granite slab–scape
Distance	6.2 miles round-trip
Total Elevation Gain/Loss	1,250'/1,250'
Hiking Time	4–5 hours
Recommended Maps	*A Guide to the Desolation Wilderness* by the US Forest Service, USGS 7.5-min. *Pyramid Peak*
Best Times	June–September
Agency	Tahoe National Forest
Difficulty	★★★

THE CRYSTAL RANGE rises southwest of Lake Tahoe, a granite landscape punctuated by lakes, peaks, and a multitude of hiking opportunities within easy striking distance of the Bay Area. The 63,960-acre Desolation Wilderness protects most of the range, a delightful pocket of wilderness laced by miles of trails.

The vacationland of Wrights Lake nestles just beyond the southwest corner of the wilderness and provides ready access for a quick foray into the naked granite slabs of the area, where hardy trees cling to life in rocky crevices and jagged peaks rise above tranquil mountain lakes.

The Hike climbs steadily above Wrights Lake over a view-rich granite landscape to reach the tranquil pair of Twin Lakes and then continues past them to reach the long waterway of Island Lake.

The hike does have a few drawbacks. First, Desolation Wilderness is one of the country's most heavily visited wilderness areas, and this hike, like most of the trails in the wilderness, receives heavy use. You will likely see dozens of hikers on the trail and may have difficulty securing parking at the trailhead during busy periods. (An overflow parking area is 1.1 miles from the trailhead.) Adding to the population pressure are a collection of vacation cabins and nearby Wrights Lake Campground. For a reduced crowd factor, start early in the morning or consider a September or early-October visit.

Second, the trail to Twin Lakes is challenging to follow at times as it travels over blank granite slabs that are often minimally marked. Add to this an abundance of small hiker-made cairns that indicate other routes and you have a potentially tricky navigation challenge. Take careful note of your route as you ascend; it's easy to make a wrong turn on the return descent.

To Reach the Trailhead Take Hwy. 50 to Wrights Rd., 4 miles east of the town of Strawberry Center and 5 miles west of Kyburz. Follow paved and twisty Wrights Rd. as it climbs 7.8 miles to reach an equestrian camp and the overflow parking area on the right. You reach a junction 0.2 mile farther, where you continue straight toward the Twin Lakes and Grouse Lake trailhead. You pass the campground entrance on the right 0.2 mile past the junction, and then turn right toward the Summer Home Tract. This bumpy and narrow road leads 0.5 mile to the trailhead, where there is an outhouse and parking for roughly 30 cars; no water is available.

Description At the trailhead (0.0/6,980'), first fill out the required day-hike permit at the kiosk, and then head through the gate and down the paved road. You pass the Lot 55 cabin and then encounter the large trailhead sign for Island Lake Trail, which bears right. The wide, flat trail initially weaves through a forest of lodgepole pines and past a meadow seasonally flush with wildflowers.

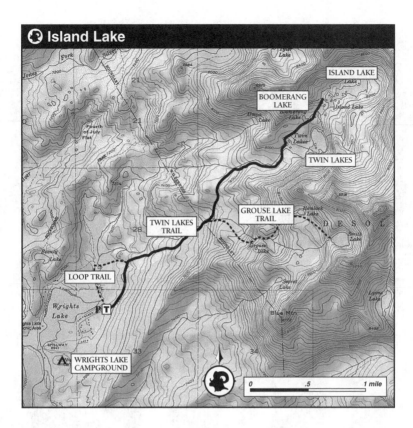

Island Lake

The splayed needles of white fir appear as you wind along the edge of granite boulder slopes and reach a posted junction for Loop Trail (0.6/6,940'). Continue straight toward Twin Lakes to immediately start rising along the edge of granite slabs. Soon the landscape abruptly transforms into bare and rocky granite, a world akin to High Sierra landscapes much farther south.

Views of the Crystal Range peaks appear ahead as the trail briefly climbs and reenters the trees. Some large western white pines now appear around you, easily recognized by their checkered bark and long, papery cones. The trail continues its steady ascent, narrowing to singletrack as it winds over rocky and bouldery terrain.

Soon you reach the first of many blank granite slabs where the trail is barely marked; as in several upcoming sections, continue to ascend in the most obvious direction and keep your eyes open for indications of the trail. If you find yourself hiking for an extended stretch without any sign, retrace your steps and try again.

After crossing open terrain, the continuing route returns to the woods, crosses an alder-lined trickle of water, and reaches the signed border of Desolation Wilderness. A short climb then brings you to the junction with Grouse Lake Trail (1.5/7,540'), which heads off to the right. Proceed straight toward Twin Lakes and immediately cruise upward over granite slabs; rocks intermittently outline the route. Look for glacial polish and gouges on the slabs around you as you ascend, indications of the ice that once buried this region.

The trail steepens and bears left to follow a clear route blasted into the rock. Views expand to the west, including the watery expanse

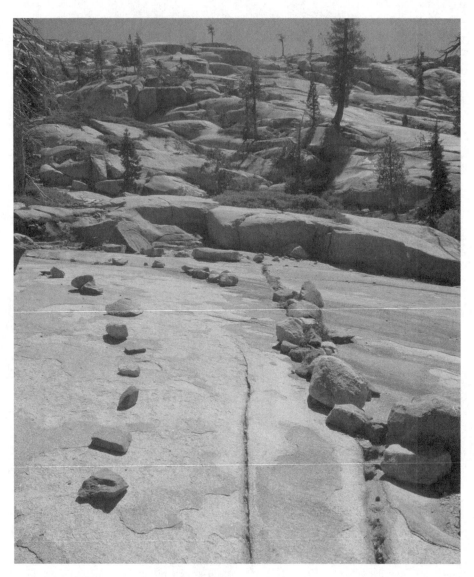

The trail to Island Lake can be hard to follow at times.

of Wrights Lake below. The trail then becomes challenging to follow as it traverses left through intermittent shrubs toward the Twin Lakes drainage. You then crest a rise and can see the remainder of the route above you, as well as views northeast toward the small bowl on the flanks of Peak 8925, which holds diminutive and off-trail Umpqua Lake.

Though the trail itself is faint and hard to follow, the route is now marked by more-regular small cairns. The climb eases as you crest another rise and drop slightly into a flat, tree-speckled area below a rubble field of granite talus. You cross a small water source by a shallow pond and hike over open slabs to reach lower Twin Lake (2.5/8,000').

The bottom of the shallow lake is visible through the crystalline water and a small island rises from its middle. Western white pine and mountain hemlock grapple for survival in the rocky surrounding landscape. The best camping options are found along the lake's north side.

Hiking onward toward Island Lake, you curve around a small inlet (the remains of an old dam can be found here) and then steadily rise and travel alongside diminutive Boomerang Lake, which shows the clear geologic transition here from granite (on its near side) to darker metavolcanic rocks (on the far side). The trail cuts left at the far end of the lake, where nearby views provide glimpses of upper Twin Lake nestled below granite cliffs. A few marginal campsites can be found there in steep lakeside terrain.

The trail then winds through one of its faintest sections yet. Stay to the left of the slender nearby pond and then cross the marshy area at its head to climb a series of tight, rocky switchbacks to Island Lake (3.1/8,170').

Several small islands punctuate this deeper lake. Views look west to the crest of the Crystal Range, and good-sized western white pines and hemlocks are scattered about the rocky landscape. Campsites are challenging, but not impossible, to find.

Spend as much time as you'd like exploring the paths that proliferate in all directions around the lake; and then return the way you came. As you descend, be careful to closely retrace your route, especially along the section that traverses back toward the Grouse Lake outlet creek—a fully marked and sometimes discernible trail continues down near the Twin Lakes outlet creek and can readily leave you astray on your way back to the trailhead (6.2/6,980').

Nearest Visitor Centers Pacific Ranger Station, 530-644-2349, is on Hwy. 50, 4 miles east of Pollock Pines. It's open daily 8 a.m.–4:30 p.m. Memorial Day weekend–Labor Day, Monday–Saturday in the fall, and Monday–Friday in winter and spring. In the Lake Tahoe area, the Taylor Creek Forest Service Visitor Center, 530-543-2674, is on Hwy. 89, 3 miles north of the Hwy. 50 junction in South Lake Tahoe. It's open daily Memorial Day weekend–October but closed the rest of the year. For year-round information, the Lake Tahoe Basin Management Unit Visitor Center, 530-543-2600, is 2 miles east of the Hwy. 50/89 junction at 35 College Dr. (Turn right on A1 Tahoe Blvd., then right at the first signal.) It's open Monday–Friday 8 a.m.–4:30 p.m.

Backpacking Information A wilderness permit is required and can be obtained from any of the above visitor centers. There is a quota of 20 people per night for this hike, in effect Memorial Day weekend–September 30. Half of the permits can be reserved up to 6 months in advance; the other half are available on a first-come, first-served basis the day of travel. Campfires are prohibited. For reservations, visit **recreation.gov** or call 877-444-6777. The permit fee is $5 per person for 1 night or $10 per person for 2–14 nights, plus a $6 reservation fee for each permit.

Nearest Campground Wrights Lake Campground (67 sites, $20), is open mid- to late June–mid-October, depending on snow conditions. Reservations are required from the Friday after July 4–Labor Day; visit **recreation.gov** or call 877-444-6777.

Additional Information www.fs.usda.gov/eldorado

HIKE 76 Mount Tallac

Highlights	Summit views encompassing all of Lake Tahoe and much of Desolation Wilderness
Distance	9.2 miles round-trip
Total Elevation Gain/Loss	3,400'/3,400'
Hiking Time	6–8 hours
Recommended Maps	*Desolation Wilderness Map & Guide* by the US Forest Service, *Desolation Wilderness & Vicinity* by Wilderness Press, USGS 7.5-min. *Emerald Bay*
Best Times	July–September
Agency	Desolation Wilderness, Eldorado National Forest
Difficulty	★★★★

MOUNT TALLAC SOARS above Lake Tahoe's southwest shore, a landmark peak beckoning fit hikers to its lofty summit. From the top, Lake Tahoe and the heart of Desolation Wilderness spread out below you.

In this land of exposed granite, Mount Tallac (9,735') is a dark, metamorphic anomaly.

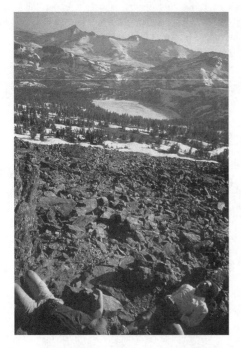

Mount Tallac view into Desolation Wilderness

A roof pendant, the mountain is a remnant of the landscape that existed prior to the intrusion of the Sierra Nevada granite. Formed near the ancient continental margin of North America 120–200 million years ago, the rocks of Mount Tallac are a complex mix of volcanic flows above metamorphosed sea-floor sediments. While these rocks once covered the surrounding landscape, erosion has exposed the underlying granite, leaving only a few small remnants on the highest peaks.

The Hike quickly and steeply ascends Mount Tallac via the most direct route from Lake Tahoe's southwest shore, passing Floating Island and Cathedral Lakes along the way. Mount Tallac is located in Desolation Wilderness, an incredibly popular area that is heavily traveled all summer long until Labor Day. In September, the weather remains delightful and crowds all but disappear—the optimal time for your "Tallac Attack." Snow lingers well into June on the trail's upper reaches and can return as early as October. No water is available at the trailhead. Cathedral Creek, about halfway up the mountain, provides a reliable trailside source.

To Reach the Trailhead Take Hwy. 89 north of the junction of Hwys. 50 and 89 in South Lake Tahoe for 3.5 miles to the posted turnoff for the Tallac Trailhead on the left. Approaching from the north on Hwy. 89, the turnoff is

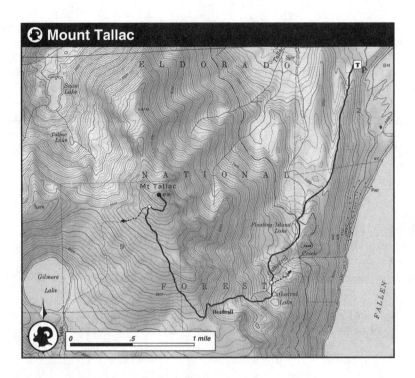

Mount Tallac

2 miles south of Eagle Point Campground. From Hwy. 89, it is a short 1.2 miles on the access road to the large trailhead parking lot—bear left at the first fork and right at the second.

Description All day-hikers are required to obtain a wilderness permit, available free at the big information sign by the start of the trail (0.0/6,500'). Immediately climbing, the trail ascends through Jeffrey pines, white firs, and manzanita to quickly reach the top of the ridge that hems in Fallen Leaf Lake, visible below you to the east. As glaciers advanced from the mountains toward Lake Tahoe in the recent geologic past, they pushed rocky debris in front of them like giant bulldozers, depositing it alongside to form lateral moraines (parallel ridges along the glacier edges) and terminal moraines at the points of farthest advance. Remaining after a glacier melted, moraines formed natural basins that filled with large lakes. Fallen Leaf Lake is an outstanding example, as is Emerald Bay, joined to Lake Tahoe because its terminal

moraine is slightly lower than Tahoe's current water level.

Views of Mount Tallac's eastern flanks are constant until the trail drops west below the ridgetop, briefly parallels Tallac Creek, and enters Desolation Wilderness a few hundred yards before reaching Floating Island Lake (1.4/7,230'). Named for the large, grassy mats that occasionally break off from its shores and float about, the shallow lake once contained a floating island buoyant enough to float six men, according to Barbara Lekisch in *Tahoe Place Names*.

The trail crosses Cathedral Creek before reaching a junction (2.3/7,580') where a steep trail climbing from Stanford Sierra Camp on Fallen Leaf Lake joins from the left. Cathedral Lake (2.5/7,620') makes a wonderful rest stop, and good views can be had from its eastern rim. Continuing, the rocky trail steepens and makes a few switchbacks on the way to a glacial cirque dotted with drooping mountain hemlocks (2.9/8,200'). A tall, wizened western white pine stands between you and the rocky slopes of Mount Tallac. The small creek here is your last opportunity to obtain water.

Snow can remain on the east-facing headwall late in the season and obscure the already difficult-to-distinguish track—the correct route runs along the headwall's northwest side. Once you're on top of the slope (3.2/8,550'), the broadly sloping southwestern flank of the mountain is revealed. Pink phlox hug the ground as the trail veers northwest parallel to the ridge, reaching the summit via a short, posted trail (4.6/9,715').

The jagged summit makes for difficult seating, but get comfortable—you'll want to savor the view. The stretch of land from Emerald Bay (Hike 77) to the Stateline casinos was once filled with rivers of ice, a spectacular scene to imagine. As you look southwest down into Desolation Wilderness, the irregular shape of island-studded Lake Aloha (8,116') sits below the peaks of the Crystal Range, and perfectly round Gilmore Lake lies immediately below you. Return the way you came.

Nearest Visitor Center Lake Tahoe Visitor Center at Taylor Creek, 530-543-2674, is 2.7 miles north of the junction of Hwys. 50 and 89 in South Lake Tahoe on Hwy. 89; it's open daily 8 a.m.–4:30 p.m. in summer, and weekends only in the fall. In the off-season, contact the Forest Supervisor's office in South Lake Tahoe, 530-543-2600; it's open Monday–Friday 8 a.m.–4:30 p.m.

Backpacking Information Campsites are extremely limited on this hike. Only a few small sites exist near Cathedral Lake; your best options are the broad southwest shoulder of Mount Tallac above the headwall and the somewhat more distant Gilmore Lake. Wilderness permits are required for all overnight stays, and there is a $5-per-person recreational fee (with an additional $5 for 2 or more nights). Permits can be obtained at the above visitor centers or at the Pacific Ranger District Office, 22 miles east of Placerville on Hwy. 50; it's open Monday–Friday 8 a.m.–4:30 p.m. and on most weekends.

Desolation Wilderness has a quota system for specific backcountry zones; 4 permits are available for the area around Cathedral Lake, 6 for the upper slopes, and 18 for the Gilmore Lake area. Thirty percent of permits are first come, first serve; 70% can be reserved anytime after the third Thursday in April by calling 530-647-5415 or visiting **recreation.gov** ($5 reservation fee).

Nearest Campground Campgrounds line Lake Tahoe's shore. The closest are Eagle Point Campground, in Emerald Bay State Park (100 sites, $235), and Fallen Leaf Campground (205 sites, $32). Note that Eagle Point Campground will be closed in 2015 for renovations.

Additional Information www.fs.usda.gov/ltbmu

HIKE 77   Lake Tahoe ✐

Highlights	Tahoe shores, Emerald Bay, and Vikingsholm
Distance	6.6 miles one-way
Total Elevation Gain/Loss	1,150'/850'
Hiking Time	3–5 hours
Recommended Map	USGS 7.5-min. *Emerald Bay*
Best Times	Mid-June–September
Agency	D. L. Bliss and Emerald Bay State Parks
Difficulty	★★

LAKE TAHOE needs no introduction. Despite the thick development elsewhere, this pristine shoreline allows you to experience the full natural majesty of the lake's shoreline.

The Hike is a one-way journey along Lake Tahoe's shoreline from D. L. Bliss State Park to Emerald Bay State Park along the Rubicon Trail. Swimming, sunning, and fishing are all possible diversions, and fairy-tale Vikingsholm awaits in enchanting Emerald Bay. While it can be completed in either direction, the hike description proceeds south from D. L. Bliss, saving Emerald Bay for the latter half of the day. A car shuttle is required for this hike.

Be aware that the trailhead is a 2.3-mile road walk from the D. L. Bliss park entrance. This trail is very crowded in summer, so arrive before 10 a.m. to get a spot in the small trailhead parking lot. After the lot has filled, check the small, unposted parking spaces 1.1 miles from the entrance—you can easily connect with the trail from there. If they too are full, the only available parking is along Hwy. 89. Water is available at the trailhead.

To Reach the Trailhead Take Hwy. 89 to the entrance for D. L. Bliss State Park. Approaching from the south, it's 4 miles past Eagle Point Campground; from the north, it's 5.5 miles past

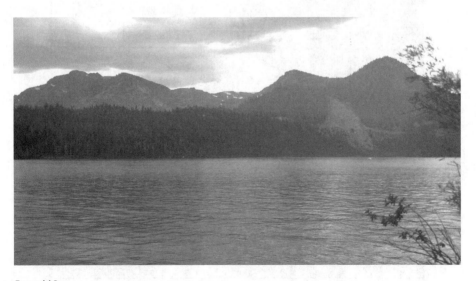

Emerald Bay

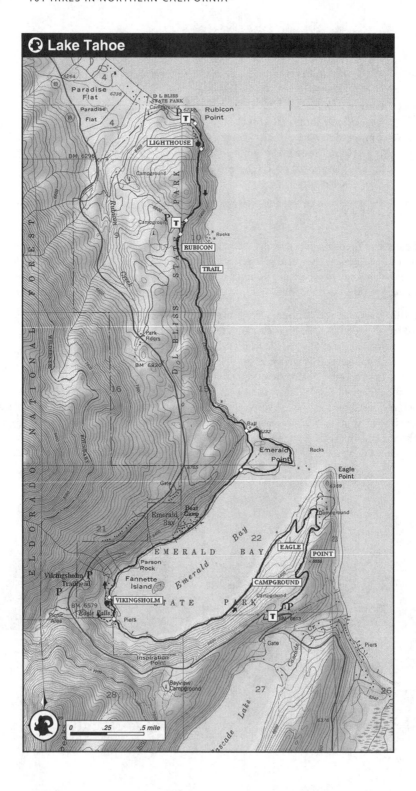

Meeks Bay Campground. From the entrance station, follow signs toward Camps 141–168 and, at the final intersection, bear right toward the Rubicon Trail parking lot. A $10 day-use fee is charged.

Description   From the parking lot (0.0/6,260'), the singletrack trail strikes south among white firs, huckleberry oaks, and manzanita. At the immediate junction for the lighthouse trail, continue straight to quickly obtain your first views of Tahoe's distinctive, clear, aquamarine-hued water below you. While reduced from its historic clarity of 120 feet deep, objects can still be seen to 75 feet in places. Along this early section of trail, numerous use paths branch down toward the lake. Lake access ends after the trail reaches a mildly precarious section protected by a chain-link fence (0.3/6,330') and slowly begins climbing. Osprey nest along this stretch and can occasionally be spotted until their departure in mid-August. By the time you reach the second junction for the lighthouse trail (0.4/6,430'), the lake is 200 feet below. Resembling a modified outhouse, the lighthouse makes for an easy 0.1-mile side trip.

Turning inland, the trail continues to climb and suddenly offers magnificent views southwest of snow-frosted Mount Tallac (see previous hike). Two large spur trails from the alternate parking lot in D. L. Bliss soon join the route in a dense forest of white firs (0.9/6,520'), just before the trail crests at 350 feet above the lake. From here the trail slowly descends, passing among the bleached debris of a 1982 avalanche before reaching the lakeshore near Emerald Point (2.5/6,230'). The trail forks: left goes around the small peninsula's perimeter to worthwhile Emerald Point and the mouth of Emerald Bay, while right shortcuts to the bay proper. The flat peninsula is the terminal moraine of the glacier that carved Emerald Bay, and pinedrops, horsetails, ferns, and large Jeffrey pines sprout in the lush, sandy soil.

Veering southwest along the shores of Emerald Bay, the trail widens, passing Boat Camp before winding through the jumbled remains of a 1980 landslide—stay along the lake—to reach the Vikingsholm complex at the head of the bay (4.4/6,230'). Considered the most authentic reproduction of Scandinavian architecture in the United States, Vikingsholm was completed in 1929 without damaging any of the site's beautiful trees. Lora J. Knight spent summers here until her death in 1945, entertaining guests both onshore and in the teahouse on Fannette Island, in the middle of Emerald Bay. Donated to the state in 1958, the site now houses a visitor center, ferry dock, and other tourist-friendly facilities. The sod roof still sprouts flowers, and regular tours inside Vikingsholm are offered daily in summer for $10. A steep trail climbs 1.0 mile and 800 feet to the Vikingsholm parking lot on Hwy. 50. From here, continue on the newly constructed trail running along the bay's southeast shore.

This quiet section is almost entirely level, climbing 300 feet only at the end to terminate at the campfire circle in upper Eagle Point Campground (6.3/6,500'). It's an easy uphill through the campground to the parking spaces on Hwy. 50.

Nearest Visitor Center   D. L. Bliss Visitor Center, 530-525-9529, is open daily 9 a.m.–4 p.m. Memorial Day–Labor Day, then intermittently until the end of September before closing for the season. Vikingsholm Visitor Center, 530-541-6498, is open daily 10:30 a.m.–4 p.m. Memorial Day–Labor Day.

Nearest Campgrounds   Eagle Point Campground, in Emerald Bay State Park (100 sites, $235), and Fallen Leaf Campground (205 sites, $32). Note that Eagle Point Campground will be closed in 2015 for renovations.

Additional Information   www.parks.ca.gov

HIKE 78 Calaveras Big Trees ○ ᛘ

Highlights	One thousand of the largest trees on Earth
Distance	5.3 miles round-trip
Total Elevation Gain/Loss	600'/600'
Hiking Time	3–4 hours
Recommended Maps	*Calaveras Big Trees State Park Map,* USGS 7.5-min. *Stanislaus* and *Crandall Peak*
Best Times	May–October
Agency	Calaveras Big Trees State Park
Difficulty	★★

THE ONLY WAY to experience this magnificent grove of giant sequoias is by foot. Unlike other popular drive-up sequoia opportunities, the South Grove of Calaveras Big Trees State Park can only be accessed by trail, providing an unparalleled opportunity to commune with the majesty of large sequoias whose gargantuan stature dwarfs the massive pines and cedars that complete the magnificent old-growth forest mosaic.

Fed by the waters of Big Trees Creek, an estimated 1,000 giant sequoias rise skyward in South Grove. It is one of two sequoia groves in the park, and by far the largest—10 times the size of the more accessible North Grove by the park entrance, which receives far more traffic and crowds.

The South Grove is remarkable for having never been logged or otherwise significantly disturbed by man, though it was at risk several times in its long and convoluted history toward conservation. Nearly logged on several occasions, it was finally purchased for permanent protection in 1954. In 1984 the South Grove was designated a natural preserve—the highest level of protection within the state park system.

South Grove is also unusual for being relatively isolated from California's other 75 groves. It is one of the northernmost in the state (only the diminutive Placer County Grove is farther north) and the next grove south is nearly 40 miles away in Yosemite National Park. Its size also makes it one of the largest groves in existence; only a handful of groves in the southern Sierra are larger.

The Hike tours much of the South Grove on South Grove Trail, a well-trod and easy-cruising path that loops through the heart of the sequoia grove. A short side excursion (1.2 miles round-trip) leads to the Agassiz Tree, the largest in the park. The fact that you must hike 1.5 miles to even reach the start of the South Grove reduces visitation significantly (though it certainly does not eliminate it—you will almost certainly see other hikers). The park is open year-round, though the access road to the South Grove is not plowed in winter. Dogs are prohibited.

To Reach the Trailhead Take Hwy. 4 to the park entrance, 3 miles north of Arnold, and follow the Walter W. Smith Memorial Parkway for 8.6 miles to the substantial trailhead parking area. An $8 day-use fee is charged.

Description From the trailhead (0.0/4,440'), your hike begins on Beaver Creek Trail. Though the giant sequoias await 1.5 miles ahead, this 0.7-mile, ADA-accessible loop trail introduces you to many fine specimens of large, ancient trees, including the deeply furrowed gray bark of incense cedars, the platy yellowish bark of ponderosa pines, and the smoother gray bark of sugar pines.

You pass a large sign detailing the many memorial groves in the park, named for significant donors whose generosity helped permanently protect the giant trees. You then quickly encounter a junction; bear right toward South Grove and Bradley Trails (Beaver Creek Trail heads left to loop back to the trailhead). Beaver Creek

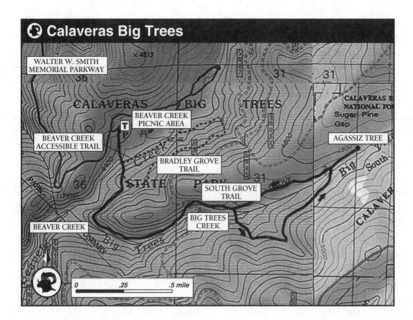

Calaveras Big Trees

becomes audible as you curve around a meadow and cross a metal bridge spanning the creek, which flows crystal clear over the smooth granite underlying the thick soil and sediment throughout the grove and park. (The creek's namesake animal is not native to the area and its naming origins are a bit of a mystery; it's possible that beavers were introduced here at one point for fur-trapping purposes.)

Fifty yards past the bridge, you pass the junction with Bradley Grove Trail on the left (0.2/4,350'). Continuing straight on South Grove Trail, you curve right and make a gently rising traverse. Some of the defining elements of old-growth forest are apparent in this section, including large standing snags and a diversity of tree ages, with many large and mature specimens. The trail then slowly curves left to enter the Big Trees Creek drainage.

Your route traverses past large white fir and sugar pine, many larger than 5 feet in diameter. You next cross an unpaved access road—a former logging railroad right-of-way and mute reminder of how close the grove came to being logged—and enter the South Grove Natural

Preserve. A slow rise leads you past an enormous fallen sugar pine before a gentle descent brings you to the start of the South Grove Loop by a huge snag (1.4/4,600').

Turn right to begin the loop, descend toward the creek, and watch for the first sequoia of the hike on the left. Though this inaugural specimen is not much larger than surrounding sugar pines, its distinctive red color makes it easy to spot.

As you cross the bridge over Big Trees Creek, take a moment to reflect in its silvery waters. Unlike most other creeks in the region, Big Trees Creek is spring fed and flows year-round, even in times of drought—one of the primary reasons this drainage is so conducive to giant sequoias. In early summer, azaleas bloom in profusion near the bridge.

Sequoias appear in abundance past the creek crossing, including a large tree with a fire scar running more than 20 feet up its trunk, blackened evidence of the regular fires that have historically swept through the area. Fire plays an essential role in the sequoia ecosystem, exposing mineral soil for seedlings to sprout and creating openings in the canopy for them to grow. Controlled burns have been done in recent years in both the north and south groves to maintain this essential balance. (Sequoias' fire-resistant bark allows them to survive the heat.)

The trail rises along the slopes and passes several fabulously old sequoias, their massive diameters and huge fire scars testament to their longevity. Mountain dogwood trees increase in the understory, festooned with snowy white flowers in the spring. (The white elements are technically bracts; the small actual flower is in the center and produces bright red berries in the fall.) Descending back toward the creek, you encounter a huge tunnel log that has fallen across Big Trees Creek—it's possible to walk through it almost entirely upright.

A bridge then leads you across Big Trees Creek and to the junction with Agassiz Trail on the right (2.2/4,700'), a worthwhile 1.2-mile side trip. The easy path leads past a standing sequoia that has been burned entirely through and rendered into a still healthy, two-legged monster. The trail then cuts between two massive sequoias and reaches the Palace Tree, another multilegged sequoia named in the 1870s for the

recently opened Palace Hotel in San Francisco. The path ends at the Agassiz Tree (2.8/4,800'). Clearly the monarch of the forest, the Agassiz Tree is larger than any other in the grove— approximately 25 feet in diameter, 250 feet tall, and weighing in excess of 5,000 tons. Though seemingly unblemished on first look, its far side reveals a huge gaping fire scar extending more than 40 feet up its trunk.

Though the trail ends here, it is possible (and permitted) to continue exploring on a challenging off-trail adventure upstream. The giant sequoias continue for roughly 2 miles farther up the drainage, where intrepid hikers can experience several remarkable groves in full wilderness solitude.

Returning to the earlier junction (3.4/4,700'), continue straight on South Grove Trail to complete the loop. Enjoy the Kansas Group in this final section, highlighted by a trio of giant sequoias. Fewer sequoias mark the last portion of the grove, replaced by an increasing number of large ponderosa pines and incense cedars. Upon returning to the start of the loop (3.9/4,600'), retrace your steps to the trailhead (5.3/4,440').

Nearest Visitor Center Calaveras Big Trees State Park Visitor Center, 209-795-2334, by the park entrance, is open daily 9 a.m.–5 p.m. Memorial Day–Labor Day, 10 a.m.–4 p.m. April and May and Labor Day–October, and weekends only November–March.

Nearest Campgrounds The park has two campgrounds, both of which have showers: North Grove Campground (74 sites, $35), by the park entrance, and Oak Hollow Campground (55 sites, $35), on Walter W. Smith Memorial Parkway roughly halfway to the South Grove. The campgrounds are open March–November and are almost always full in summer; reservations are essential. Visit **reserveamerica.com** or call 800-444-7275.

Additional Information www.parks.ca.gov, bigtrees.org

HIKE 79   Grouse Lake

Highlights	Splitting granite gorges and remote Grouse Lake
Distance	11.0 miles round-trip
Total Elevation Gain/Loss	2,500'/2,500'
Hiking Time	6–8 hours
Recommended Maps	*A Guide to the Mokelumne Wilderness* by the US Forest Service, USGS 7.5-min. *Pacific Valley* and *Mokelumne Peak*
Best Times	Mid-June–September
Agency	Mokelumne Wilderness
Difficulty	★★★★

UNLIKE MOST OF the High Sierra, the little-traveled Mokelumne Wilderness is a land more renowned for its deep river gorges than its soaring mountains. Experience here the sweep and variety of a rolling granite landscape topped with volcanic peaks and sliced by canyons thousands of feet deep.

The Hike follows a ridge west from the popular Blue Lakes to isolated Grouse Lake, perched in a magnificent granite bowl near the chasm formed by Summit City Creek. The trail passes Granite

Lake in 1.8 miles, a somewhat traveled fishing destination for the numerous anglers that ply the waters of the Blue Lakes area. Fishing is possible at both lakes. Snow usually clears by late June, with July and August the best months for wildflowers. While no water is available at the trailhead, faucets can be found in the nearby campgrounds around the Blue Lakes.

To Reach the Trailhead Take Blue Lakes Rd. (FS 015) south from Hwy. 88—the posted turnoff is 6.6 miles east of Carson Pass. The

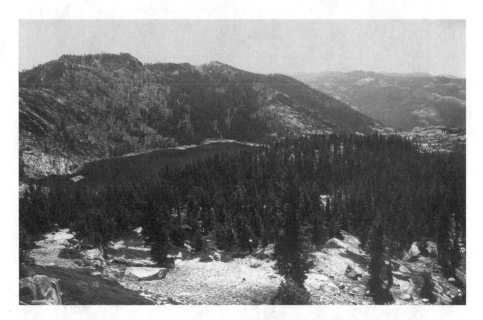

Deep valleys dissect the ridge-lined landscape of Mokelumne Wilderness.

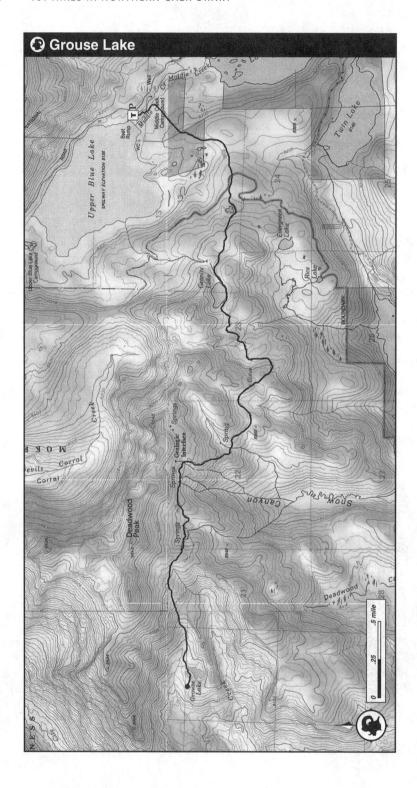

paved road ends in 7.3 miles, and you reach the junction for the Tamarack Lake Trailhead 3.7 miles farther—go straight. When you reach the Mokelumne Hydroelectric Project 1 mile later, the road becomes paved again; bear right and drive 1.9 miles toward Upper Blue Lake dam. The trailhead lot is on your left, past Lower Blue Lake Campground (within sight of Upper Blue Lake dam).

Description From the parking lot (0.0/8,140'), the trail immediately passes along a seasonal creek beneath a thick cover of lodgepole pine and mountain hemlock. Corn lilies, alpine asters, and a variety of other seasonal wildflowers decorate the moist understory along this early section of trail. Veering west, the trail crosses a stream and diverges in three directions: Go left (downstream), paralleling the stream briefly before angling away from it. As you gradually climb to Granite Lake, western white pines replace the lodgepole pines and you soon cross into Mokelumne Wilderness. Behind you, the Nipple (9,342') is visible immediately northeast, the rocky turret of Jeff Davis Peak (8,960') east-northeast, and the dark brown ridge of pyramidal Raymond Peak (10,014') and more distant Reynolds Peak (9,679') southeast. All these darker peaks are remnants of ancient volcanic flows that intermittently coursed over the rolling granite landscape of Mokelumne Wilderness during the past 30 million years. Today's rivers have eroded through most of these overlying volcanic rocks to reach the granite bedrock, but the higher peaks remain capped by these reddish-brown flows.

Ringed by broken hills of granite, pretty Granite Lake (1.8/8,700') is a pleasant spot for a breather and offers good fly-fishing. Passing its western edge, the trail forks—head away from the lake. Cresting a small rise, you get the first views of the deep canyon of North Fork Mokelumne River. A few Sierra junipers can be identified as the now undulating trail slowly climbs to a distinct granite/volcanic interface near the ridgetop, passing several easy side trips to spectacular views south. Immediately prior to reaching the darker volcanic rocks (4.0/9,220'), the trail passes below a striking illustration of the local geology. Along the interface above, granite boulders can be seen protruding from an eroding shell of loose volcanic rock, graphic evidence that the first lava flows pooled around and covered earlier existing features.

Traversing above meadow-filled Snow Canyon, the trail crosses several lush gullies, fed by springs emerging from the interface. Approaching the edge of the Snow Canyon watershed, the trail becomes indistinct; you encounter a triangular meadow bordered by several springs. Follow the farthest spring approximately 50 feet before crossing it near the edge of the exposed granite. The route is marked with small rock piles where it crests a slight ridge into the Grouse Creek drainage. Grouse Lake soon becomes visible more than 600 feet below you. The trail descends quickly to meet it (5.5/8,540'), passing through a healthy forest of western white pine and mountain hemlock on its way down. Note your route as you descend; it looks considerably different on the ascent.

Go beyond the west shore of Grouse Lake for views southwest of Mokelumne Peak (9,334') and the tantalizing upper cliffs of the Summit City Creek gorge. Return the way you came.

Nearest Visitor Center The local Chamber of Commerce runs an excellent visitor center in Markleeville, 530-694-2475, that's open daily 8 a.m.–4 p.m. April–November, with reduced hours the rest of the year. A closer source of information is the US Forest Service Carson Pass Information Center, located at the pass itself. It's open daily approximately 9 a.m.–5 p.m. during the summer.

Backpacking Information There are campsites at Grouse Lake. Wilderness permits are required and can be obtained at the trailhead, at Carson Pass during open hours, or anytime at the register outside of the Markleeville Visitor Center.

Nearest Campgrounds Pacific Gas and Electric runs four campgrounds around Upper and Lower Blue Lakes (78 sites, $23); call 916-386-5164 for additional information, or visit **recreation.pge.com.**

Additional Information **www.fs.usda.gov/eldorado**

HIKE 80   Mokelumne River 🏃 🚶 🐕

Highlight	A remote, challenging, magnificent granite gorge
Distance	15.6 miles round-trip
Total Elevation Gain/Loss	5,100'/5,100'
Hiking Time	10–14 hours
Recommended Maps	*A Guide to the Mokelumne Wilderness* by the US Forest Service, USGS 7.5-min. *Mokelumne Peak* and *Spicer Meadow Reservoir*
Best Times	June–September
Agency	Mokelumne Wilderness, Stanislaus National Forest
Difficulty	★★★★★

MOKELUMNE WILDERNESS is quite likely the grandest California wilderness you've never heard of. Sandwiched between Hwys. 108 and 4 south of Lake Tahoe, the 105,165-acre wilderness encompasses much of the upper section of the Mokelumne River watershed and protects a land of raw and continuous granite sliced into a canyon more than half a mile deep.

The Mokelumne River canyon is remote, challenging to access, and exceptionally scenic—perfect for fit, adventurous hikers looking to get away from it all.

The Hike descends to the Mokelumne River at Camp Irene, in a pocket of old-growth forest at the bottom of the canyon. Unless you have a four-wheel-drive, high-clearance vehicle (see directions below), you'll need to begin this epic journey from Hwy. 4 on Bee Gulch Trail, which ascends 3 miles and 1,500 feet before plummeting 3,500 feet to the river. This is not a hike for the faint of feet—excellent stamina is required.

The trail is little used and faint in spots, especially in the middle section. Careful route finding is sometimes required; small cairns often indicate the route. Though it can be done as a (very long) day hike, this trip is best done as an overnight journey, especially since enticing opportunities for exploration await along the river from trail's end. Water is scarce on much of this hike—carry ample supplies, especially for the return ascent.

To Reach the Trailhead Take Hwy. 4 to the turnoff for Bear Valley Ski Area (Hwy. 207) and continue 1.7 miles on Hwy. 4 to a small dirt parking area on the right by Lake Alpine. Alternatively, if you have a four-wheel-drive, high-clearance vehicle, turn left on Hwy. 207 and then take an immediate right in 0.1 mile onto FS 7N93. In approximately 1.2 miles, this rough

Mokelumne River

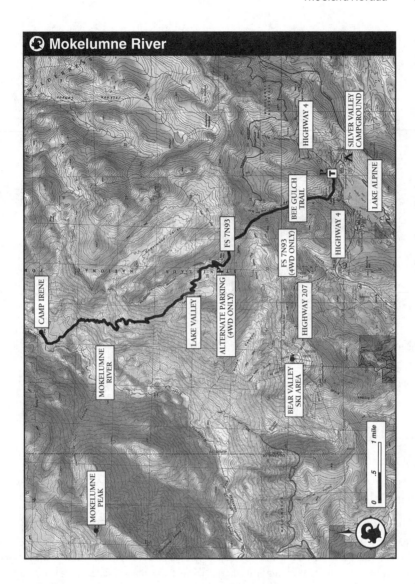

road climbs steeply to attain the ridgecrest, which it then follows for 0.6 mile. It then curves left to traverse the upper slopes for 0.8 mile—do not ascend to the nearby ridgeline above—to reach the trailhead at road's end.

Description From the parking lot, cross the road to find the signed Bee Gulch trailhead (0.0/7,340'). The well-trod and dusty single-track trail steadily climbs past granite boulders protruding from the hillside and traverses the slopes above the lake. Views south look toward bare volcanic ridges, part of nearby Carson-Iceberg Wilderness (Hike 81). Remnants of long-ago volcanic activity, these rocks cap deep stores of granite beneath them. In Mokelumne Wilderness, most of the volcanic layers have been cut through, appearing only on the high ridges ahead.

You undulate through a lodgepole pine forest punctuated by red fir and reach Bee Gulch

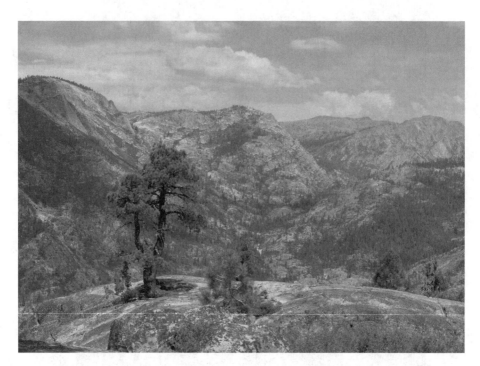

The Upper Mokelumne River watershed. Camp Irene awaits at the bottom of the canyon.

stream (0.4/7,400'), a thin water source that often dribbles late into the season. Crossing the small stream, you turn uphill and ascend by an old wooden water tank that collects water from a spring. The trail passes another trickling spring and reaches a junction, signed for the Tahoe–Yosemite Trail. Your route continues straight and soon crosses through a primitive gate by old barbed wire. The less-trod trail makes a slow rise through shady forest, steepening as it enters more open terrain blanketed with abundant mule's ear. You cross a small flowing creek lined with willows and lupine, and views open of the upper Bee Gulch drainage.

The trail steadily steepens over open slopes, eventually returns to shady woods, and then makes the steepest climb yet toward the rounded ridgeline above you. The route curves left to make a rising traverse among increasing red fir. Western white pine makes its first appearance in this section, readily identified by the distinctive checkerboard pattern on its trunk.

Upon attaining the crest, you immediately encounter a four-wheel-drive road (FS 7N93) at a fork (2.0/8,420'). Proceed straight—not uphill—to reach a posted junction for Lake Valley. Go right, enjoying views for the first time of the lower Mokelumne River canyon. The road traverses upward to another unposted fork, where you go left to continue the traverse. A steady rise over exposed slopes leads you to the ridgecrest, where the road ends at a clearing with 360-degree views (2.8/8,750'), including Mount Mokelumne (9,334') across the canyon and Bear Valley Ski Area to the southwest.

The journey into the Mokelumne River canyon now begins. From the ridgecrest, the path cuts downhill to the right, with views into Lake Valley below. Though faint in places, the trail is clearly discernible as it traverses downward and makes three switchbacks on its continuing descent. Enjoy the views of Mount Mokelumne, noting the dark pyramid of volcanic rock on the summit—part of the same geologic layer as the prominent volcanic fin visible on the ridge just ahead.

The trail next crests over a low rise and drops below the dark outcrops, passing large black and gray boulders en route. You pass through a flattish area of red fir and cross an unmarked path on the far side; your route continues straight and immediately crosses back into granite country, where a ledge viewpoint soon peers down over the rapidly steepening slopes below.

The path traverses among granite boulders, makes a few switchbacks downward over increasingly exposed ledges, and then begins a dusty and more direct descent. A confusing collection of cow paths appear as you approach the bottom of Lake Valley; several head left toward a large flat area with potential camping opportunities. Your route follows along the edge of the flat (4.0/7,950') and then close to a diminutive creek, which runs thin late in the season.

You soon encounter the hike's first grove of quaking aspens, their bright green leaves fluttering brightly. The trail winds through the aspens to continue its traverse and soon reaches the hike's first—but far from last—brushy section, where manzanita and other shrubs encroach. The route switchbacks left, then curves back to the right to pass over granite slabs marked by glacial grooves.

The descent steepens and passes through brushy and occasionally rocky terrain, with some spots nearly overgrown by the surrounding vegetation. You reach a potentially confusing section in a young aspen grove, where a deep-cut trail abruptly drops off toward the flats in lower Lake Valley below. Your continuing route instead proceeds straight through the grove on a nearly level traverse.

A shady descending traverse curves right to lead you out of the Lake Valley drainage and onto the slopes high above the Mokelumne River, visible far below at the bottom of the canyon. The magnitude of the steep, deep drop ahead of you is now apparent.

The trail traverses above sheer slopes and offers exceptional views down-canyon that slowly expand to include the raw landscape up-canyon

as well, where the sheer drainage of Summit Creek can be seen joining from the northeast. The trail remains obvious, despite abundant knee-high brush, and travels through a lush, flatter area before climbing slightly to round a corner and crest at an exceptional overlook of the upper canyon (5.7/7,030').

The serious descent now begins. The trail weaves down through the granite landscape and then drops steeply directly alongside a long ridgeline slab. The route curves left to pass through a lusher, brushier area, then bears right by a pair of large Jeffrey pines. You pass through mixed terrain—thick brush, loose rock, open granite—and then approach the lip of the canyon once again (6.1/6,650').

The continuing faint trail traverses to the right over solid granite and then near the edge of open slabs. The route now descends via a series of steep switchbacks before traversing right toward nearby Underwood Creek. Looking down into the canyon below, you can spot your destination at Camp Irene, in the largest pocket of trees along the river.

The route finding now becomes easier—a rough and clearly discernible path has been blasted from the smooth rock underfoot, and small rock piles regularly mark the route. You reach the end of a long rock slab on the edge of some trees highlighted by the deep red bark of incense cedars.

The continuing descent stays to the right side of the small adjoining ridge (at one point 6.7/6,100'), a distinct trail splits left but dead-ends at a sheer drop). You descend close to the adjacent creek bottom and then complete a series of steep, steady, tight switchbacks downward. Manzanita shrubs increase, and then the landscape abruptly shifts from shrubs and granite slabs to a lush forest environment (7.0/5,800').

Sugar pine and black oak rise around you as the trail switches from rocks to packed dirt and weaves through a shady, mostly level forest. The descent resumes down a rocky gully, passes some very large sugar pines, and then makes several steep switchbacks before finally easing near the bottom.

Gorgeous old-growth forest surrounds you in this sylvan oasis. Huge and ancient pines are joined by incense cedars so large they resemble giant sequoias. Substantial black oak, white fir, canyon live oak, and juniper trees complete the mosaic. Soon the river becomes audible as you wind north through the woods, then abruptly

emerge at an established camping area near the river's edge (7.8/5,290'). Several other sites can be found upriver. Deep pools provide swimming opportunities in the area. The terrain up-canyon is an explorer's delight.

Revel in this magical location, and then return the way you came (15.6/7,340').

Nearest Visitor Centers Alpine Ranger Station, 209-753-2811, 1.3 miles east of Bear Valley Rd. in a small hut by Hwy. 4, is open sporadically in season Thursday–Monday 8:30 a.m.–5 p.m. A more reliable information source is the Calaveras Ranger District Office, 209-795-1381, in Hathaway Pines on Hwy. 4; it's open Monday–Friday 8 a.m.–5 p.m. and Saturday 8 a.m.–2 p.m.

Backpacking Information A wilderness permit is required and can be obtained from either ranger station above. Campsites are limited for most of the hike, with water being a major concern. The best option is at Camp Irene at canyon bottom. Lake Valley is an option for a late-day start, though it is heavily used by roaming cows and the water source is questionable as a result.

Nearest Campgrounds Five developed campgrounds are in the immediate vicinity of Lake Alpine; an additional overflow campground also opens when they are full. The turnoff for Silver Valley and Pine Marten Campgrounds (21 and 36 sites, respectively) is nearly adjacent to the trailhead. All sites are first come, first served ($22).

Additional Information www.fs.usda.gov/stanislaus

HIKE 81 Hiram Peak 🥾 🧍 🐐

Highlights	The summit of Hiram Peak and the heart of Carson-Iceberg Wilderness
Distance	2.4 miles round-trip
Total Elevation Gain/Loss	1,250'/1,250'
Hiking Time	2–3 hours
Recommended Maps	*A Guide to Carson-Iceberg Wilderness* by the US Forest Service, USGS 7.5-min. *Dardanelles Cone*
Best Times	Mid-June–September
Agency	Carson-Iceberg Wilderness, Stanislaus National Forest
Difficulty	★★★

FORGOTTEN Carson-Iceberg Wilderness is a little-visited landscape of volcanic peaks that straddles the central Sierra between Yosemite and Lake Tahoe. Set apart, Hiram Peak (9,795') provides summit views extraordinaire of the high wilderness heartland.

The Hike is a short, steep, easy-to-follow cross-country route from Highland Lakes Campground to the top of Hiram Peak. The region receives light use with the majority of visitors fishing at Highland Lakes. Snow usually clears by late June; July and August are

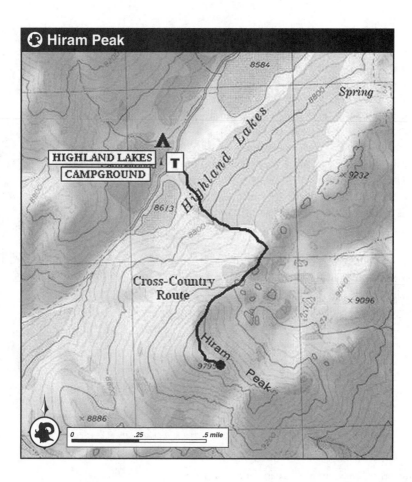

⊘ Hiram Peak

the best for wildflowers. Water is available at the trailhead.

To Reach the Trailhead Take Hwy. 4 toward Ebbetts Pass and bear south on Highland Lakes Rd.—the posted turnoff is 17 miles east of Bear Valley Road and 1.3 miles west of Ebbetts Pass. Approaching from the east, the turn is an easily missed hairpin on the left, so pay close attention. Unpaved Highland Lakes Rd. is passable for all vehicles and winds for 5.8 miles to its terminus at Highland Lakes Campground. Hiram Peak is plainly visible southeast of the campground on the opposite side of lower Highland Lake. Behind Site 31 in the eastern half of the campground, the trailhead is indicated by a small wooden trail sign.

Description From the trailhead (0.0/8,670'), follow the obvious route upward through red firs and western white pines before breaking out onto an open hillside. Seasonal wildflowers here include mariposa lilies, explorer's gentian, wild carrots, lupine, and mule's ears. Weaving along the forest edge, the trail begins to fan out and disappear as the summit of Hiram Peak comes into view to the south. Continue to the ridgetop above you (0.5/9,130'), and then traverse south to the base of the talus slopes. As you begin your ascent, use paths make clambering up the slopes somewhat easier. You soon reach the ridge that bends southeast and leads you to the summit (1.2/9,795'). You pass a few stumpy, twisted whitebark pines along the way to the top.

Beginning some 30 million years ago, intermittent volcanism covered the land of today's Carson-Iceberg Wilderness in layers of lava, mudflows, and volcanic debris; the region surrounding Hiram Peak is a complex composite of these flows. Feast on the view and admire the headwaters of three major California rivers. Looking east, the closest mountain is Arnot Peak (10,054'), part of the Sierra Divide. Its northeastern slopes are the headwaters of Wolf Creek, whose glacially carved valley can be seen trailing off northeast to join the Carson River. Flowing to the Stanislaus River, Disaster Creek drains the western flanks of Arnot Peak and is visible in the tarn-dotted open basin below you to the northeast. Looking south, the towering massif of Airola Peak (9,942') and mostly hidden Iceberg Peak (9,781') split the headwaters of Arnot Creek (east) and Highland Creek (west). Highland Creek flows into visible Spicer Meadows Reservoir before also joining the Stanislaus River. The two Highland Lakes to the north actually mark a significant watershed between the Mokelumne River, fed by the upper lake, and the Stanislaus River, fed by the lower lake. On the horizon, the peaks of Mokelumne Wilderness (Hikes 79 and 80) lie northwest, and the mountains of Emigrant Wilderness (see next hike) rise southeast. Return the way you came.

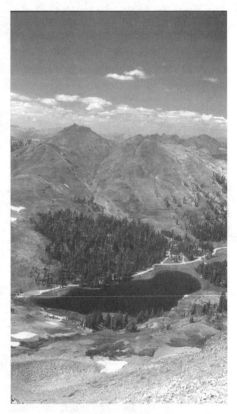

The road ends at lower Highland Lake on the edge of Carson-Iceberg Wilderness.

Nearest Visitor Centers Alpine Ranger Station, 209-753-2811, 1.3 miles east of Bear Valley Rd. in a small hut by Hwy. 4, is open sporadically in season Thursday–Monday 8:30 a.m.– 5 p.m. A more reliable information source is the Calaveras Ranger District Office, 209-795-1381, in Hathaway Pines on Hwy. 4; it's open Monday–Friday 8 a.m.–5 p.m. and Saturday 8 a.m.–2 p.m.

Backpacking Information A wilderness permit is required; get it at the Calaveras Ranger District Office during business hours or outside the Alpine Ranger Station at any time. While there are no campsites along this hike, options do exist east of Hiram Peak along the cross-country route toward Arnot Creek.

Nearest Campground Highland Lakes Campground, at the trailhead, has 35 sites ($12).

Additional Information www.fs.usda.gov/stanislaus

HIKE 82 Deadman Lake 🐾 🏃 🐐

Highlights	The volcanic High Sierra—solitude among falls, creeks, lakes, and peaks
Distance	4.5 miles round-trip
Total Elevation Gain/Loss	1,700'/1,700'
Hiking Time	3–5 hours
Recommended Maps	*A Guide to the Emigrant Wilderness* by the US Forest Service, USGS 7.5-min. *Sonora Pass*
Best Times	July–September
Agency	Emigrant Wilderness
Difficulty	★★★

EMIGRANT WILDERNESS receives only the smallest fraction of the hordes that descend upon neighboring Yosemite National Park. Blue Canyon lies in a most remote corner of the wilderness. Solitude, anyone?

Above 9,000 feet near the Sierra Divide, Blue Canyon exists in a landscape of volcanic rubble unusual in this land of naked granite. Roughly 10 million years ago, a period of volcanism centered east of today's Sonora Pass smothered the landscape beneath numerous flows of mud and molten rock. Today these looser volcanic sediments have largely been eroded away, but sections still remain north of Yosemite near the Sierra Crest. The layered, multihued bands exposed in the rocks and cliffs of Blue Canyon are part of these geologic remnants.

The Hike winds upward through Blue Canyon along the headwaters of Blue Canyon Creek, passing starkly beautiful waterfalls en route to a couple of vibrantly blue lakes—Blue Canyon Lake and Deadman Lake. The singletrack trail is steep and rocky, the lakes are surrounded by loose talus slopes, and the final mile to Deadman Lake is cross-country. Due to the high elevation, snow lingers deep into June and can return as early as October. While no water is available at the trailhead, Blue Canyon Creek is regularly accessible.

To Reach the Trailhead Take Hwy. 108 toward Sonora Pass. The unposted trailhead is accessed from a small pullout on the south side of Hwy. 108. Approaching from the west, it is 2.1 miles past Chipmunk Flat dispersed camping area; your landmark is the distinctive waterfall where Blue Canyon Creek joins Deadman Creek, and the pullout is immediately after the falls disappear from view. Approaching from the east, the trailhead is 2.8 miles past Sonora Pass (the pullout is 0.1 mile after the road begins its steepest descent from Sonora Pass). A dozen small lodgepole pines line the edge of the pullout, bare granite blocks sit across Hwy. 108 from it, and there is space for four cars.

Description From the pullout (0.0/8,920'), a discernible trail drops 40 feet to cross both Deadman Creek and the granite/volcanic geologic divide before quickly ascending the steep opposite slope to enter Blue Canyon. A few wilderness signs indicate you're on the right track as the trail winds through lodgepole pines and begins to offer views up-canyon. A use trail converges from the west side immediately before you cross a small feeder creek. Western white pines begin to appear, easily identified by the deep red of their plated bark. The trail then swings away from the creek and begins steeply climbing, soon crossing the most significant feeder creek yet (0.8/9,520'). Shortly thereafter, you come to a very sheer section of trail where the main path diverges in two directions—drop down to the creek and follow the obvious path

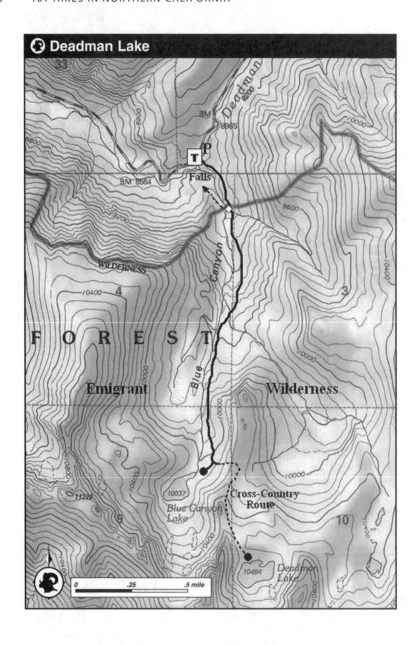

alongside it. The trail next curves away from the creek and peters out immediately before reaching Blue Canyon Lake (1.5/10,037'). At the bottom of a rubble-filled glacial cirque, the sapphire lake offers a few exposed campsites. Looking down-canyon, the peaks of Carson-Iceberg Wilderness (see previous hike) are visible on the skyline.

Begin your cross-country adventure to Deadman Lake from here by ascending east toward the col of the long ridge, which lies between the small shark's-fin peak seen from the early sections of trail and the thumb-like peak that juts from the ridge. Having reached the ridgetop (1.8/10,300'), you traverse north around the thumb on its east side and then scramble down over the tinkling piles of loose rock to reach the lake (2.2/10,484'). Barren, brilliantly blue, and ringed by naught but snow, rock, and lichen, Deadman Lake has a desolate beauty. Looking east, the nearby ridge marks the Sierra Divide and the routing of the Pacific Crest Trail. Return the way you came.

Nearest Visitor Centers Summit Ranger District Office, 209-965-3434, in Pinecrest on Hwy. 108, is open daily 8 a.m.–5 p.m. and closed weekends and holidays October–May. Volunteer-staffed Brightman Flat Visitor Center is occasionally open, too, and is 7 miles west of the Kennedy Meadows turnoff on Hwy. 108.

Backpacking Information A wilderness permit is required and is available at the above visitor centers. The few campsites along this hike are bare and exposed, with Blue Canyon Lake offering the best sites. No quota is in effect for this trailhead.

Nearest Campgrounds Chipmunk Flat dispersed camping area (free, river water only) is 5 miles east of the turnoff for Kennedy Meadows on Hwy. 108. Numerous other campgrounds line Hwy. 108, including Baker and Deadman Campgrounds at Kennedy Meadows (44 and 17 sites respectively, $20).

Additional Information www.fs.usda.gov/stanislaus

HIKE 83   Green Creek 🥾 🧍 🐐

Highlights	Rugged mountains and lakes east of the Sierra Crest
Distance	9.0 miles round-trip
Total Elevation Gain/Loss	1,700'/1,700'
Hiking Time	5–7 hours
Recommended Maps	*Hoover Wilderness Map and Guide* by the US Forest Service, USGS 7.5-min. *Dunderberg Peak*
Best Times	June–September
Agency	Hoover Wilderness, Humboldt-Toiyabe National Forest
Difficulty	★★★

GREEN CREEK SLICES eastward from the high peaks along Yosemite's northeast border, tumbling deeply through the rugged landscape of Hoover Wilderness. Multiple lakes nestle in its mountainous watershed, striking specimens of Jeffrey pine stand fast on the surrounding slopes, and the wilderness offers a quieter alternative than the backcountry bustle of Yosemite and the eastern Sierra farther south.

Yosemite National Park protects land up to the divide of the Sierra Nevada. Hoover Wilderness protects the mountains and upper watersheds on the far eastern side of the Sierra Crest just north and east of Mono Lake. The

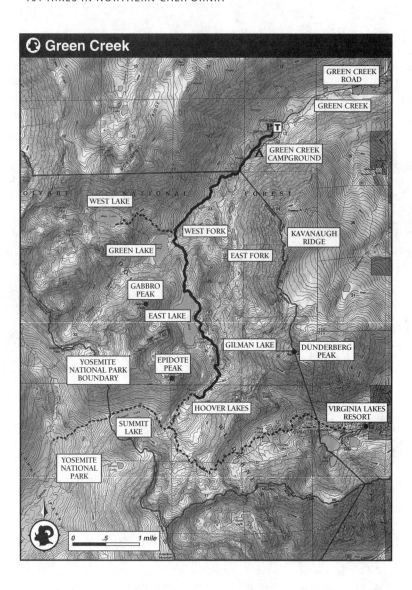

128,000-acre wilderness area has long been protected. Established as a primitive area in 1931, it later became one of the inaugural wilderness areas designated by the Wilderness Act in 1964.

The Hike ascends the Green Creek drainage in the central portion of the wilderness and visits Green and East Lakes en route; both offer overnight opportunities and provide good base camps for exploring the other lakes in the area.

The region feels remote, a quality enhanced by the long drive in from Hwy. 395, and the distinctive surrounding peaks are composed of complex metavolcanic rocks that add a distinct red hue to the rubbly peaks—a striking contrast to the granite that characterizes most of Yosemite. Note that both East and Green Lakes are used as a seasonal water supply for dry areas farther east; late-season drawdowns can noticeably lower lake levels.

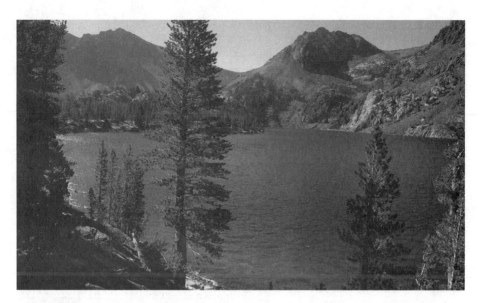

East Lake

To Reach the Trailhead Take Hwy. 395 north of the Hwy. 120 (Tioga Pass) junction for 21.2 miles to the unposted turnoff on the left for unpaved Green Creek Road—it's 2.2 miles north of the turnoff for Bodie. Approaching from the north, the turnoff is 3.8 miles south of the Bridgeport Ranger Station.

Follow Green Creek Rd. and bear left in 0.9 mile where Upper Summers Meadow Rd. splits left. In 2.5 miles, bear right to remain on Green Creek Road at the junction with Dunderberg Meadow Road. Continue for another 6 miles, including a long stretch along the creek valley (dispersed camping permitted). You reach the substantial trailhead parking area on the right, a short distance before Green Creek Campground at road's end. The road is easily passable for low-clearance vehicles. Water is available at the trailhead.

Description From the trailhead (0.0/8,020'), note the Jeffrey pine and Sierra juniper that surround the parking lot, telling indicators of your position on the margin between mountain forest and high desert environments. The flowing water of nearby Green Creek can be heard as you strike out on the singletrack trail,

quickly passing a huge and gnarly Jeffrey pine on the right—the first of many ancient and impressive specimens on this hike.

Fluttering aspens and lodgepole pines appear as you slowly rise, briefly spotting the road below that continues to the campground. Glimpses appear of the high ridges that hem in this watershed—Monument Ridge to the north, Kavanaugh Ridge south—soaring high above 10,000 feet. A prominent avalanche path scars the flanks of Kavanaugh.

You reach your first open view up-canyon—Virginia Pass crosses the saddle at the head of the valley; Gabbro Peak (11,033') is to its left—and then encounter the final stretch of Green Creek Road, which you follow as it approaches bubbling Green Creek and passes a private cabin (0.5/8,110'). The road narrows to a wide trail, immediately crosses a small water source, and then climbs a nicely laid rock path to run along a short bluff above the river.

The trail narrows further to wide singletrack and begins a steadier climb, returning to the now rushing creek. A series of switchbacks then climb through a bouldery area before leveling out to offer the first view down-valley. You can trace the transition to drier conditions by the rapid disappearance of trees farther east; trees on the sunnier south-facing slopes diminish more rapidly than their counterparts on shadier north-facing slopes.

A steady, traversing rise leads you to a massive and gnarled Jeffrey pine just before you cross a small creek and reach the boundary of Hoover Wilderness (0.9/8,380'). You cross a pair of water sources among thicker aspen and enjoy your first view of striking Dunderberg Peak (12,374') to the south, its red volcanic summit contrasting with the pale granite that composes most of Kavanaugh Ridge.

The route winds through a lush aspen grove, reenters the bare slopes above, and then returns to thick forest and makes a slow, steady ascent. The hulk of Gabbro Peak looms ahead and good views down-valley accompany you as you hike again over open terrain to reach the posted junction for West Lake (2.2/8,920'), a scenic but strenuous side trip that climbs a steep 1.5 miles and 950 feet to the lake.

Bear left instead toward East and Green Lakes, dropping briefly to rock-hop across Green Creek and reach the shores of Green Lake. Dammed on its eastern shore, the lake level can be influenced by human activity when water is released downstream for agricultural purposes (a long-standing use almost certainly grandfathered in when the wilderness was established).

The trail forks just as the lake comes into view. Right leads along the lakeshore to several campsites; left marks your continuing route, which completes a quick series of switchbacks to bring you close to the audible stream emanating from East Lake above. The trail ascends the rocky landscape and crosses the stream on some nicely placed boulders (2.5/9,100').

Western white pines appear, along with some sizable hemlocks in a mature forest lush with corn lilies and lupine. A steady climb returns you parallel to the trickling stream, and then back across it. As you climb the slopes here, notice the collection of jumbled rocks that surround you. This is a terminal moraine,

bulldozed into position by the glacier that once filled this valley.

A slow rise leads you through a field of large boulders, some car-sized. Whitebark pine appears just before the lake, and the surrounding peaks loom above. You cross the stream once more and reach East Lake by another old dam and outflow gate (3.3/9,460'). A large and heavily used lakeshore campsite is posted as NO CAMPING, though it makes for a pleasant rest stop.

The trail now winds along the steep east shore of the lake, which offers excellent views of the lake as its depths range from green to dark blue. Three prominent peaks hem in the lake to the west. From left to right (south to north), they are Epidote Peak (10,964'), Page Peaks, and Gabbro Peak (11,033'). Behind you to the east is the striking massif of Dunderberg Peak (12,374').

The trail reaches level terrain punctuated by flat granite slabs near the shore—some of the best camping potential is in this area—and then turns inland, passing a small tarn and climbing steeply to emerge above the far shore of East Lake. Views down-canyon extend the length of Monument Ridge; the distinctive U-shape of this glacially carved valley is clearly apparent.

The route crests briefly, then passes above tiny Nutter Lake and drops to reach its far shore (4.2/9,510'). Continuing, you soon hit views of Gilman Lake far below (4.5/9,500'). Surrounded by steep slopes with challenging access, the lake marks a scenic endpoint for the hike.

Though this hike description ends here, the trail continues beyond Gilman Lake to ascend through an increasingly rubbly landscape to reach Hoover Lakes—a small, twinkling pair nestled in the rocks—in just over a mile and a bit over 400 feet of climbing. Beyond, 1.7 miles past Gilman Lake, is a junction for the trail from Virginia Lakes. Bearing right here leads you in a half mile to long Summit Lake; its far side marks the Sierra Divide and boundary with Yosemite National Park.

Nearest Visitor Center Bridgeport Ranger Station, 760-932-7070, on the east side of Hwy. 395 just south of Bridgeport, is open daily 8 a.m.–4:30 p.m. Memorial Day–September, and weekdays only the rest of the year.

Backpacking Information A wilderness permit is required June–mid-September and can be picked up only at a Humboldt-Toiyabe ranger station. There is a quota of 40 people per day from this trailhead. Half of the permits can be reserved beginning March 1 by mailing in a wilderness-permit reservation application (available at **www.fs.usda.gov/htnf**; $3 per person); reservations are not accepted online or by phone. The other half of permits are available on a first-come, first-served basis. A bear canister is required for the wilderness; you can rent one at Ken's Sporting Goods in Bridgeport, 760-932-7707, or try the Mono Basin Visitor Center on Hwy. 395 in Lee Vining, 760-647-6331.

Nearest Campgrounds Green Creek Campground (10 sites, $17) is just past the trailhead at road's end and is first come, first served. Dispersed camping is also available along Green Creek Road on the drive in.

Additional Information www.fs.usda.gov/htnf

HIKE 84 Mono Lake ○ 👭

Highlights	Magical tufa-scapes
Distance	1.5 miles
Total Elevation Gain/Loss	Negligible
Hiking Time	1 hour
Recommended Map	USGS 7.5-min. *Lee Vining*
Best Times	May–October
Agency	Mono Lake Tufa State Reserve
Difficulty	★

EXPLORE THE wild wonderland of Mono Lake, with its salty water, tufas, and wildlife. It sits in a natural basin where the sun evaporates 45 inches of freshwater annually, leaving large quantities of dissolved solids behind. Ongoing for more than 700,000 years, this process has left Mono Lake exceptionally salty and alkaline—at present, with the lake being two times saltier than the ocean and 100 times more alkaline, 10% of it is dissolved solids. The water has a greasy, slippery feel and provides enough buoyancy to easily float a person.

Mono Lake currently has a surface area of approximately 70 square miles with an average depth of only 50 feet and a maximum depth of 150 feet. In 1941 the water-hungry city of Los Angeles began diverting four of the five streams that feed Mono Lake, which caused the lake level to drop more than 40 feet and upset the natural ecological balance. Concerned citizen groups took initiative in the 1980s to save the shrinking lake; in 1994 the State Water Resources Control Board ordered that Mono Lake be protected and its level be raised 17 feet over the ensuing decades. With the lake recovering (the level still varies from year to year depending on the weather), current efforts now focus on how best to rehabilitate the lake environment.

Mono Lake's receded shoreline has exposed many of the spectacular tufa formations

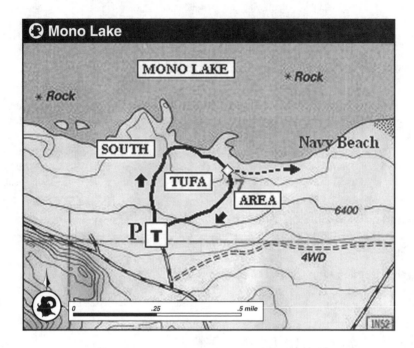

previously hidden beneath the surface. Formed by a reaction between calcium-bearing fresh-water springs that bubble up beneath the lake and the carbonate-rich water, the tufas are composed of solid calcium carbonate (limestone). A tufa tower grows upward from the bottom around the mouth of the spring until exposed above the surface of the lake. The towers of the South Tufa Area were completely submerged prior to 1941 and will gradually return to the lake with rising water levels. Numerous active tufa towers continue to grow unseen beneath the lake today.

The wildlife is as bizarre as the surrounding tufa-scapes. While the inhospitable water precludes the survival of most aquatic life (there are no fish in Mono Lake), a few species thrive here in mind-boggling numbers. The winter algae bloom provides sustenance for the brine shrimp, which begin to hatch in the spring. By midsummer, an estimated 4 trillion tiny brine shrimp are swimming in the lake; thousands of pounds are harvested annually for sale as tropical fish food. Brine-fly pupae, the lake's other primary denizen, also depend on the algae for sustenance. During the summer, mature flies blanket the lakeshore and produce harmless knee-high swarms when disturbed. The Kuzedika ("Fly-Pupae Eaters"), a band of the Paiute Tribe who once lived by the lake, harvested the fly pupae for food and trade. The size and color of brown rice grains, the prepared pupae taste like bacon bits. By late summer the algae is gone and the lake is once again clear and blue. Millions of birds pass through Mono Lake annually as they migrate or winter here, consuming shrimp and flies as they go. Osprey nest on top of a few exposed tufa towers. Safe from predators, the osprey hunt in the nearby creeks and lakes.

The Hike is an easy stroll on the lake's south shore through surreal tufa formations. The trail is open and accessible during the snow-free months of the year, with heavy visitation throughout the summer months. Due to the area's popularity, this is not a hike for solitude seekers. No water is available at the trailhead or anywhere along the route. A swim in Mono Lake can be an unforgettable experience. Nearby

Navy Beach offers the best opportunity and can be accessed either by hiking along the lakeshore or driving from the South Tufa Area. Avoid getting water in your mouth or eyes and be prepared for a salty, crusty coating on your body—no showers are available.

To Reach the Trailhead Take Hwy. 395 south from Lee Vining for 6 miles to the Hwy. 120 junction. Follow Hwy. 120 east for 5 miles to the posted turnoff on your left for the South Tufa Area; a mile-long dirt road leads to the large trailhead parking lot. A $3-per-person entrance fee is charged.

Description A 7-foot-wide asphalt path leads from the kiosk to the lakeshore, passing numerous tufa towers and soon providing your first opportunity to touch the lake water. The now-singletrack clay trail heads east from shore, winding through odd configurations of tufa and seasonal swarms of brine flies. While numerous paths wind through the brush, your route is clearly indicated. After turning away from the lake, the trail forks. Bearing left takes you on a longer return loop (an extra 0.5 mile) to the parking lot. Going straight brings you directly back.

Nearest Visitor Center The outstanding Mono Basin Scenic Area Visitor Center, 760-647-3044, is on Hwy. 395 near Lee Vining, 1.3 miles north of the Hwy. 120 junction. It's open daily 8 a.m.–5 p.m. mid-May–mid-October, with reduced hours until it closes for the season in early November.

Nearest Campgrounds While there are no campgrounds around Mono Lake itself, numerous options exist south of Mono Lake along Hwy. 120 in Lee Vining Canyon and Hwy. 158 (the June Lake loop).

Additional Information monolake.org

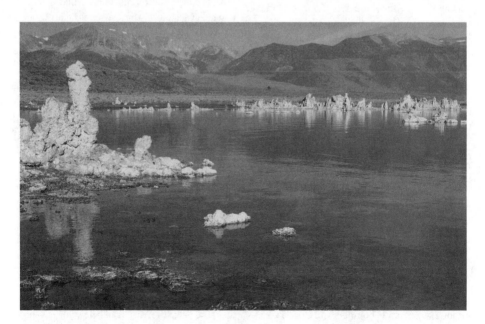

Tufas rise above the waters of Mono Lake.

HIKE 85   Nevada and Vernal Falls ⬈

Highlights	The raging river, incredible waterfalls, and spectacle of Yosemite
Distance	5.9 miles round-trip
Total Elevation Gain/Loss	1,900'/1,900'
Hiking Time	5–7 hours
Recommended Maps	*Map of Yosemite Valley* by Tom Harrison Maps, USGS 7.5-min. *Half Dome*
Best Times	Mid-May–June
Agency	Yosemite National Park
Difficulty	★★★

AH, YOSEMITE. Despite the crowds, despite the hassle, there is no other place on Earth like it. Go.

The Hike climbs from Yosemite Valley to the top of Nevada Fall, passing Vernal Fall along the way via the Mist Trail and returning on the John Muir Trail. The more water there is in the river, the more spectacular the hike—snowmelt typically increases its flow until the end of June, at which point it begins to decrease considerably. Exploding spray courses over the trail below Vernal Fall for much of the season, making good raingear and waterproof boots useful but not essential. Crowds are unavoidable and, for some, perhaps overwhelming. Winter routes are available, and much of the hike can be done year-round—check the latest conditions at the visitor center (see box page 289). Water is available at the trailhead.

To Reach the Trailhead Park in one of Yosemite Valley's day-use parking lots and take the free Yosemite Valley Shuttle Bus to Happy Isles Nature Center. A $20-per-vehicle entrance fee is charged for Yosemite National Park, valid for seven days.

Description From the bus stop (0.0/4,030'), cross the Merced River bridge and head upriver on the 15-foot-wide superhighway of packed dirt to quickly reach the gigantic trailhead sign. Just beyond the sign, the trail winds up among huge granite boulders and closely parallels the now violent river. As you ascend, look

for two of Yosemite's other landmark waterfalls—Upper Yosemite Fall is briefly visible behind you down-canyon before being cut off from view by Glacier Point, and the wispy fall of Illilouette Creek to the Merced River can be momentarily seen cross-canyon.

Vernal Fall Bridge (0.8/4,400') provides your first views of the waterfall. Its smooth, foaming curtain of water drops 317 feet and is dominated by two towering granite peaks—Mount Broderick (6,706') on the left and Liberty Cap (7,076') just beyond it. Restrooms and a drinking fountain are available. Postings around the bridge indicate that, yes, the strong current can batter you to death against the rocks. Here, as everywhere along this hike, *do not go in the water.*

Climbing from the bridge, the trail quickly reaches a junction for the John Muir Trail (JMT) (1.0/4,440')—continue straight up the Mist Trail. Billowing clouds of spray soon wash over the trail as it climbs through a lush garden of dripping greenery. You will get wet, so protect your camera. Just where the mist tapers out, you can peer into the heart of the fall over the top of a glistening rainbow, an unforgettable sight. Climbing to the top of the fall, the trail becomes steep and narrow; it traverses the face of a granite cliff, where hikers are protected by a metal guardrail. Surmounting this section, you reach a wide, open space above the fall where hikers dry out or sunbathe (1.5/5,050'). Look over the lip of the fall at the Mist Trail below you. Do not be tempted to go in the river—almost every year, some unfortunate soul is swept over the fall and killed.

Continuing to Nevada Fall, parallel the river on any one of the many use paths to rejoin the main trail. Passing another short connector to the JMT, the trail crosses the river and climbs gradually to near the base of Nevada Fall. Here the mist is blown down-canyon rather than over the trail and forms a towering wall of spray visible through the trees. A short scramble would take you into the mist, but the fall itself is obscured if the river level is high.

With the sheer cliffs of Liberty Cap looming overhead, the trail then climbs 600 feet via nearly two dozen ever-tightening switchbacks to reach another junction with restroom facilities (2.3/6,000'). To return to the trailhead go right on the JMT. In 0.2 mile you reach the top of Nevada Fall, where another restroom is available. You can access the cascade's protected lip via a short spur trail before the river crossing. Nevada Fall explodes, its water blown into swirling clouds that flow like an airborne river. Peering over the edge, buffeted by its winds, marvel at the torrent plummeting 571 feet to the rocks below.

The trail continues across the river and soon reaches a fork—go right. Traversing below the escarpment of Panoramic Cliffs, the JMT provides outstanding views of Liberty Cap and Nevada Fall, before descending along seemingly endless switchbacks to rejoin your earlier trail just above Vernal Fall Bridge (5.1/4,440'). Halfway down, you have the option of retracing your steps on the Mist Trail by taking the posted connection to the top of Vernal Fall. Return to Happy Isles to conclude your day on the trail.

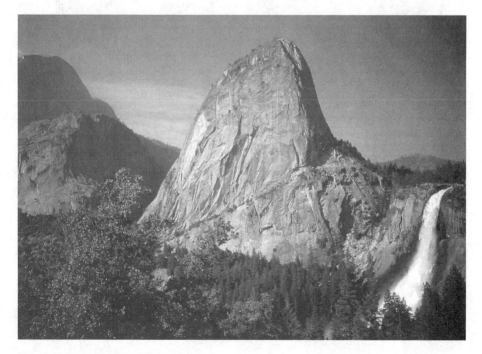

Nevada Fall explodes below Liberty Cap.

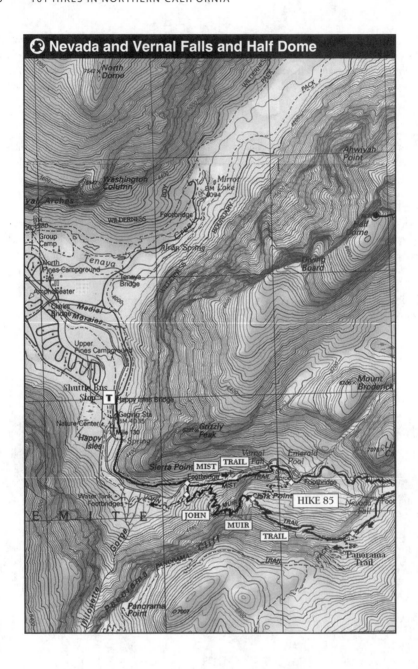

● Nevada and Vernal Falls and Half Dome

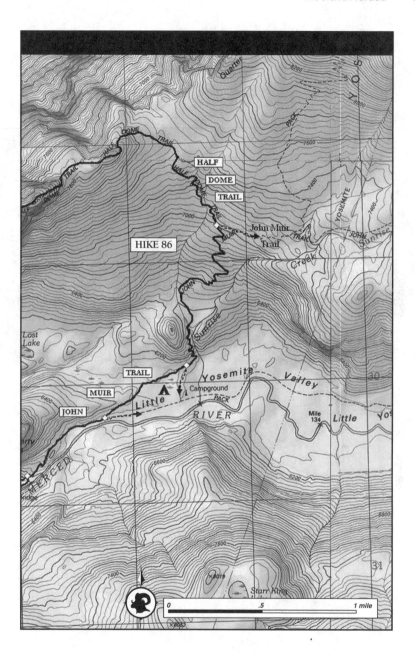

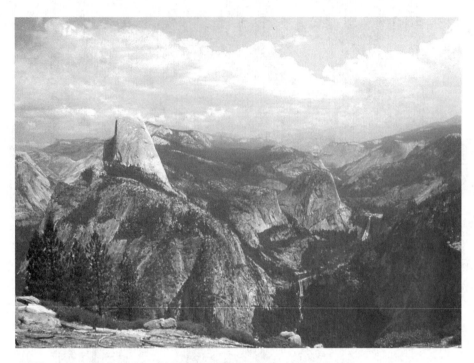

Half Dome from Glacier Point, with Vernal and Nevada Falls visible to the right

Nearest Visitor Center Valley Visitor Center, in Yosemite Village (Shuttle Bus Stops 5 and 9), is open 365 days a year. In summer it's open daily from approximately 9 a.m. to 7 p.m. (hours may vary depending on budget and staffing), with reduced hours the rest of the year. For general recorded information, call 209-372-0200.

Backpacking Information The closest backcountry camping is in Little Yosemite Valley, 0.5 mile past the top of Nevada Fall. See the next hike for more information about the wilderness-permit system.

Nearest Campgrounds Reservations are required mid-March–November for the 3 car campgrounds (each $20 per night) in Yosemite Valley: Upper Pines (238 sites), Lower Pines (60 sites), and North Pines (81 sites). Reservations are available up to 5 months in advance, in blocks of 1 month at a time, with the next block becoming available on the 15th of each month. (For example, reservations for June 15–July 14 become available on February 15.) To make reservations, call 877-444-6777 between 7 a.m. and 9 p.m. (7 a.m.– 7 p.m. November–February), or visit **recreation.gov**—you should reserve as early as possible on the 15th.

If you arrive without reservations in the Valley, try first-come, first-served Camp 4, a walk-in camping area (no individual sites; smaller groups will likely share the 6-person sites with others; $5 per person). Otherwise, head outside the Valley—try Tuolumne Meadows or Bridalveil Creek Campgrounds in the morning, and the US Forest Service campgrounds just west of the park in the afternoon and evening.

Additional Information nps.gov/yose

HIKE 86 Half Dome 🥾🚶

Highlight	Scaling Half Dome by cable with dizzying vertigo
Distance	16.4 miles round-trip
Total Elevation Gain/Loss	4,800'/4,800'
Hiking Time	10–12 hours
Recommended Map	USGS 7.5-min. *Half Dome*
Best Times	Mid-June–September
Agency	Yosemite National Park
Difficulty	★★★★★

(See map on page 286.)

THERE IS NO OTHER hike in the world like this one.

The Hike is an extremely strenuous, all-day affair that climbs to the summit of Half Dome from Yosemite Valley. (It is a dramatic extension of Hike 85.) The final stretch to the top is by a cable route so steep that you need to pull yourself up with both arms. Hikers should be in good shape and not suffer from acrophobia. Installed by the park once conditions allow, the cable route is usually up by Memorial Day and removed in early to mid-October. It is closed during the winter months. Sunscreen is essential for this hike, because the bare rock of Half Dome provides no protection against the sun's burning rays.

Though arduous, the biggest challenge of ascending Half Dome is obtaining the permit needed to do so—permits to hike to the top are required seven days per week when the cables are up. In order to protect wilderness character and natural resources and reduce crowding, a maximum of 300 hikers are allowed each day beyond the base of the subdome (roughly 225 day-hikers and 75 backpackers).

Permits are distributed by lottery at **recre ation.gov,** with one preseason lottery (applications due in March, results announced in mid-April) and daily lotteries during the hiking season. During the preseason lottery, 225 permits are available for each day. During the hiking season, approximately 50 permits are available each day by lottery. Applications must be submitted two days before the hiking date between midnight and 1 p.m. Pacific time; results are sent later that night. (For example, to hike on Friday, you would apply early in the day on Wednesday and receive e-mail notification of the results that night.)

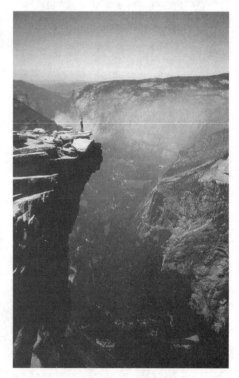

Dance with vertigo a vertical mile above Yosemite Valley.

If you have flexibility in your schedule, you have much better odds of securing a permit for a weekday than a weekend. Don't be tempted to climb Half Dome without a permit—rangers are stationed at the base of the subdome and will turn you away without one. To apply for a permit, visit **recreation.gov** or call 877-444-6777 between 7 a.m. and 9 p.m. Pacific time. A nonrefundable application fee is charged, plus an additional per-person fee if you do receive a permit.

To Reach the Trailhead Park in one of Yosemite Valley's day-use parking lots and take the free Yosemite Valley Shuttle Bus to Happy Isles Nature Center. There is a $20 entrance fee per vehicle for Yosemite National Park, valid for seven days.

Description From the bus stop (0.0/4,030'), cross the Merced River bridge and head upriver to quickly reach the gigantic trailhead sign. Just beyond the sign, the trail winds up among huge granite boulders and closely parallels the now violent river. Vernal Fall Bridge (0.8/4,400') provides your first views of the waterfall. Its smooth, foaming curtain of water drops 317 feet and is dominated by two towering granite peaks—Mount Broderick (6,706') on the left and Liberty Cap (7,076') just beyond it. Restrooms and a drinking fountain are available. Postings around the bridge indicate that, yes, the strong current can batter you to death against the rocks. Here, as everywhere along this hike, *do not go in the water.*

Climbing from the bridge, the trail quickly reaches a junction for the John Muir Trail (JMT; 1.0/4,440')—continue straight up the Mist Trail. Billowing clouds of spray soon wash over the trail as it climbs through a lush garden of dripping greenery. You will get wet, so protect your camera. Just where the mist tapers out, you can peer into the heart of the fall over the top of a glistening rainbow, an unforgettable sight. Climbing to the top of the fall, the trail becomes steep and narrow; it traverses the face of a granite cliff, where hikers are protected by a metal guardrail. Surmounting this section, you reach a wide, open space above the fall where hikers dry out or sunbathe (1.5/5,050'). Look over the lip of the fall at the Mist Trail below you. Do not be tempted to go in the river—almost every year, some unfortunate soul is swept over the fall and killed.

Continuing to Nevada Fall, parallel the river on any one of the many use paths to rejoin the main trail. Passing another short connector to the JMT, the trail crosses the river and climbs gradually to near the base of Nevada Fall. Here the mist is blown down-canyon rather than over the trail and forms a towering wall of spray visible through the trees. A short scramble would take you into the mist, but the fall itself is obscured if the river level is high.

With the sheer cliffs of Liberty Cap looming overhead, the trail then climbs 600 feet via nearly two dozen ever-tightening switchbacks to reach another junction with restroom facilities (2.3/6,000'). To continue toward Half Dome, head left, immediately passing the restroom on your way toward Little Yosemite Valley.

Now gently climbing, the trail crests a small rise; it loses elevation for the first time where the top of Half Dome becomes visible northwest. Wide and sandy, the path rejoins the much calmer river before arcing away from it and passing the designated campground and seasonal ranger station on the right, as well as burn marks and other evidence of a 2014 wildfire that burned portions of this area. Bear left at all junctions. *Little Yosemite Valley is your last reliable opportunity to get water for the rest of the hike.*

Turning north, your trail ascends through a dense red fir forest to reach the junction with the Half Dome Trail (4.8/7,000'). While the JMT bears east here on its long journey to Mount Whitney, you continue north to begin the ultimate ascent. You soon encounter a seasonal spring on the left where a small pipe conveniently diverts water for easy fill-up during the spring and early summer. Views across Tenaya Canyon open up through the trees where the trail heads west to the base of the open slopes on the ridgetop (6.3/7,900').

Signs in many languages warn of the danger of lightning strikes. Take them seriously and do not proceed if thunderstorms are threatening. With your horizon clear, continue upward on the zigzagging stairway of granite blocks. As you pass twisted trees clinging to life in the nooks and crannies of bare rock, the trail gets progressively steeper. It soon crests a small rise and then drops to the subdome at the bottom of the cable route (7.3/8,410').

With both arms needed to pull yourself along, hand protection is important for preventing cable burn—a pile of mangled gloves is often found at the base of the cable route, though bringing your own is recommended. The climb steepens on the upper section before finally reaching the end of the line (7.5/8,810'). The actual summit (8,838') is at the north end.

Experience the dizzying vertigo of Half Dome as you creep toward the edge, staring almost 5,000 feet down to the valley floor. Half Dome's northwest face is a vertical, 2,000-foot sheer wall

of granite, on which climbers can often be spotted. With unparalleled views from here, most of the southern half of the park is visible. Almost due north is Mount Hoffman (10,850'), below which runs Tioga Road. Looking east beyond Little Yosemite Valley, the peaks of the Cathedral Range line the horizon. Southeast are the spires of the Clark Range, all of which exceed 11,000 feet. Closer by, Clouds Rest (Hike 88) is immediately northeast along the ridge, with the bulges of Quarter Domes between it and Half Dome. If you look west down Yosemite Valley, many of the valley's most prominent landmarks can be identified—Glacier Point is across the Merced River canyon, and Cathedral Spires, El Capitan, and Yosemite Village are all visible.

Done reveling in this awe-inspiring place? Go back the way you came. For an alternate (and easier) descent, follow the JMT from Nevada Fall back to the Vernal Fall Bridge.

Nearest Visitor Center Valley Visitor Center, in Yosemite Village (Shuttle Bus Stops 5 and 9), is open 365 days a year. In summer it's open daily from approximately 9 a.m. to 7 p.m. (hours may vary depending on budget and staffing), with reduced hours the rest of the year. For general recorded information, call 209-372-0200.

Backpacking Information Turning the marathon ascent of Half Dome into an overnight trip makes for a more leisurely journey. Wilderness permits are required, and there is a quota for this trailhead that always fills up. While 60% of the permits are subject to reservation, the other 40% are available on a first-come, first-served basis.

First-come, first-served permits are available beginning at 11 a.m. the day before your hike, or you can reserve up to 24 weeks in advance by fax (recommended), by mail, or by calling 209-372-0740 Monday–Friday, 8:30 a.m.–4:30 p.m. ($5 reservation fee plus $5 per person). To learn more—and to download the reservation form for fax or mail—visit **nps.gov/yose.**

Permits can be obtained at the wilderness center adjacent to the Valley Visitor Center and from permit stations at Tuolumne Meadows, Wawona, Big Oak Flat (just past the west entrance station on Hwy. 120), and Hetch Hetchy. Bear canisters are required and can be rented from the permit stations. In Little Yosemite Valley, camping is allowed only at designated sites. Sleeping on Half Dome is prohibited.

Note that you must also request a Half Dome permit as part of the wilderness-permit application process—if Half Dome permits are available, you will receive a wilderness permit that includes them. If not, you can still apply for a permit via the daily Half Dome permit lottery (see above, page 290).

Nearest Campground Reservations are required mid-March–November for the 3 car campgrounds (each $20 per night) in Yosemite Valley: Upper Pines (238 sites), Lower Pines (60 sites), and North Pines (81 sites). Reservations are available up to 5 months in advance, in blocks of 1 month at a time, with the next block becoming available on the 15th of each month. (For example, reservations for June 15–July 14 become available on February 15.) To make reservations, call 877-444-6777 between 7 a.m. and 9 p.m. (7 a.m.– 7 p.m. November–February), or visit **recreation.gov**—you should reserve as early as possible on the 15th.

If you arrive without reservations in the Valley, try first-come, first-served Camp 4, a walk-in camping area (no individual sites; smaller groups will likely share the 6-person sites with others; $5 per person). Otherwise, head outside the Valley—try Tuolumne Meadows or Bridalveil Creek Campgrounds in the morning and the US Forest Service campgrounds just west of the park in the afternoon and evening.

Additional Information nps.gov/yose

HIKE 87 Sentinel Dome and Taft Point ◖

Highlights	Head-spinning verticality and excellent Half Dome views
Distance	5.2 miles round-trip
Total Elevation Gain/Loss	1,150'/1,150'
Hiking Time	2–3 hours
Recommended Maps	*Map of Yosemite Valley* by Tom Harrison Maps, USGS 7.5-min. *Half Dome*
Best Times	June–September
Agency	Yosemite National Park
Difficulty	★★

TAFT POINT PROTRUDES over an overhanging abyss that will send your vestibular system into stomach-churning overdrive. Sentinel Dome is a delightful and easily accessible landmark that exemplifies the park's geology and spectacular views, including excellent vistas of Half Dome. Combining this hike with a visit to nearby Glacier Point makes for an excellent day trip.

The Hike loops counterclockwise from Glacier Point Road, first visiting the bare summit of Sentinel Dome before circling back to Taft Point via a less traveled section of trail. As is true throughout most of Yosemite, this is a popular destination and you will likely see dozens to hundreds of people. Parking can be a hassle during busy times, especially during the height of the summer. Come early or later in the day for a more relaxing experience. Note

that the hike to Sentinel Dome is a good outing for children, but Taft Point is surrounded by precipitous and unprotected cliffs—not the best place for young wanderers. No water is available at the trailhead.

To Reach the Trailhead Take Glacier Point Rd. 6 miles east of the Bridalveil Creek Campground turnoff to reach the trailhead, 2.2 miles before road's end at Glacier Point. Parking is limited, and the overflow can stretch for some distance in both directions.

Description From the trailhead (0.0/7,730'), strike out among large western white pines, red firs, and Jeffrey and lodgepole pines. You immediately reach a junction, where you turn right toward Sentinel Dome (you'll return from the left). You cross a small dry drainage and then rise briefly through a mature forest.

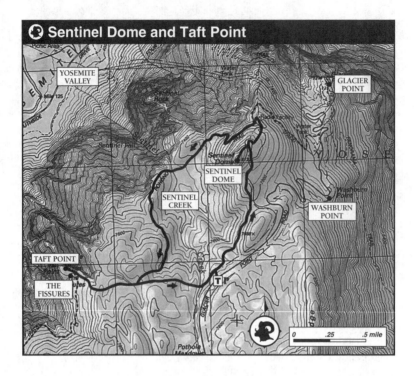

The trail travels over rockier terrain, and soon the rounded form of Sentinel Dome comes into view. A gentle, traversing rise leads you past an enormous Jeffrey pine more than 4 feet in diameter and then winds slowly upward toward Sentinel Dome ahead. You emerge on open granite slabs and reach a junction by old pavement, which you follow as it curves around Sentinel Dome. Half Dome begins to loom through the trees as you reach a junction for Glacier Point (0.9/7,960'); bear left to quickly reach the posted junction for the summit of Sentinel Dome (1.1/8,000').

The views expand as you make the short, heart-boosting climb to the top (1.2/8,120'), where a sweeping 360-degree vista awaits. Major landmarks (including Half Dome, Liberty Cap, Nevada Fall, and Yosemite Falls) are identified on a helpful metal disc at the summit.

To continue on the loop, descend to the previous junction and bear left (1.3/8,000'). The crowds immediately diminish as the wide dirt trail descends and crosses an access road, which switchbacks down on either side of the trail to reach a cell and radio tower facility.

The trail now cuts left and passes views of El Capitan, its sheer granite walls soaring upward above lower Yosemite Valley. At the next trail junction for Glacier Point (1.7/7,800'), continue left toward Taft Point. The narrow trail traverses gently through the woods, passes intermittent views of Yosemite Falls and El Capitan, and makes a pair of switchbacks among some substantial fir trees.

The quiet woods and lack of crowds offer a delightful respite from the park bustle as you descend to reach flowing Sentinel Creek (2.5/7,420'), where a nearby ledge offers an excellent view of the lower valley, including El Capitan and Cathedral Spires.

Continuing, you cross the creek and ascend through mature forest with a few intermittent views. The trail next winds between two 20-foot-high rocks and into a striking boulder landscape. Sentinel Dome reappears behind you as the trail turns inland, climbs slowly, and passes many grizzled Jeffrey pines.

The path narrows on its steeper, final ascent to Taft Point Trail (3.5/7,770'), where you go right. This superhighway of a trail cruises past lush corn lilies, ferns, and a small wildflower-filled meadow, then makes a gentle descent on the rock-lined path.

The open granite slabs of Taft Point become visible ahead and soon you reach the area known as the Fissures, where large cracks in the granite provide glimpses of the drop-dead vertical cliffs beside you. Belly out to the edge for a heart-racing peer into the abyss.

Beyond the Fissures, just before Taft Point, you pass the continuing trail to Inspiration and Dewey Points on the left before heading upward to your final stop at Taft Point itself (4.1/7,503'). It's an intense and stomach-churning spot, where a small railing offers a modicum of protection and allows you to lean out and peer down over the overhanging lip at several thousand feet of vertical drop.

After testing your mettle against verticality, retrace your steps to the earlier junction (4.7/7,770') and proceed back to the parking lot on the wide and easy-cruising trail (5.2/7,750').

Nearest Visitor Center Valley Visitor Center, in Yosemite Village (Shuttle Bus Stops 5 and 9), is open 365 days a year. In summer it's open daily from approximately 9 a.m. to 7 p.m. (hours may vary depending on budget and staffing), with reduced hours the rest of the year. For general recorded information, call 209-372-0200.

Nearest Campground Bridalveil Creek Campground (110 sites, $14) is on Glacier Point Rd., approximately 8 miles from its junction with Hwy. 41. All of the sites are first come, first served and typically fill by early afternoon. The campground is open July–early September, depending on conditions.

Additional Information nps.gov/yose

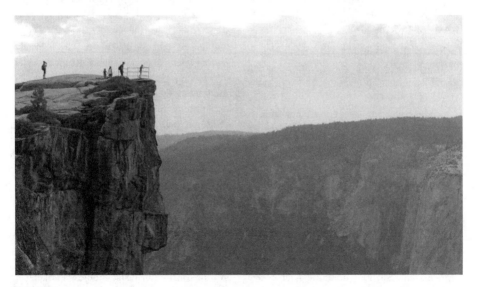

Taft Point

HIKE 88   Clouds Rest 🥾 🚶

Highlight	Half Dome minus the madness
Distance	14.0 miles round-trip
Total Elevation Gain/Loss	2,500'/2,500'
Hiking Time	8–10 hours
Recommended Maps	*Yosemite National Park & Vicinity* by Wilderness Press, USGS 7.5-min. *Tenaya Lake*
Best Times	Mid-June–September
Agency	Yosemite National Park
Difficulty	★★★★

LET'S FACE IT: Yosemite Valley is crazy. If the congestion there is too much for you, then you should be on Tioga Road. And if you're on Tioga Road, you should be climbing Clouds Rest.

The Hike ascends Clouds Rest (9,926') from Tenaya Lake, a steady climb with rewarding summit views of Half Dome and much of the national park. As throughout Yosemite, there will be people on the trail with you. However, there will be far fewer people than you would encounter on trails emanating from the Valley. Snow generally clears by mid-June, although it can linger into early July in years of deep snowpack. Water is unavailable at the trailhead, and sources beyond Tenaya Creek can be nonexistent late in the season.

To Reach the Trailhead Go east on Tioga Rd. (Hwy. 120) to just west of Tenaya Lake in central Yosemite National Park, and park in the Sunrise Trailhead lot, 33 miles east of Crane Flat and 9 miles west of Tuolumne Meadows Campground. A $20-per-vehicle entrance fee is charged for Yosemite National Park, valid for seven days.

Description At the trailhead, by the food-storage lockers, the trail immediately splits—go left toward Sunrise High Sierra Camp. Passing among lodgepole pines, the wide concrete path soon becomes dirt. Skirting a pleasant meadow before crossing Tenaya Creek, the trail quickly reaches a junction for Tuolumne High Sierra Camp—bear right toward Sunrise. After briefly

paralleling the creek, the trail curves south and passes on a long, level stretch, weaving through boulders, lodgepole pines, and clearings seasonally flush with tiger lilies and other wildflowers. Red firs and western white pines appear as the trail climbs again; you soon find yourself switchbacking steeply to the top of a forested saddle. There is a four-way junction here—continue straight ahead. The unmarked trail that comes in from the right leads to surprise viewpoints of upper Tenaya Canyon. Left leads to the nearby Sunrise Lakes.

Descending south, the trail passes a shallow pond before crossing a small tributary of Tenaya Creek, which can run dry late in the season. This is your last source for water. Your route is a gentle rise from here to the next junction, where you continue straight ahead. The trail drops briefly before making a quick ascent to a broad saddle where views south are obscured by the trees . . . but not for long.

Continue along the ridgeline. Suddenly nothing impairs your view of the naked flanks of Clouds Rest shearing 4,000 feet into Tenaya Canyon below. Sheets of exfoliating granite peel away from the slopes. The trail becomes indistinct the final 200 feet to the summit; take the broad granite runway directly along the ridgeline to the top (9,926').

Visible for the first time, Half Dome immediately draws your attention southwest. Those with binoculars can pick out the cable route's ant line on the northeast shoulder (Hike 86). Yosemite Valley winds away west below it all.

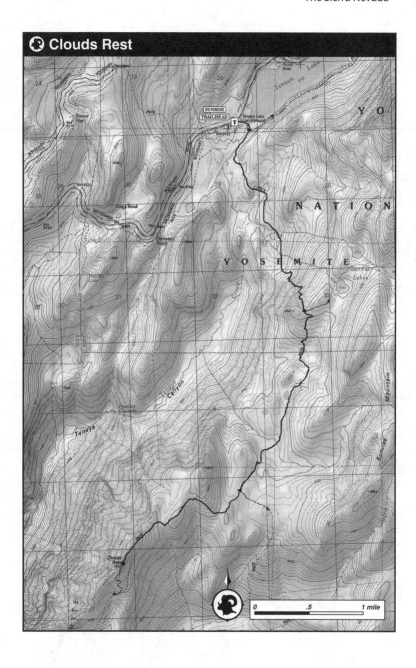

Clouds Rest

Southeast beyond Little Yosemite Valley, the peaks of the Clark Range can be seen. Northeast on the skyline are the jagged pinnacles of the Cathedral Range. North is Mount Hoffman (10,850'), below which the Tioga Road winds around Tenaya Lake. Return the way you came.

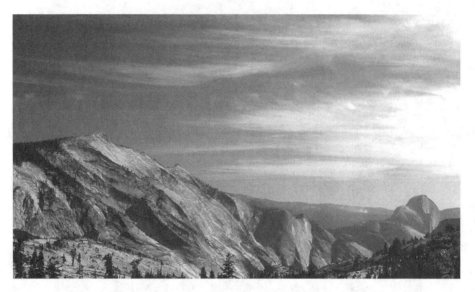

Clouds Rest (left) and Half Dome in the distance

Nearest Visitor Center Tuolumne Meadows Visitor Center, 209-372-0263, is open approximately 8 a.m.–5 p.m. daily mid-June–mid-October, with occasional extended hours during peak times. For general Yosemite information, call 209-372-0200.

Backpacking Information Numerous campsites exist along or near this hike, although few have convenient access to water; try Sunrise Lakes. No legal options are available on the summit. A wilderness permit is required, and there is a quota for this trailhead that almost always fills. Permits can be obtained on a first-come, first-served basis beginning at 11 a.m. the day before your hike, or you can make a reservation up to 24 weeks in advance by fax (recommended), by mail, or by calling 209-372-0740 Monday–Friday, 8:30 a.m.–4:30 p.m. ($5 reservation fee plus $5 per person). To learn more—and to download the reservation form for fax or mail—visit **nps.gov/yose.**

Permits can be obtained at the wilderness center at Tuolumne Meadows as well as in Yosemite Valley adjacent to the Valley Visitor Center and from permit stations at Wawona, Big Oak Flat (just past the west entrance station on Hwy. 120), and Hetch Hetchy. Bear canisters are required and can be rented from the permit stations.

Nearest Campground Tuolumne Meadows Campground (304 sites, $20) opens once snow conditions allow, typically late June or early July, and usually closes in late September. Half the sites are subject to reservation; the other half are first come, first served and typically fill by early afternoon. Reservations can be made up to 5 months in advance, in blocks of 1 month at a time, with the next block becoming available on the 15th of each month. To make reservations, call 877-444-6777 between 7 a.m. and 9 p.m. or visit **recreation.gov.** Try to reserve as early as possible.

Additional Information nps.gov/yose

HIKE 89 Ireland Lake ◯ 🚶

Highlight	An emerald jewel in Yosemite's high country
Distance	22.4 miles round-trip
Total Elevation Gain/Loss	3,300'/3,300'
Hiking Time	12–16 hours
Recommended Maps	*Yosemite National Park & Vicinity* by Wilderness Press, USGS 7.5-min. *Vogelsang Peak*
Best Times	July–September
Agency	Yosemite National Park
Difficulty	★★★★

TUOLUMNE MEADOWS is the primary gateway to Yosemite's high country, offering a constellation of trails that radiate in all directions. The Cathedral Range jags skyward to the south, a collection of striking and rugged mountains that cradle several beautiful lakes in their arms. Ireland Lake is one of the most scenic, a large disc flanked by expansive green heather evocative of its namesake locale.

The Hike completes a long loop from Tuolumne Meadows, traveling first along broad Lyell Canyon on the John Muir Trail (JMT) and then climbing west across the northern flanks of the Cathedral Range, including a 3-mile side trip to Ireland Lake. After reaching scenic Vogelsang High Sierra Camp, the journey descends Rafferty Creek Trail to return to the trailhead.

This is a very long hike that only the überfit can complete in a single day. Turning it into an overnight journey is recommended (though it does require navigating the park's wilderness-permit system). If you are interested in a more manageable day hike, consider just hiking along Lyell Canyon, which offers mostly level hiking and increasingly grand scenery the farther you go. Alternatively, make the 14.6-mile out-and-back to Vogelsang High Sierra Camp via Rafferty Creek; it's an exceptionally scenic spot, backed by jagged cliffs of soaring granite.

Note that mosquitoes can be thick in Lyell Canyon and the Ireland Creek drainage early in the season; bring insect repellent.

To Reach the Trailhead Take Tioga Rd. (Hwy. 120) to Tuolumne Meadows and turn right 0.7 mile after the general store. You pass the Wilderness Center in 0.1 mile and reach the JMT trailhead parking area on the left in 0.5 mile. Overnight hikers can park at either location; store any food in the bear boxes around the parking area.

Description From the JMT trailhead (0.0/ 8,720'), cross the road and strike out on the broad trail as it runs parallel to the pavement and along flowing Dana Fork, one of the headwater streams of the Tuolumne River. Flowing into Hetch Hetchy Reservoir in the northwestern portion of the park, the Tuolumne River watershed encompasses much of Yosemite, draining 51% of the park.

The JMT bears right shortly after the park ranger station (0.3/8,720'), quickly crosses Dana Fork on a sturdy footbridge, and runs alongside the wide stream. You soon reach the next junction (0.5/8,740'), where you bear right toward Lyell Canyon. The wide and level path travels through woods and soon reveals views of Mammoth Peak and Kuna Crest to the southeast, which hem in Lyell Canyon to the east.

You next cross Lyell Fork on two distinctive bridges spanning granite slabs. The river runs green and enticing, with deep opportunities for a refreshing dip. Immediately past the bridges, bear left at the junction for Tuolumne Meadows Campground to remain on the JMT

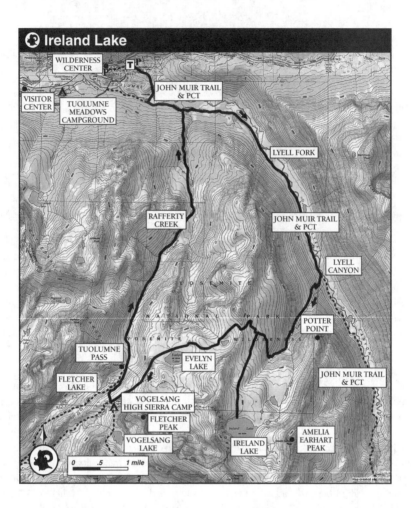

Ireland Lake

(1.1/8,720'). You travel through dense, lush woods on a wide path and cross granite slabs, where boulders mark the edge of the trail. Note the large pink crystals that pimple these boulders. These are feldspar, one of the constituent minerals of granite.

You next reach the junction with Rafferty Creek Trail by its namesake stream (1.6/8,760'), your return trail (or direct route for the day hike to Vogelsang). The continuing hike remains on the JMT, crossing the creek on a bridge and beginning a rockier, viewless section through the trees. You eventually break out in a large meadow, where you can see the dark pyramid of Mount Dana (13,057') looming to the west-northwest and Kuna Crest to the southeast.

Lyell Fork soon comes into sight for the first time. Running close to the river, the trail turns a corner to the southeast to reveal far-reaching views up-canyon. The trail winds along the river and by broad meadows, and soon the distinctive profile of Potter Point appears up-canyon to the right. The rugged profile of Amelia Earhart Peak (11,974') rises to its south, a regular companion over the upcoming miles (it hems in Ireland Lake).

Views of Amelia Earhart Peak expand as you continue up-canyon, weaving closer and then farther away from the river. You rise briefly into the woods as the river drops in sheets of water over bare rock ledges, curve inland, then return close to the river and reach the junction for Ireland Lake and Vogelsang (5.8/8,900').

Turn right toward Ireland Lake to make a steady ascent on a singletrack, rocky trail that climbs via multiple switchbacks before traversing over toward increasingly audible—but still out-of-sight—Ireland Creek. The climb continues among increasingly thick lodgepole pines; a brief glimpse of the nearby rushing creek provides a rare view of the waterway.

You cross a small tributary joining from the right and then quickly reach the first convenient access to Ireland Creek. The gradient eases soon thereafter as the trail runs close to the creek and then enters a nice open meadow. Ireland Lake lies beyond the saddle above; you can also spy Ireland Creek, which drains the lake, sheeting over the rocks.

The trail next curves away from the creek and resumes a steady ascent up a narrowing canyon. The flow audibly diminishes as you climb through dense woods, switchback right, and then traverse away from the stream. You pass through a boulder-studded section and then curve left to make one final rise to the Ireland Lake junction (8.6/10,420').

Don't be put off by the erroneously signed distance to Ireland Lake (3.0 miles)—it refers to the round-trip distance. To make the highly recommended side trip, follow the easy singletrack trail toward Ireland Lake, which slowly climbs to soon offer views of the upper valley. Amelia Earhart Peak looms immediately to the southeast, while more distant Mount Florence (12,561') rises south.

Trees diminish as you pass into boulder-studded meadows laced by a small stream. You crest a rise and see the final ridge guarding Ireland Lake, which you attain after a short ascent. From here, it's a long walk across a vast

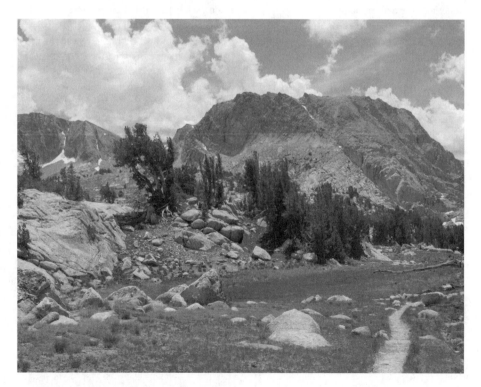

Approaching Vogelsang High Sierra Camp

meadow, a soft and emerald landscape devoid of trees and resonant of its Gaelic namesake. One last rise brings Ireland Lake into view. The trail peters out near the lake's northwest shore; from here it's a choose-your-own-adventure across the landscape to reach the shore (10.1/10,780').

The lake's crystalline blue-green water entices for a brisk swim, or you can simply enjoy the dramatic views of the mountain peaks that surround you. Admire the varied geology here. The peaks on the western side of the bowl are composed of distinctive layered metavolcanics, while those on the east are pale granite. Views also reach into the northern distance toward the peaks that define the Sierra Crest and park's boundary, including the bare granite of Mount Conness and more distant Matterhorn Peak.

If you're considering spending the night here, be aware that this vast and treeless meadow is very exposed to the elements. More shelter— and better potential camping options—can be found among the trees and rocks near the lake's outlet on the northeast shore.

After reveling in this beautiful spot, return to the earlier junction (11.6/10,420') and head west toward Vogelsang. You cross a small creek, make a level traverse, and then curve left to start a steadier climb. A pair of switchbacks leads you higher and to views east of the twin summits of Kuna Peak (13,002') and Koip Peak (12,962'). The boulder-lined path winds among increasing granite slabs and offers ever-more-expansive views west.

The route leads down to a scenic, unnamed pond backed by cliffs and talus fields. You cross the pond's outlet, climb briefly on a rock-lined trail, and then make a slow descent toward Evelyn Lake, which soon comes into view ahead. You descend to cross a large boulder-studded meadow lining the idyllic lakeshore, cross the outlet stream (13.6/10,350'), and enjoy excellent views, including vistas north toward the peaks that define the Sierra Crest and park boundary.

A section of nice trail and steps leads you beyond Evelyn Lake and toward the striking nearby cliffs and peaks of Fletcher and Vogelsang Peaks. The route descends to run along a ledge far above Rafferty Creek to your right (your return route), its deep valley backed by the crenulated ridge of Rafferty Peak.

A slow drop returns you to the trees, where the towering granite flanks of nearby Fletcher Peak loom imposingly, and then you abruptly emerge at the head of pleasant Fletcher Pond. Just beyond is a four-way junction by Vogelsang Camp (15.1/10,200'). To the right, by an old outhouse in the meadow, is the designated backpacker overnight area. To the left are the Vogelsang tent cabins and small camp store, which sells a few small sundries and snacks. The sheer cliffs of adjacent Fletcher Peak and farther jags of Vogelsang provide an exceptional backdrop.

To return to the trailhead, bear right toward Tuolumne Meadows to quickly begin a sustained drop on a rocky traverse. Small Booth Lake becomes visible below, the gradient eases, and you reach the junction with Rafferty Creek Trail in the broad saddle of Tuolumne Pass (15.9/10,050'). Continuing toward Tuolumne Meadows, you pass two small tarns and then commence a steady descent over a wide and much-used trail. The first trickles of Rafferty Creek appear as the trail levels briefly to pass through a smaller and then larger meadow.

The beautifully maintained trail, complete with granite steps and a continuous rock border, resumes its descent and leaves the dramatic views of Fletcher and Vogelsang Peaks behind. Nearby Rafferty Creek becomes increasingly audible, though there is no trailside access at this point, as you cross several small flowing water sources and eventually emerge in another small meadow. The gradient eases as the trail winds past many standing snags—remnants of a past wildfire— and then briefly runs alongside Rafferty Creek.

The descent ultimately deposits you at the earlier junction with the JMT (21.2/8,760'), where you turn left to return to the trailhead (22.4/8,720').

Nearest Visitor Center Tuolumne Meadows Visitor Center, 209-372-0263, is open approximately 8 a.m.–5 p.m. daily mid-June–mid-October, with occasional extended hours during peak times. For general Yosemite information, call 209-372-0200.

Backpacking Information Numerous campsites exist along this hike—in Lyell Canyon, at Ireland Lake, and at Vogelsang's designated backpacker area—though you must travel at least 4 miles from Tuolumne Meadows before setting up camp.

A wilderness permit is required, and there is a quota for this trailhead that almost always fills. Permits can be obtained on a first-come, first-served basis beginning at 11 a.m. the day before your hike, or you can reserve up to 24 weeks in advance by fax (recommended), by mail, or by calling 209-372-0740 Monday–Friday, 8:30 a.m.–4:30 p.m. ($5 reservation fee plus $5 per person). To learn more—and to download the reservation form for fax or mail—visit **nps.gov/yose.**

Permits can be obtained at the wilderness center at Tuolumne Meadows as well as in Yosemite Valley adjacent to the Valley Visitor Center and from permit stations at Wawona, Big Oak Flat (just past the west entrance station on Hwy. 120), and Hetch Hetchy. Bear canisters are required and can be rented from the permit stations.

Nearest Campground Tuolumne Meadows Campground (304 sites, $20) opens once snow conditions allow, typically late June or early July, and usually closes in late September. Half the sites are subject to reservation; the other half are first come, first served and typically fill by early afternoon. Reservations can be made up to 5 months in advance, in blocks of 1 month at a time, with the next block becoming available on the 15th of each month. To make reservations, call 877-444-6777 between 7 a.m. and 9 p.m. or visit **recreation.gov.** Try to reserve as early as possible.

Additional Information nps.gov/yose

HIKE 90 Mariposa Grove ☾

Highlights	The largest living things on Earth
Distance	5.8 miles
Total Elevation Gain/Loss	1,100'/1,100'
Hiking Time	3–4 hours
Recommended Map	USGS 7.5-min. *Mariposa Grove*
Best Times	May–October
Agency	Yosemite National Park
Difficulty	★★

INCOMPARABLE, indescribable, unbelievable, the giant sequoias must be experienced first-hand. Visit the Valley only and you have seen but half the wonders of Yosemite.

The Mariposa Grove is one of the most northerly of 75 recognized giant sequoia groves that dot the western slopes of the Sierra Nevada. It is also the most heavily visited. Not a spot for solitude, the grove receives hundreds to thousands of visitors daily. Most walk but a short distance to the Grizzly Giant before returning, leaving the trails—and the magnificent upper grove—to far fewer people.

The Hike explores the entire grove by trail and allows you moments to briefly escape the Yosemite bustle and peacefully commune with these giant trees. Mariposa Grove is open daily from approximately late April until late October, when snow closes the 2-mile access road. Crowds are lightest in the evenings and early mornings. Water is available at the trailhead.

Note: In 2015–16, significant changes will take place in Mariposa Grove as the park implements a comprehensive restoration plan. Two changes in particular will affect the visitor experience. First, the grove's paved roads, which have long provided access for the open-air tram tours, will be converted largely to walking trails. (Tram tours will no longer be offered as of 2015.) This may have some implications for the hike description below. Second, the current parking area in the lower grove will be removed to prevent long-term damage to the surrounding sequoias; on-site visitor parking will no longer be available. To access the grove, visitors will instead park at a newly constructed lot by the park's south entrance and take free and regular shuttle buses to the grove. The grove will be intermittently closed in 2015 and 2016 during this work, so check with the park for current information.

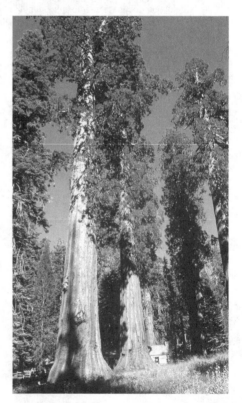

Upper Mariposa Grove and the Mariposa Grove Museum

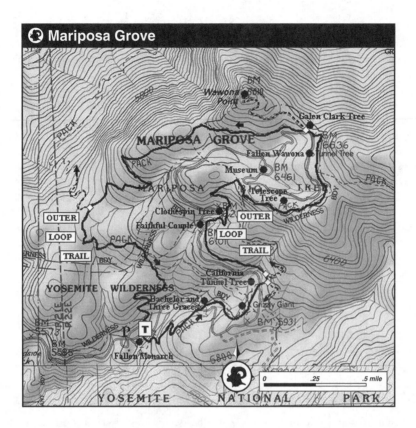

Mariposa Grove

As a result of this work, this heavily visited natural wonder will be better preserved for the future—with the added bonus of making the spectacular upper grove (once accessible by tram tour) now open only to those who hike there.

To Reach the Trailhead Proceed to the park's South Entrance Station on Hwy. 41 and park as directed. From Yosemite Valley the roughly 35-mile drive takes approximately 75 minutes, depending on conditions and traffic. A $20-per-vehicle entrance fee is charged for Yosemite National Park, good for seven days.

Description First, a reminder: To preserve the grove for future generations of trees (and visitors), do not take cones as souvenirs. The trail begins beside a kiosk where free brochures printed in multiple languages are available (0.0/5,600'). First head to the nearby Fallen Monarch, believed to have toppled more than

300 years ago. Crossing the road, you ascend numerous oversized steps before recrossing the old roadbed by the Bachelor and Three Graces (0.5/5,760'). Swelling in size near its base, the Bachelor provides a good example of what is known as a buttressed trunk.

The Grizzly Giant, the fifth-largest living thing on Earth, is next. Blackened and scarred, huge and grizzly indeed, its estimated age of 2,700 years makes it one of the oldest living sequoias known. Just beyond it is the California Tunnel Tree, one of two trees in the grove tunneled by man; how the tree remains upright is an interesting physics problem of torque and balance. Walk through the tree, cross the former roadbed, and bear left at both trail junctions. The trail follows the route of the old roadbed and soon reaches the Faithful Couple (1.5/6,140'), a pair of enormous trees sutured together for more than 50 feet.

The posted trail continues across the road to the Clothespin Tree, so named because of the enormous symmetrical gash that runs through it. Climbing into the Upper Grove, the trail reaches the road again near four magnificent specimens. Paths split off in all directions—continue right on the posted Outer Loop Trail, following the former road's upper loop. The Mariposa Grove Museum is visible beyond the restrooms and has informative displays, books, and a welcome drinking fountain when open (2.2/6,460').

Continuing on the Outer Loop Trail, take time for a quick side trip inside the Telescope Tree. Though without blemish on the outside, it is hollow inside; blue sky can be seen through the opening on top. The trail next loops to the famous Wawona Tunnel Tree (2.8/6,600'), lying on its side below the trail. The final landmark tree on this hike is the Galen Clark Tree, named for the man who tirelessly promoted the grove and urged its protection in the late 1850s and 1860s.

Immediately past the Galen Clark Tree is the junction for Wawona Point Vista, which offers simple views across the South Fork Merced River to Wawona Dome. The return to the parking lot on Outer Loop Trail leaves the sequoias behind and passes instead through a quiet forest of sugar pines, incense cedars, white firs, and Jeffrey pines. Those wishing to return through the sequoias should backtrack to the museum and descend from there. Otherwise, continue straight at all junctions in the upper grove. Halfway down to the parking lot (4.5/6,120') the trail to Wawona splits off west, but you continue straight and bear right at the remaining junctions to reach the lot.

Nearest Visitor Center Wawona Information Station, 209-375-9501, is open daily in summer from approximately 8:30 a.m. to 4:30 p.m., depending on staffing. From Hwy. 41 in Wawona, take Chilnualna Falls Rd. to the first right-hand turn past the stables. For general recorded park information, call 209-372-0200.

Backpacking Information Camping is prohibited in the grove from roughly April through October, when the access road is open. Once snow closes the road, the grove becomes designated wilderness and intrepid cold-weather backpackers can hike, ski, or snowshoe the access road and camp beneath the sequoias. A wilderness permit is required, available from the Wawona Information Station. Note that Hwy. 41 from Wawona to Yosemite Valley is closed during the winter.

Nearest Campground Wawona Campground (93 sites, $20) is near Wawona and is open year-round. Reservations are required mid-April–mid-October and can be made up to 5 months in advance, in blocks of 1 month at a time, with the next block becoming available on the 15th of each month. To make reservations, call 877-444-6777 between 7 a.m. and 9 p.m. or visit **recreation.gov.** Try to reserve as early as possible on the 15th.

Additional Information nps.gov/yose

HIKE 91　Ediza Lake ⚲ 🧍 🐕

Highlight	The mountainous heart of Ansel Adams Wilderness
Distance	15 miles round-trip to Ediza Lake, 18 miles round-trip to Iceberg Lake
Total Elevation Gain/Loss	2,100'/2,100'
Hiking Time	8–12 hours
Recommended Maps	*Devils Postpile* by Tom Harrison Maps, USGS 7.5-min. *Villa Creek* and *Burro Mountain*
Best Times	July–September
Agency	Ansel Adams Wilderness, Inyo National Forest
Difficulty	★★★

THE TWIN MASSIFS of Mount Ritter and Banner Peak soar as the defining pinnacles of Ansel Adams Wilderness. Ediza Lake nestles below their sheer eastern flanks, an alpine gem in a rugged and beautiful landscape of mountains, lakes, and wilderness adventure.

The Hike begins at Agnew Meadows Trailhead west of Mammoth Lakes and visits Shadow Lake en route to Ediza Lake. Access and crowds are perhaps the biggest challenges of this hike. Agnew Meadows is an extremely popular trailhead and requires some effort to reach during most of the hiking season, when a shuttle-bus trip is required to proceed past Minaret Summit (see directions below).

A post–Labor Day visit is recommended if possible; crowds diminish and you have the option of driving directly to the trailhead. Regardless of when you come, you will see dozens of other hikers, though their presence is vastly overmatched by the stunning scenery around you. Dogs are allowed, but must be muzzled and leashed for the shuttle-bus ride. Snow typically lingers until early to mid-June depending on the season. Mosquitoes can be ferocious in early summer. Water is available at the trailhead.

To Reach the Trailhead During the summer, you'll need to catch the mandatory shuttle bus from Mammoth Mountain Lodge and Adventure Center, 5 miles west of Mammoth on Hwy. 203. Buses depart every 30 minutes from approximately 8 a.m. until 5 p.m.; the final return trip from Agnew Meadows is at 6 p.m.; check the current schedule for the latest information. Tickets are $7 per adult, $4 for children. Get off the shuttle bus at Stop 1, 2.7 miles west of Minaret Summit, and walk 0.4 mile down the turnoff to the Agnew Meadows trailhead.

After Labor Day—or if you're spending the night at one of the campgrounds past Minaret Summit—you can drive to the trailhead, though you'll have to pay a $10 entrance fee (in addition to any campground fees). The turnoff to Agnew Meadows is on the right, 2.7 miles past Minaret Summit. Follow the short road 0.4 mile past the pack station to the trailhead parking area on the left, and proceed to the trailhead on the south side of the parking area, signed for the Pacific Crest Trail (PCT).

Description From the trailhead (0.0/8,320'), strike out on the PCT toward Shadow Lake Trail. The trail immediately hops over two small creeks flowing through a forested landscape of lodgepole pines and then winds among huge piles of trees leveled by a ferocious windstorm in November 2011. The trail passes by an open meadow with views up-valley and then curves around the edge of the meadow to provide a look at the slopes above Agnew Meadows.

You cross a pretty stream flowing out of the meadow, where large red firs begin to appear in the forest mix. The flat, sandy trail runs close to the lip of a small valley below and then

Ediza Lake

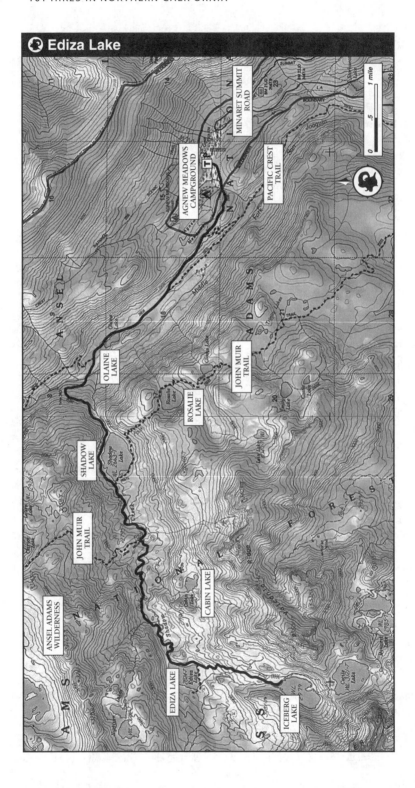

MINARET SUMMIT ROAD

AGNEW MEADOWS CAMPGROUND

PACIFIC CREST TRAIL

OLAINE LAKE

ROSALIE LAKE

JOHN MUIR TRAIL

SHADOW LAKE

JOHN MUIR TRAIL

ANSEL ADAMS WILDERNESS

CABIN LAKE

EDIZA LAKE

ICEBERG LAKE

1 mile

.5

0

starts to descend, immediately reaching a junction where the PCT turns left (0.9/8,300')—go straight toward Shadow Lake. The route now makes a rocky, traversing descent. Views ahead reveal your upcoming route—the prominent cleft in the slopes ahead and to the left. Sierra juniper mixes into the forest, and soon you reach a trail junction at valley bottom by a striking and large western white pine (1.5/8,050'), where you bear right.

The trail heads north past the wooded shores of Olaine Lake (2.1/8,080') to reach the junction with Shadow Lake Trail (2.4/8,100'). Rushing water becomes audible as you turn left to head toward Shadow Lake, drop toward the river, and cross it on a stout wooden bridge. Cottonwoods and aspens line the lush riparian alley.

The trail soon makes a switchback right and begins the ascent over slopes dotted with large and mature Sierra juniper. A long traverse rises above the rapidly steepening river valley, the ascent aided by many excellent stone steps. The trail makes several tight switchbacks and then curves left on a rising traverse toward the cleft above. Nice views look back down the valley; Mammoth Mountain can be spotted rising above the nearby ridge.

The surrounding rocks show clear evidence of past glacial activity here; smooth glacial polish and linear gouges are readily apparent and indicate the direction of past glacial flow. Next up are the roaring cascades that pour out of Shadow Lake, tumbling through a narrow gash in the rocks. Here the trail goes right along its edge more than a hundred feet above the water, where large rocks stand guard like a railing and views look deep into the crevasse; in one spot, an enormous, RV-sized boulder wedges between the walls.

The trail turns a corner, abruptly encounters the fast-rising creek, and reaches the outlet to Shadow Lake. A stunning alpine view awaits here, including the knife-edge summit of towering Mount Ritter (Banner Peak still hides from sight). The crystalline water of Shadow Lake rapidly deepens from shore in a spectrum of alpine green and blue.

The trail winds through dusty lodgepole woods along the northern shore, where smooth-faced rocks fin downward into the nearby lake. On the far side of the lake, you encounter another major bridge where the John Muir Trail (JMT) joins the trail from the left (4.3/8,760'). A surprisingly substantial amount of water flows through here.

The continuing route approaches the rushing stream, climbs briefly alongside it, and then rises to traverse on the edge of the valley floor. The trail winds intermittently along the idyllic valley floor as it continues, passing some falls and a few heavily used camping areas—nice spots for a break. (Note that no camping is allowed between the trail and the creek from Shadow Lake to Ediza Lake.)

You next reach a junction (5.2/8,180') where the JMT goes right toward Garnet Lake. Your route bears left toward Ediza Lake on a level, easy cruising section of trail that winds along a broad meadow on the left; the river is on its far side. Prominent Volcanic Ridge looms across the valley; several distinct avalanche paths can be seen on its slopes.

The level trail eventually returns to the river and travels directly alongside the placid waterway. Large hemlock trees now appear, readily identified by their lacy needles, small cones, and drooping tops. The parade of waterfalls soon resumes as the trail traverses steeply upward through a citadel of stone, where looming rocks on both sides punctuate a section of exceptional trail work and steps.

The jagged shards of the Minarets come into view on the left as the trail levels and soon emerges at the base of naked rock cliffs towering to the right. You cross a railless two-log bridge over a stream (the outlet from off-trail Nydiver Lakes above you to the north) and make a rising traverse away from and then back toward the stream. A steady ascent leads to a final curve into the amphitheater of Ediza Lake (7.2/9,300'), where the surrounding mountain theater opens in all its glory. Most striking are Mount Ritter and Banner Peak towering over the lake's south shore and the striking Minarets, which rise across from Mount Ritter.

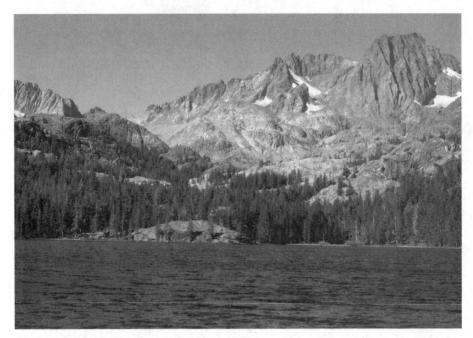

The striking massif of Mount Ritter rises above Ediza Lake.

The best camping options around the aquamarine lake are along the northwest shore, which is best accessed by proceeding clockwise around the lake (going counterclockwise is shorter but requires crossing a rubbly rockslide and is not recommended).

To continue to Iceberg Lake (or explore the far shores of Ediza Lake), follow the continuing trail above the east lakeshore. Approximately a third of the way around the lake, you reach the signed junction for Iceberg Lake (7.5/9,320'), where a path splits right toward the northern shores of Lake Ediza. A left turn leads you toward Iceberg Lake; switchbacks immediately rise upward on a narrower, but still well-trod, trail.

The scenery is stunning as you rise quickly above Lake Ediza on a steep traverse among willow bushes, then via switchbacks and rock steps. The gradient then eases in a level area, where flowing rills run among the rocks. The trail runs through beautiful meadows, curves back toward the main creek at an emerald pool, and then makes the final rise into the Iceberg Lake basin.

Perched at the base of the Minarets rising more than 2,000 feet above, Iceberg Lake (9.0/9,774') is exposed, windy, and scenic. It also marks the end of this hike, though a challenging continuation climbs the steep and loose scree and boulder field on the lake's far side to reach remote Cecile Lake. Limited camping options are available in the terrain near the outlet stream, though finding protection from the wind can be a challenge.

Retrace your steps from here to the trailhead, savoring the magnificent scenery once again as you go.

Nearest Visitor Center Mammoth Lakes Visitor Center, 760-924-5500, a few miles west of Hwy. 395 on the way into Mammoth Lakes, is open daily year-round, 8 a.m.–5 p.m., for current backcountry and shuttle-bus information, wilderness permits, and more.

Backpacking Information A wilderness permit is required from May through October. There is an overnight quota of 30 people per day for this trailhead, which always fills. Eighteen permits can be reserved in advance; 12 are available on a first-come, first-served basis beginning at 11 a.m. the day before your hike. Reservations can be made up to 6 months in advance at **recreation.gov** or by calling 877-444-6777 ($6 reservation fee plus $5 per vehicle).

Bear canisters are required on this hike; they can be rented for a nominal fee at Mammoth Lakes Visitor Center. Note that no camping is permitted within a quarter mile of Shadow Lake or between the trail and creek between Shadow and Ediza Lakes.

Nearest Campgrounds Five Forest Service campgrounds and 1 National Park Service campground are available west of Minaret Summit on the road to Devils Postpile National Monument. They are all first come, first served; check availability at the visitor center or the Minaret Summit entrance station. Note that Agnew Meadows Campground sustained significant damage from the November 2011 windstorm and may be closed in 2015 or beyond.

Additional Information www.fs.usda.gov/inyo

HIKE 92 Balloon Dome ⚴ 🚶 🐐

Highlights	Monolithic Balloon Dome and the mighty San Joaquin
Distance	9.9 miles round-trip
Total Elevation Gain/Loss	2,300'/2,300'
Hiking Time	8–10 hours
Recommended Map	USGS 7.5-min. *Balloon Dome*
Best Times	May–October
Agency	Ansel Adams Wilderness
Difficulty	★★★★

A NAKED BUBBLE of granite rising nearly 3,000 feet from canyon bottom, Balloon Dome stands—a monolith, an inspiration, a companion on your descent to the sandy banks of the mighty San Joaquin River. Carving the Sierra Nevada between well-trod Yosemite and Kings Canyon National Parks, the river pours through a delightful, less visited landscape of abundant wildlife.

The Hike begins at the western border of Ansel Adams Wilderness and follows Cassidy Trail as it descends steadily to the San Joaquin River. A lower-elevation hike, it makes an exciting option in spring and late fall when snow has closed the higher regions. Fishing and swimming are possible in the San Joaquin. Bring sun protection. Water is available at the trailhead from Granite Creek.

To Reach the Trailhead Go 4.5 miles north on Hwy. 41 from the Hwy. 49 junction in Oakhurst, and turn east on Bass Lake Rd. In 6 miles, turn left on Beasore Rd. (FS 7), which you'll follow

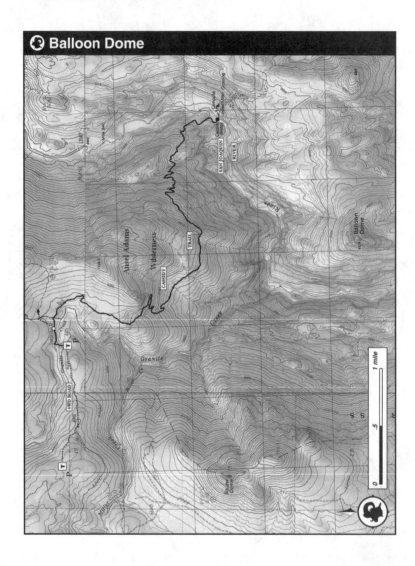

⊙ Balloon Dome

for the next 30-plus miles (a 60- to 90-minute drive).

Cold Springs Summit is reached in 12.1 miles, where the road becomes a US Forest Service Scenic Byway. Paved FS 6S01 branches right 2.7 miles later—continue straight. The pavement ends 5 miles later just past a posted junction for Mugler Creek and Grizzly Rd. Continuing for another 11 miles on increasingly rough road, you reach a stop sign and the end of FS 7. Go straight on FS 5S30 for 1.1 miles, and turn right at the posted turnoff for Cassidy Trail. The first

1.7 miles is very rough but passable for all vehicles; then the access road drops steeply down a granite ramp. Park here if you can't go farther. The final 1.3 miles requires a high-clearance vehicle and reaches the trailhead in an open parking area just before the road switchbacks down toward Granite Creek.

Description From the parking area (0.0/ 6,550'), descend north on Cassidy Trail to cross Granite Creek on a seasonal footbridge. The path curves right (downstream), traverses slowly upward, and then passes a trail junction on the left. You next cross above a gully and head southwest, passing through a dense forest of large Jeffrey pines, sugar pines, white firs, and incense cedars. The bald hump of Squaw Dome (7,818') appears directly ahead before the trail begins to descend slowly and bend southeast. Suddenly you see Balloon Dome between the trees.

A granite dome occurs when a huge block of fracture-free granite is exposed at the surface after overlying layers have eroded away. Freed from the pressure of overlying rock, the dome begins slowly shedding giant curved layers of rock in a process known as exfoliation. Such an unusually solid mass of rock takes a long time to wear away and will stand sentinel over the landscape for eons. Half Dome (Hike 86) is the most famous example.

Changing views of Balloon Dome finally disappear as the trail begins a long, arcing traverse to the east. Look for Sitting Hen Rock on the left, posted with the only sign you will encounter on this hike. At the upper elevation of

their range, black oaks appear along this section. At the end of the traverse (2.7/5,950'), the trail begins its 1,500-foot descent to the river. Looking northeast, the Middle Fork San Joaquin can be seen curving west from Mammoth Crest on the horizon. The South Fork flows just south of Balloon Dome, and, although you can't see it, the northern headwaters drain the peaks of the Silver Divide on the east skyline.

The descent to the river is rocky, often exposed to the sun, and has more than 40 switchbacks. Poison oak appears near the bottom. Finally a metal bridge comes into view and river sounds fill your ears (4.9/4,410'). Helicoptered to this site in 1956, the bridge has sustained recent flood damage: its bent central girders testify to the river's mind-boggling height that day. Exploration up- and downriver is easy, and there are fishing holes aplenty. While Cassidy Trail continues across the bridge toward Rattlesnake Lake, to keep this a day hike you must return the way you came.

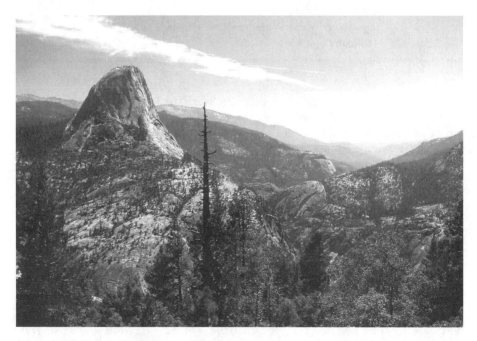

The land of the Balloon Dome

Nearest Visitor Centers The tiny Clover Meadow Ranger Station, 559-877-2218. ext. 3136, is 0.6 mile past the turnoff for Cassidy Trail on FS 5S30 and open daily 8 a.m.–noon and 1–5 p.m. mid-June–mid-September. In the off-season, try the Bass Lake Ranger District Office, 559-877-2218, which is open year-round, Monday–Friday 8 a.m.–4:30 p.m.

Backpacking Information Wilderness permits are required and can be obtained at the above ranger stations. There is a quota of 10 people for Cassidy Trail, though it rarely fills. Permits can be reserved up to 1 year in advance by mail only; visit **www.fs.usda.gov/sierra** for more information and to download the application form.

Nearest Campground Clover Meadow (6 sites, free) almost always has space.

Additional Information www.fs.usda.gov/sierra

HIKE 93 Kaiser Peak 🐾 🚶 🐐

Highlight	A panoramic view of the central Sierra Nevada
Distance	10.0 miles round-trip
Total Elevation Gain/Loss	3,200'/3,200'
Hiking Time	6–8 hours
Recommended Maps	*A Guide to Kaiser Wilderness* by the US Forest Service, USGS 7.5-min. *Kaiser Peak*
Best Times	Mid-June–September
Agency	Kaiser Wilderness, Sierra National Forest
Difficulty	★★★★

KAISER PEAK STANDS ALONE—a western spur of the towering Sierra ridge that bounds the San Joaquin River. Ascend this peak and stand upon the lip of a great divide.

The Hike climbs steadily up the southern slope of Kaiser Peak (10,310') and offers increasingly expansive views of the Huntington Lake basin, before reaching the summit crest and superlative vistas north. Despite its immediate proximity to popular Huntington Lake, Kaiser Wilderness attracts few hikers. A visit in late June or September will provide an unusual degree of solitude. Potable water is available at the pack station near the trailhead, and there are two sources along the trail—Deer Creek near the beginning and Bear Creek near the goal.

To Reach the Trailhead Take Hwy. 168 east from Clovis to its end along the east shore of Huntington Lake; turn left at the T-junction. In 1 mile turn right at the posted turnoff for the D&F Pack Station (just before the entrance to Deer Creek Campground). Bear right on Upper Deer Creek Lane after 0.1 mile and right again onto Deer Lane after another 0.5 mile. While the dirt road horseshoes over a creek and into the pack station, you should park in the small lot before the creek. The trailhead is at the north end of the pack-station customer parking lot.

Description At the trailhead (0.0/7,200'), two trails split off—bear left toward Kaiser Peak. Ascending among large Jeffrey pines, you reach

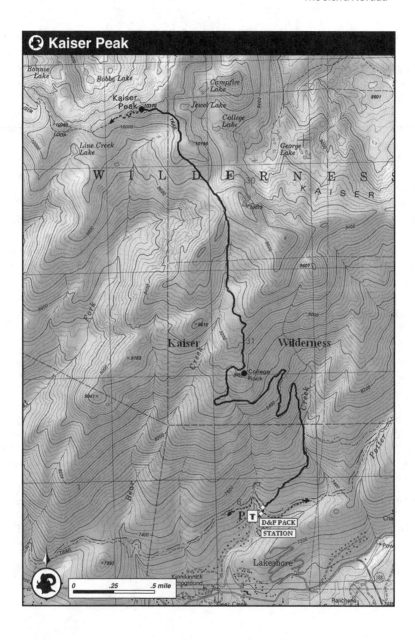

Kaiser Peak

another junction 100 yards along—continue straight ahead. The trail narrows to single-track and slowly climbs to meet Deer Creek on the right (0.5/7,600'). Briefly paralleling the creek, the trail then begins a long, switchbacking ascent to College Rock among enormous, fantastically shaped granite boulders. Flowers abound in season, including lupine, paintbrush, and western hound's-tongue. The red cones of snow plants protrude from the litter of the forest floor.

An ideal picnic spot, College Rock (2.5/ 9,055') can be surmounted with a bit of scrambling for some exciting views. Ringed by mountains, Huntington Lake is spread out below. If you look southwest into the Great Central Valley, the Coast Range outline often appears above the haze—a distance of more than 100 miles.

From here, several tight switchbacks lead up 200 feet before the trail slowly traverses to Bear Creek, joining it at a large flat meadow (3.0/9,340') among lodgepole and western white pines. Weaving to and from creekside, the trail passes below a massive fortress of granite as it ascends to a crest (4.0/9,800'). Suddenly, the strange moonscape of upper Kaiser Ridge comes into view, devoid of all trees and only occasionally matted with plant life. Traversing around a false summit, you reach a small cleft below now-visible Kaiser Peak, with Jewel Lake (closer) and Campfire Lake (farther) several hundred feet below. You reach the summit (5.0/10,310') via a very short, posted spur trail.

The view is exceptional. Before you drains the mighty San Joaquin. The prominent granite knob to the north poking out of the river valley is Balloon Dome (Hike 92). Farther north, the sawtoothed Minarets of the Ritter Range are easily identified, with the North Fork San Joaquin draining west below them. The Middle Fork wraps east around them, curving north below Mammoth Crest. The high peaks west of the Minarets form the southern border of Yosemite National Park. East-southeast, the South Fork San Joaquin drains the distant mountains of northern Kings Canyon National Park, visible along the skyline. Just below to the northwest is Bonnie Lake. The small twins of Bobby Lake lie nearly 1,000 feet beneath you. Don't be so distracted by the view that you leave your food unattended—several marmots that make the summit rocks their home love to pilfer. Return the way you came.

Nearest Visitor Center High Sierra Ranger District Office, 559-855-5355, is in Prather on the way up Hwy. 168 and is open daily 8 a.m.–4:30 p.m.

Backpacking Information A wilderness permit is required and is available in Prather during business hours. Due to a lack of good campsites on this hike, there is a quota of 12 people in effect for this trailhead from the last Friday in June through mid-September, though it rarely fills outside of holiday weekends. Permits can be reserved up to 1 year in advance by mail only; visit **www.fs.usda.gov/sierra** for more information and to download the application form.

Nearest Campground Six campgrounds ($28) line the shores of Huntington Lake.

Additional Information **www.fs.usda.gov/sierra**

HIKE 94   Little Lakes Valley   🥾 👥 🐐

Highlight	Direct access to the roof of the Sierra Nevada
Distance	7.0 miles round-trip
Total Elevation Gain/Loss	1,150'/1,150'
Hiking Time	3–5 hours
Recommended Maps	*Trail Map of the Mono Divide High Country* by Tom Harrison Maps, USGS 7.5-min. *Mount Abbot* and *Mount Morgan*
Best Times	July–September
Agency	John Muir Wilderness, Inyo National Forest
Difficulty	★★

IF YOU WANT TO access the incredible high-elevation scenery and soaring alpine peaks of the Eastern High Sierra, Little Lakes Valley is hard to beat. Surrounded by a multitude of sheer peaks rising above 13,000 feet, Little Lakes Valley offers nearly level walking past a multitude of small, tranquil lakes that reflect the alpine grandeur all around you.

The Hike explores the length of Little Lakes Valley from the Rock Creek trailhead—one of the highest-elevation trailheads in the state—on a wide path that gently undulates through the valley before rising steeply near the end to crest above 11,000 feet at Morgan Pass. The easy access and spectacular scenery attract crowds, but are well worth the effort. At this elevation, snow lingers late in the season and can easily persist deep into June and return as early as late September.

To Reach the Trailhead Take Hwy. 395 to the Rock Creek Lake turnoff, 24 miles north of Bishop, and follow the paved road 10.4 miles as it ascends more than a vertical mile to the large trailhead parking area at road's end. Past Rock Creek Pack Station, the road passes an overflow parking area and narrows to one lane for its final 1.2 miles.

Description From the trailhead (0.0/10,250'), strike out past a bridge on the left leading to Mosquito Flat Walk-In Campground (backpackers with permits only). The wide, easy-walking superhighway of a trail runs parallel to willow-lined Rock Creek and provides access to its briskly flowing water. You quickly reach the posted boundary of John Muir Wilderness (0.3/10,300') and wind among aspens and whitebark and lodgepole pines.

The thin, high-elevation air becomes apparent to your lungs on the trail's first ascent, which is aided by a series of nice granite steps that lead you to the junction for Mono Pass (0.5/10,440'). Bear left to continue toward Little Lakes Valley, soon reaching the first incredible view of the surrounding alpine peaks.

Bear Creek Spire is the most prominent peak, straight up the valley. To its left is a striking, unnamed triangular peak, below which is the deep and narrow gash of Morgan Pass. To the right of Bear Cap Spire is a serrated divide of peaks. Going from south to north (left to right), they are Mount Dade (13,600'), Mount Abbot (13,704'), and Mount Mills (13,451').

You next reach the junction for aptly named Marsh Lake (1.0/10,430'), where a path leads to a sandy beach, and then cross a pair of streams flowing into nearby Heart Lake. The trail curves around the grass-lined shore of shallow Heart Lake (1.5/10,440') and then rises briefly through a rare viewless section before emerging above Box Lake. Descending to the lake's far side (1.6/10,480'), you parallel the stream, enter a meadow area, and then cross the stream to reach the shore of deep, green Long Lake (2.0/10,580'), another pleasant stop.

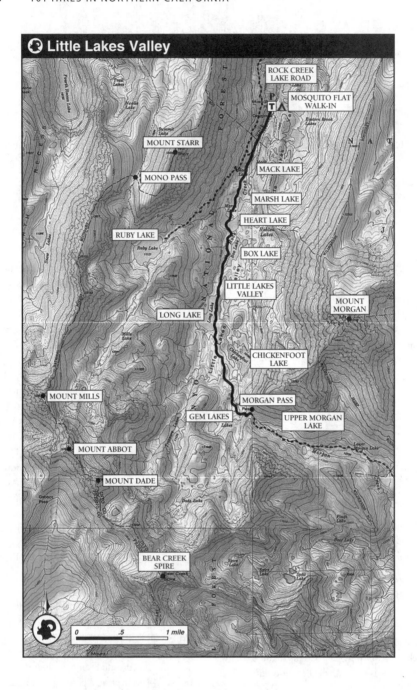

⊙ Little Lakes Valley

The Treasure Lakes basin is straight ahead below Bear Creek Spire, but you follow the continuing trail as it bears left and winds below the base of another striking cliff formation. The path rises steadily past Long Lake and reaches the junction for Chickenfoot Lake (3.0/10,780'), which requires a short ascent to access.

Morgan Pass—the prominent cleft above you—comes into view as the continuing trail crests and then descends into a meadow.

Looking back, you can see Chicken Foot Lake, ringed by trees near their elevation limit; the treeline here hovers just above 11,000 feet.

Continuing, you climb momentarily then level briefly as the pass rapidly looms close. The trail drops briefly to pass among several small ephemeral tarns, where a use path from Chickenfoot Lake joins. The outlet stream from nearby Gem Lake can be spotted flowing through an adjacent meadow, and then you begin the final climb with the help of impressive stone steps.

You pass the posted junction for Gem Lakes (3.3/10,870'), a scenic and worthwhile detour, and then continue across a bridge over a small trickle. The very wide trail makes a rising traverse, switchbacks twice near a large granite talus field, and attains the divide (3.5/11,120'), where you can spot Gem Lakes below and enjoy great views across the valley. Return the way you came to the trailhead (7.0/10,250').

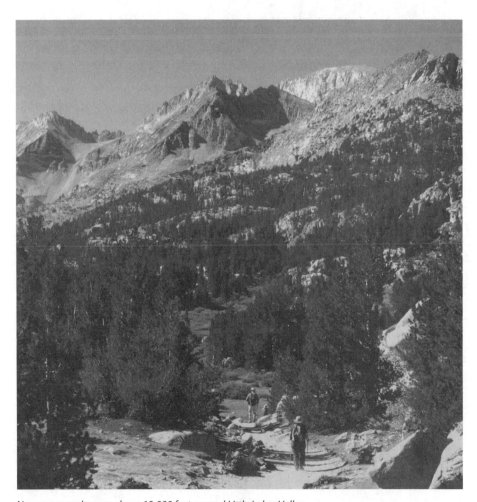

Numerous peaks soar above 13,000 feet around Little Lakes Valley.

Nearest Visitor Centers Mammoth Lakes Welcome Center, 760-924-5500, a few miles west of Hwy. 395 on the way into Mammoth Lakes, is open daily 8 a.m.–5 p.m. year-round. White Mountain Ranger Station Visitor Center, 760-873-2500, in Bishop at 798 N. Main St., is open daily 8 a.m.–5 p.m. May–October, and Monday–Friday 8:30 a.m.–4:30 p.m. November–April.

Backpacking Information Campsites are abundant in the valley, though special care should be taken in this high-use area to leave no trace and stay out of sight as much as possible. A wilderness permit is required, and there is an overnight quota of 25 people per day from this trailhead that almost always fills; 60% of permits can be reserved up to 6 months in advance, with the remainder available on a first-come, first-served basis beginning at 11 a.m. the day before your trip.

To make a reservation, visit **recreation.gov** ($6 reservation fee plus a per-person fee). Both reserved and first-come, first-served permits can be picked up at the White Mountain Ranger Station in Bishop, at the Mammoth Lakes Visitor Center, or at the Mono Basin Scenic Area Visitor Center. For additional information, call the wilderness-permit office at 760-873-2483 (open daily 8 a.m.–4:30 p.m.), or visit **www.fs.usda.gov/inyo.** The wilderness-permit process can be challenging to navigate—do your research.

Note also that bear canisters are required for overnight trips and can be rented for a nominal fee at any of the above visitor centers; they must be returned to the location where you rented them.

Nearest Campgrounds More than 10 campgrounds can be found along the road to the trailhead. Most are first come, first served, though 3—East Fork, French Camp, and Tuff—have sites that can be reserved. Visit **recreation.gov** or call 877-444-6777. Note that Mosquito Flat Walk-In Campground, by the trailhead, is designated for use only by those who have a backcountry wilderness permit for the next day for Little Lakes Valley or Mono Pass.

Additional Information www.fs.usda.gov/inyo

HIKE 95 Methuselah Grove ○

Highlights	Phantasmagoria and the oldest living things on Earth
Distance	4.2 miles
Total Elevation Gain/Loss	1,000'/1,000'
Hiking Time	2–3 hours
Recommended Map	USGS 7.5-min. *Westgard Pass*
Best Times	Mid-June–September
Agency	Ancient Bristlecone Pine Forest, Inyo National Forest
Difficulty	★★★

GNARLED AND TWISTED, sculpted and sublime, the bristlecone pines endure. In the Methuselah Grove, you can commune with trees more than 4,000 years old.

The rocks of the White Mountains were deposited as sea-floor sediment approximately 600 million years ago, making them the oldest rocks described by this guidebook. Thrust into mountains about 350 million years ago, the rocks today contain numerous exposed pockets of dolomite, a form of metamorphic limestone that is highly alkaline and inhospitable to most plants. In this soil, at elevations from 9,000 to 11,000 feet, the hardy bristlecone pine sets its roots.

Pinus longaeva (long-lived pine) is readily identified by its curved branchlets resembling long foxtails; its dark green, short needles growing in clusters of five; and its gooey sap-laden purple cones. The small bristle that appears at the end of mature cones gives the tree its name. Precipitation is minimal in the White Mountains. Between 12 and 15 inches fall annually, limiting the trees to only six to eight weeks of growth each year. The short growth cycle, coupled with the nutrient-poor dolomitic soil, allows the trees to produce only very small amounts of wood each year. Extremely dense and resinous, the wood is highly resistant to rot, pests, and fire. Ironically, the oldest trees grow in the most inhospitable sites: steep slopes of poor soil that retain little water. These restricted conditions cause slower than normal growth, producing denser (up to 150 rings per inch) and more durable wood than trees growing in better spots. During times of adversity, a bristlecone

can also let entire limbs die, often maintaining adequate nutrient flow to only a single branch. Dead branches take thousands more years to decay, becoming sculpted into fantastical shapes by windblown sand and ice crystals. Tree roots are seldom deeper than 2 feet, and despite the slow rate of slope erosion (less than 1 foot per 1,000 years), death by toppling over is a common end for the most ancient trees. Fallen trees can remain on the ground for up to 7,000 years. A dendrochronologist's delight, bristlecone pines provide a nearly complete chronology of the

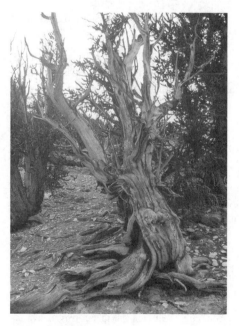

A gnarled bristlecone pine

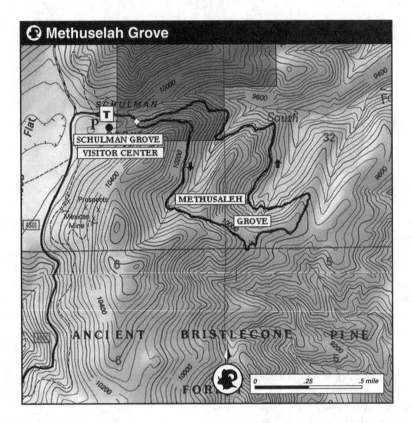

past 10,000 years through living and dead wood samples.

The Hike winds down to Methuselah Grove, location of more than 20 trees older than 4,000 years and home of Methuselah—at 4,700 years the world's oldest living thing. In order to protect Methuselah, its exact location is kept secret. Throughout this hike, it is critical that you stay on the trail—off-route hiking greatly increases the rate of erosion and can damage the root systems of the trees. Additionally, the removal of any wood, living or dead, is strictly prohibited. Because the trail elevation hovers around 10,000 feet, altitude sickness is a real concern, especially for those driving straight up from Owens Valley, 6,000 feet below. A morning start is best for solitude on the trail, as many day-trippers arrive in the early afternoon from Owens Valley. Weather can range unpredictably from cold to sudden thunderstorms to scorching sun. It can snow year-round.

To Reach the Trailhead Take Hwy. 168 east from Hwy. 395 in Big Pine—the turnoff is 0.5 mile north of the Texaco station. After 13.5 miles, turn left onto White Mountain Road. With the exception of small bottles of water and basic snacks at the visitor center, water and supplies are unavailable past this point—be prepared. The trailhead is at the Schulman Grove Visitor Center parking lot, a steep 10.7 miles past the entrance station, where a per-vehicle day-use fee is collected ($3 or $5).

Description The trail begins left of the picnic tables, where a self-guiding trail brochure can be picked up for a nominal fee (0.0/10,100'). After a short 0.2 mile, bear right at the fork. (You'll return from the left.) Curving along the south slopes of a deep creek gully, the trail climbs to the first rest bench (0.5/10,220'), which provides views east far into Nevada. The trail brochure's Stop 7, past the second bench, overlooks Methuselah Grove, occupying a small, distinctly white ridgelet in the valley below. As you hike there, you cross a vegetation zone where sagebrush and mountain mahogany dominate, due to more hospitable sandstone soils.

Descending from the ridge, you soon begin passing through the ancient Methuselah Grove.

With many of these trees predating the pyramids of Egypt, there is an impalpable feeling of time. Are you walking softly? Departing the grove at the trail's lowest point (2.3/9,730'), the trail bends west and gradually switchbacks up the creek canyon to return to the parking lot (4.2/10,100').

Nearest Visitor Centers Schulman Grove Visitor Center is located at the trailhead and is open daily 10 a.m.–5 p.m. Memorial Day–mid-October, with reduced hours in spring and fall. For general information, contact the White Mountain Visitor Center in Bishop, 530-873-2500.

Camping Information There is no backpacking or backcountry camping allowed in the Methuselah Grove or anywhere within the designated Ancient Bristlecone Pine Forest, a 44-square-mile area straddling the White Mountains above 9,000 feet. The closest developed campground is Grandview Campground (no water), a donation-based facility 5.1 miles beyond the entrance station on White Mountain Rd. (which doesn't quite live up to its name).

Additional Information www.fs.usda.gov/inyo

HIKE 96 Palisade Glacier 🥾 🧍 🐕

Highlights	Emerald lakes and the Sierra Nevada's largest glacier
Distance	17.0 miles round-trip
Total Elevation Gain/Loss	5,200'/5,200'
Hiking Time	12–16 hours
Recommended Maps	*John Muir Wilderness* by the US Forest Service; USGS 7.5-min. *Split Mountain, North Palisade, Mount Thompson,* and *Coyote Flat*
Best Times	Mid-July–September
Agency	John Muir Wilderness
Difficulty	★★★★★

STRIDE THE EAST SIDE. Less than 5 miles from the trailhead, above an idyllic basin studded with emerald lakes and naked granite, the Sierra Divide splits the sky. Continuing upward to attain the edge of Palisade Glacier as a dayhike is one of the greatest challenges this book offers. It is a mile of vertical gain to an active glacier below a serrated ridge of 14,000-foot peaks. In this highest mountain zone, life is left behind for a land of rock and ice.

The Hike follows North Fork Big Pine Creek into a substantial basin and visits five spectacular lakes. From there, it climbs 1,800 feet along an increasingly thin trail to reach the glacier. The final 700 feet of ascent are cross-country, and the hike tops out at more than 12,000 feet. Due to the hike's high elevation, altitude sickness can be a problem and snow can linger deep into the summer, sometimes beyond mid-July. Wear your sturdiest and stiffest hiking boots for

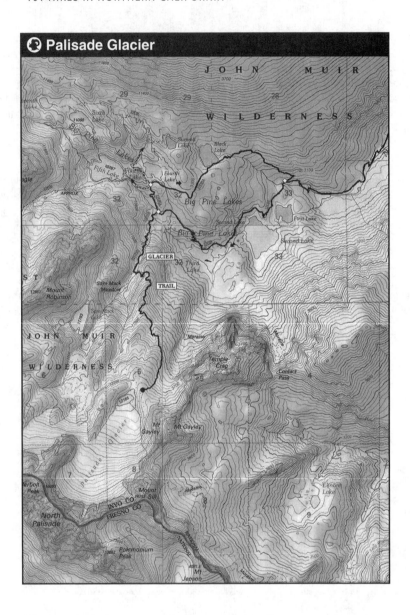

Palisade Glacier

this hike, as loose rock and constant boulder-hopping can wreak havoc on your feet.

The limited trailheads of the Sierra's eastern slopes tend to funnel crowds into small geographic areas, and this hike is no exception. Obtaining a wilderness permit for overnight trips can be challenging (see box page 329), and the best time to visit is September when summer crowds begin to dwindle. Even then, don't expect solitude. Fishing is possible at all the lakes. No water is available at the trailhead, but the river is regularly accessible after the first mile.

To Reach the Trailhead Take Crocker St. west from Hwy. 395 in Big Pine. Crocker St. becomes Glacier Lodge Rd., snaking upward 10 miles to the trailhead lot on the right, immediately past

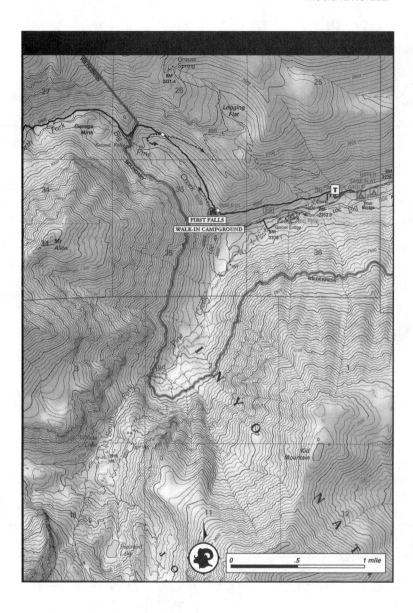

Upper Sage Flat and Sage Flat campgrounds. The road continues another 0.3 mile to Big Pine Creek Campground, but all hikers must leave their vehicles in the designated trailhead lot.

Description Beginning by the outhouse (0.0/7,750'), the singletrack trail strikes west through open sage and passes above the Glacier Pack Station before gently climbing to First Falls Walk-In

Campground (0.9/8,250'). The free campground is a short drop below the trail and has five sites with picnic tables and fire rings, though firewood is nonexistent. Unseen and inaccessible because of the brush, First Falls itself can only be heard.

On the next section, from First Falls to the base of Second Falls, you have two options. The more scenic route traverses the creek's partly

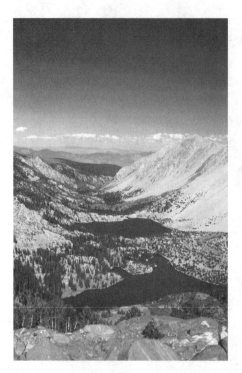

Big Pine Basin

exposed northeast slopes, offering good views up-canyon. The alternative—along the valley floor from First Falls Campground—provides easy walking on a wide path before it climbs steeply to rejoin the main trail. It is shadier and has regular access to water. The trails join at a junction for Baker Lake (1.7/8,580')—continue straight ahead toward impressive Second Falls. The trail switchbacks tightly near the top of the falls, where numerous overlooks let you view the tumbling river.

Now almost level, the trail winds through a dense riparian corridor of lodgepole pines, cottonwoods, and alders, with a few Jeffrey pines. Big Pine Wilderness Ranger Camp (2.6/9,160'), an impressive granite building soon encountered on the left, once belonged to actor Lon Chaney. The fluted massif of Temple Crag comes into full view south as the trail enters more open terrain. You soon reach the posted junction beginning your loop (4.2/10,000')—continue straight toward First Lake.

The surreal color of First Lake (4.4/9,960') can be spotted through the trees, and numerous use paths lead to the rocky shore. Like Second and Third Lakes, First Lake is fed by meltwater from Palisade Glacier. Extremely fine sediment ground by the glacier (glacial flour) is suspended in the water, causing the startling green hue of the three lakes. From shore you can identify the rounded summits of Mount Gayley (13,510') and—farther—Mount Sill (14,153'), just west behind landmark Temple Crag. The serrated ridge visible on the southwest skyline includes, from south to north, North Palisade (14,242'), Mount Winchell (13,775'), and Mount Agassiz (13,893').

The trail traverses some 100 feet above Second Lake (10,059'), the largest, before passing near Third Lake (10,249'). While both are readily accessed via a number of use paths, Second Lake provides the more impressive lakeshore. Paralleling much-diminished Big Pine Creek above Third Lake, the trail climbs quickly to a large meadow, where posted Glacier Trail splits off (6.0/10,640').

To head to Palisade Glacier, cross the creek and follow Glacier Trail upward on numerous tight switchbacks. Paralleling an oft-hidden stream coursing beneath granite rubble, the trail eventually crests into Sam Mack Meadow (6.8/11,050'). Waving with shooting stars and paintbrush, the meadow contains a shallow creek whose blue-gray tint indicates its glacial origin. While an obvious trail continues through the meadow to a few high-elevation campsites, you should rock-hop across the creek near the foot of the meadow. Continue climbing on the opposite slope, where the trail is marked.

Increasingly rough and rocky, the trail passes krummholz whitebark pines, marking the upper limit of tree growth. As you attain the top of a small ridge and continue traversing upward on the far side, incredible views downcanyon of First, Second, and Third Lakes open up. The distinctive linear heap of small stones and loose scree now visible above you is a lateral moraine left behind by receding Palisade Glacier. Wrapping around the base of the moraine (8.0/11,780'), the trail fades completely after

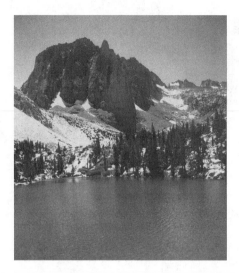

Temple Crag rises above First Lake.

crossing the loosest (and most maddening) rock of this trip. Indicated by numerous small cairns, the now completely cross-country route ascends the former glacier path, an undulating, polished-granite ramp. Sucking enough oxygen from the thin air is now the hardest part. When you finally crest the rubble of the terminal moraine (8.5/12,300'), you behold the great amphitheater of Palisade Glacier.

The glacier's snout terminates in an ice-choked pond 150 feet below you; the towering peaks scrape the sky 2,000 feet above. Hidden from all angles but this one, Palisade Glacier gouges a barren alpine landscape. Time and energy permitting, scramble down the loose moraine slopes to walk on the glacier itself. Unlike its larger relatives, Palisade Glacier generally lacks crevasses or cracks that would pose serious risk—especially on its lower, boulder-strewn surface—but always exercise caution. The notable features from south to north above the glacier are Mount Sill (14,153'), the prominent dome-shaped summit; V-notch and U-notch, two neighboring gaps in the ridge clearly resembling these letters; North Palisade (14,242'), though small and rounded immediately north of U-notch, the highest point; and Thunderbolt Peak (14,003'), the incisor-sharp spires above the glacier's far northwest corner. North beyond the glacier basin are the summits of Mount Winchell (13,775') and Mount Agassiz (13,893').

Savor the thickening air as you retrace your steps downward to the earlier junction in Big Pine Basin (11.0/10,640'). Bear left and ascend briefly to Fourth Lake (11.3/10,760'). Fed by snow rather than glacial ice, its water contrasts sharply with the Technicolor of the first three. The long descent home begins here. After dark Black Lake (11.8/10,680'), the trail then descends 500 feet via nine switchbacks to join the earlier trail. Return the way you came.

Nearest Visitor Center White Mountain Visitor Center, 760-873-2500, on Hwy. 395 in downtown Bishop (across the road from Burger King), is open daily 8 a.m.–5 p.m. mid-June–mid-September. The rest of the year it's open Monday–Friday 8 a.m.–noon and 1–4:30 p.m.

Backpacking Information A wilderness permit is required, and there is an overnight quota of 25 people per day from this trailhead that almost always fills; 60% of permits can be reserved up to 6 months in advance, with the remainder available on a first-come, first-served basis beginning at 11 a.m. the day before your trip.

To make a reservation, visit **recreation.gov** ($6 reservation fee plus a per-person fee). Both reserved and first-come, first-served permits can be picked up at the White Mountain Ranger Station in Bishop, the Mammoth Lakes Visitor Center, or the Mono Basin Scenic Area Visitor Center. For additional information, call the wilderness-permit office at 760-873-2483 (open daily 8 a.m.–4:30 p.m.), or visit **www.fs.usda.gov/inyo.** The wilderness-permit process can be challenging to navigate—do your research.   *(continued)*

Note also that bear canisters are required for an overnight trip and can be rented for a nominal fee at any of the above visitor centers; they must be returned to the location where you rented them.

Nearest Campgrounds Big Pine Creek Campground (30 sites, $22) is located at the road's end. Also try Upper Sage Flat and Sage Flat Campgrounds (20 and 28 sites, respectively; $22) near the trailhead. Reservations are recommended; visit **recreation.gov** or call 877-444-6777.

Additional Information www.fs.usda.gov/inyo

HIKE 97 Yucca Point 🥾🏕

Highlight	The deepest canyon in North America
Distance	3.4 miles round-trip
Total Elevation Gain/Loss	1,150'/1,150'
Hiking Time	2–3 hours
Recommended Maps	USGS 7.5-min. *Hume* and *Wren Peak*
Best Times	Spring and fall
Agency	Sequoia National Forest
Difficulty	★★★

THOUGH HWY. 180 winds a stunning course above the Kings River, gaining perspective from your car on the immense depth of Kings Canyon is difficult. Luckily, your descent to the river below Yucca Point will remedy this.

The Hike descends quickly to the confluence of the Middle and South Forks of the Kings River and provides spectacular views up both river canyons. Due to the lower elevation here, spring and fall provide the most agreeable temperatures and May offers the best wildflowers. Summer months can be sweltering. The trail is also a popular access point for anglers, although there are strict regulations governing this stretch of river. In order to protect its population of large wild trout, catch-and-release fishing applies and only artificial lures with barbless hooks may be used. Current regulations should be posted by the trailhead. The river is usually not fishable until July, when the raging waters of melting snowpack subside. No water is available at the trailhead.

To Reach the Trailhead Take Hwy. 180 east from Grant Grove Visitor Center for 15 miles. On the left, a US Forest Service sign for Yucca Point and a dirt lot with space for four vehicles mark your trailhead. This hike is located in Sequoia National Forest, but access requires passage through Kings Canyon National Park, where a $20-per-vehicle entrance fee (valid for seven days) is collected.

Description From the trailhead (0.0/3,380'), descend among manzanita, canyon live oaks, cottonwoods, California buckeyes, and California bays until you reach the first switchback (0.5/2,900'). From here, views of the South Fork canyon open up; the Windy Cliffs are visible where the river bends out of sight. Look for wildflowers as you descend west to the second switchback. Along with the ubiquitous flowering yucca you can find western wallflower and farewell-to-spring—two wildflowers rarely seen at higher elevations.

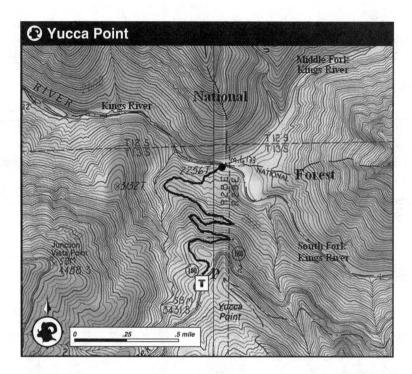

⊘ **Yucca Point**

Views along the upper section of trail are more expansive than from canyon bottom. Spanish Mountain (10,051'), rising nearly 8,000 feet from the opposite bank, offers a neck-craning exercise in topographic relief. The Middle Fork tumbles southwest through nearly 10 miles of inaccessible gorge and is overshadowed south by Monarch Divide, a steep ridge ushering the two forks together.

At the third switchback (0.9/2,600') a cottonwood tree can be readily identified by its heart-shaped leaves. Below the fourth switchback (1.3/2,430'), an unexpected and beautiful stream races over seven visible cascades—each one becoming progressively larger. Finally the water pours over a smooth granite face into a deep pool full of brook trout. This is Tenmile Creek, which drains the Hume Lake Reservoir 4 miles upstream. While pleasant in May and June, the water here gets funky as the flow decreases and Hume Lake receives its thousands of summer-camp visitors in July and August. Ten yards beyond where the falls first become visible, an unmarked spur trail leads down to a vantage point and a short scramble to the flat rocks at the base of the waterfall.

As you continue to Kings River, poison oak appears everywhere. The trail ends among the granite jumble of the riverbank (1.7/2,250'). Many boulders include excellent examples of inclusions (overlying rocks absorbed and partially melted by rising molten bubbles of granite), some 100 million years old. Sparrows dart above the river in search of insects. Return the way you came.

Nearest Visitor Center Kings Canyon Visitor Center at Grant Grove, 559-565-4307, 2 miles past the park entrance station along Hwy. 180, is open 365 days a year. Hours vary depending on the season, but it's generally open 9 a.m.–5 p.m. May–June and 8 a.m.–5 p.m. July–Labor Day, with reduced hours the rest of the year.

Backpacking Information Backpacking is permitted, but the lack of good campsites makes it a less appealing option. A campfire permit is required.

Nearest Campgrounds There are more than a dozen campgrounds in Kings Canyon National Park and adjacent Sequoia National Forest. Most are first come, first served. Check at the visitor center for current information.

Additional Information nps.gov/seki, www.fs.usda.gov/sequoia

HIKE 98 Redwood Canyon ○ 🥾

Highlight	Enchanted groves whose patriarchs dwarf your mind
Distance	10.0 miles
Total Elevation Gain/Loss	1,900'/1,900'
Hiking Time	5–7 hours
Recommended Map	USGS 7.5-min. *General Grant Grove*
Best Times	June–September
Agency	Kings Canyon National Park
Difficulty	★★★

REDWOOD CANYON provides the opportunity to peacefully commune with giant trees in the largest sequoia grove on earth. One-on-one with these magnificent trees, while your mind gropes at scales of time and size, you feel the insignificance of humankind.

The Hike loops around the canyon slopes and ridges, dropping briefly to Redwood Creek and passing through numerous stands of giant sequoias. While it can readily be completed in either direction, this description covers the route clockwise. (A shorter, 7.5-mile loop can be created by using the trail that heads directly downcanyon.) Late June offers abundant flowering lupines and dogwoods as well as fewer people; it is the ideal time to visit. While no water is available at the trailhead, an ample number of streams are encountered along the way.

To Reach the Trailhead Take Hwy. 180 east from Fresno to Kings Canyon National Park. Continue 1 mile past the entrance station to a Y-junction—bear right onto Generals Hwy. heading south toward Sequoia National Park. In 3.8 miles you reach the posted turnoff for Hume Lake on the left. Instead, make a right here onto what appears to be a small dirt cul-de-sac. The bumpy dirt road to Redwood Canyon begins at this dirt lot and is easily navigable for all cars, although trailers and RVs are definitely not recommended. Immediately beyond an ENTERING KINGS CANYON NATIONAL PARK sign, the road gradually descends 1.9 miles to the posted turnoff for the trailhead. A $20-per-vehicle entrance fee is charged for Kings Canyon and Sequoia National Parks, valid for seven days.

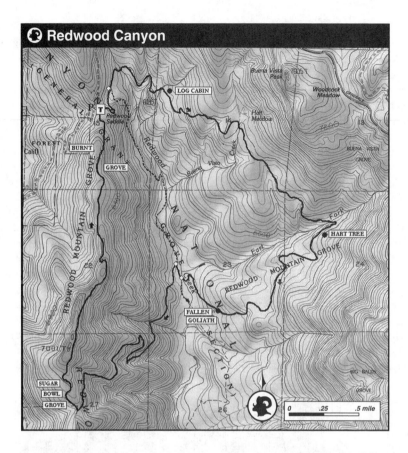

Description The trail begins at the information sign by the far end of the parking lot (0.0/6,250'). Your return path winds in from the right but you head left down a loamy, 3-foot-wide trail, immediately passing a fire hydrant and sign for REDWOOD CANYON–HART TREE TRAIL. You soon find yourself enveloped in the primeval giant sequoia forest, whose numerous large specimens dwarf the white firs, sugar pines, Jeffrey pines, and dogwoods also found here. The trail descends steadily via several lazy switchbacks and comes to a posted junction (0.4/6,070'); bear left toward the Hart Tree. (Right takes you directly down-canyon to connect with the midpoint of the hike, shaving 2.5 miles off the hike.) From here the trail traverses the eastern slopes of the canyon, crossing three small tributaries of Redwood Creek before reaching a log cabin (1.1/6,100').

Nothing more than a single fallen sequoia log, the cabin was originally owned by woodcutter John Crose. Used in the 1890s for equipment storage, the log was modified in the early part of the century by Crose's son Jack and nephew Willis. Upon scraping out the log's insides, the pair enclosed it with shakes, a door, and a fireplace and chimney. The Barlow family purchased Crose's holdings in the late 1920s, and both families lived in the area well into the 1930s, inhabiting both Crose's log and a tiny cabin (now long gone) built atop a large sequoia stump. The federal government acquired the property in the late 1930s, bringing an end to this unique lifestyle.

From here you briefly leave the sequoias and ascend 400 feet among black oaks, incense cedars, and alders. The trail tops out at a large open space of bare granite, offering the only vista from the canyon's eastern slopes. Another undulating trail mile takes you past boggy Hart Meadow (and through another hollow sequoia log) to the East Fork Redwood Creek. Although it's too small to be fishable, keep an eye out for the small, native brook trout that populate its crystalline waters. A brief climb out of the creek gully brings you to a posted 100-yard spur trail to the Hart Tree (3.4/6,200').

Once thought to be the world's 4th-largest tree, the Hart Tree is now recognized as only the 16th-largest on Earth. As of 1990 it was 278 feet tall, had a ground perimeter of 75.3 feet, had a diameter of 21 feet, and was estimated to contain 34,407 cubic feet of wood. Back on the main trail, a gradual descent brings you to the Fallen Goliath (4.8/5,700'), just beyond view from the trail. Moist, covered in moss, and nurse log to young sequoias sprouting from its crest, the Fallen Goliath probably sprouted more than 3,000 years ago; it provides an excellent example of the incredible decay resistance of sequoia wood.

The trail now descends to Redwood Creek (5.3/5,400'). Clear as glass, the creek flows through level surroundings studded with impressive sequoias. From mid-June through July, a sea of purple lupine washes the area, lapping at the cinnamon sequoia trunks. Just across the creek a signed junction indicates the route up-canyon to the right.

A short 0.1 mile upstream, the trail reaches another junction; head west up the canyon slope toward Sugar Bowl Grove. (Those tired or short of time can take the shorter, more direct route up-canyon to reach the parking lot.) Climbing gradually to the ridgetop, the trail quickly breaks out of the dense forest after two quick switchbacks. The result of a recent fire, the clearing lets you see the proliferation of young sequoias whenever openings occur in the forest canopy. Extending spiny branches into the air, the young trees outgrow their neighbors to maximize sunlight. Extremely shade-intolerant, the trees shed any sickly yellow-green branches and will rapidly perish if

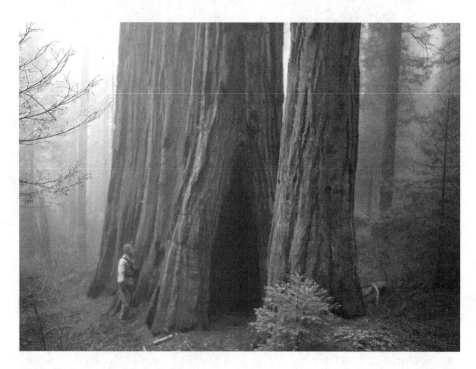

Giant sequoias dwarf your mind.

overtopped by another tree. Beyond this clearing, thimbleberry, bear clover, paintbrush, and green-leaf manzanita are abundant, as the trail steadily climbs to the ridgetop.

Before attaining the ridgetop, you enter Sugar Bowl Grove (7.5/6,600'), a thick stand of mature sequoias interspersed with several gnarled, ancient specimens of stupendous size. A cluster of more than 20 stand sentinel within a 75-yard radius at the heart of this enchanted grove. From here the trail follows the ridgetop, soon reaching its highest elevation of 1,500 feet above the canyon floor. Now slowly descending, you begin passing through Burnt Grove. Another thick stand of sequoias, Burnt Grove parallels the trail to the parking lot for the final mile.

Nearest Visitor Center Kings Canyon Visitor Center at Grant Grove, 559-565-4307, 2 miles past the park entrance station along Hwy. 180, is open 365 days a year. Hours vary depending on the season, but it's generally open 9 a.m.–5 p.m. May–June and 8 a.m.–5 p.m. July–Labor Day, with reduced hours the rest of the year.

Backpacking Information Redwood Canyon offers one of the few giant sequoia groves open to backpackers. A wilderness permit is required and can be obtained at Kings Canyon Visitor Center; there is a fee of $15 per permit. There is a quota of 15 people per day for this trailhead, though it seldom fills. You must camp at least a mile from the trailhead, and you may spend no more than 2 nights in the grove. Fires are prohibited.

Nearest Campgrounds There are more than a dozen campgrounds in Kings Canyon National Park and adjacent Sequoia National Forest. Check at the visitor center for current availability.

Additional Information nps.gov/seki

HIKE 99 Pear Lake ✐ 🜚

Highlights	Shattered granite basins and the Watchtower
Distance	12.4 miles round-trip
Total Elevation Gain/Loss	2,750'/2,750'
Hiking Time	8–12 hours
Recommended Map	USGS 7.5-min. *Lodgepole*
Best Times	July–September
Agency	Sequoia National Park
Difficulty	★★★★

PEAR LAKE's frigid green waters fill a granite bowl ringed by crenellated cliffs of fractured stone. En route are three choice Sierra lakes and the Watchtower, a titanic granite tower rising 2,000 feet above Tokopah Valley.

The Hike climbs steeply to the Watchtower before making a gradual traverse above impressive Tokopah Valley to reach the lakes. For those seeking a shorter hike, the round-trip to the Watchtower is 7 miles, gains 1,700 feet of elevation, and can be completed in four to six hours. Snow usually clears from the trail by late June and returns in November. July provides spectacular wildflowers. Water is available at the trailhead in the nearby restrooms.

To Reach the Trailhead From Generals Hwy. in Sequoia National Park, take the road to Wolverton east to the parking lot at the road's end—your turnoff is 1.7 miles south of the one for Lodgepole Visitor Center and 0.7 mile north of the General Sherman Tree parking lot. The trail begins midway along its northern edge. Lockers provide the only safe storage of your food-stuffs while you're on the trail, because bears break into vehicles here all the time.

Description Striking first through a forest dominated by white firs, the trail is quickly joined on the left by a small feeder trail from the Lodgepole complex (0.1/7,400'), and then on the right by a short spur from the Wolverton area. The trail now slowly gains elevation, traversing a forest whose lush understory includes

numerous wildflowers: lupine, phlox, tiger lilies, shooting stars, and paintbrush. Beyond a junction for Alta Peak Trail (1.8/8,060'), the path recrosses a small spring-fed creek before reaching the junction for the Hump (2.1/8,160'). A right turn, taking you over the Hump, provides a slightly shorter, more direct route to Heather Lake. But this shortcut is steeper and more strenuous, and lacks the exceptional views of the main trail. If you bear left instead, a gradually rising traverse leads you to the Watchtower (3.5/8,973').

Take a memorable break on the Watchtower by scrambling to the top of this towering granite pillar, skirting its precipitous chasm. With Tokopah Valley visible in its entirety, even Lodgepole Visitor Center can be spotted down-canyon. Below where the Marble Fork Kaweah River tumbles down 1,000 feet of granite chutes and faces is Tokopah Falls. Up-canyon, the high peaks on the southern rim overshadow your unseen destinations: Emerald and Pear Lakes.

Views lost as the trail continues east become sweeping vistas as it heads southeast, now offering views of the Heather Lake basin. The lake remains hidden until you pass the junction where the Hump shortcut rejoins the main trail (4.1/9,260'). Lodgepoles and western white pines are scattered about this day-use-only lake. Like the others on this hike, Heather Lake brims with brook trout up to 8 inches in length.

Continuing to even prettier lakes, the trail briefly climbs before descending into

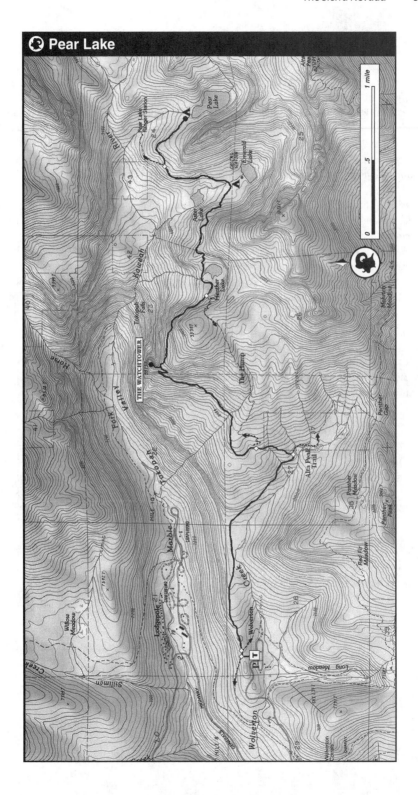

⊙ Pear Lake

the granite amphitheater of the Emerald Lake basin. Aster Lake can be seen north of the trail, but there is no established access trail. Approaching Emerald Lake, you reach the organized campsites near its north shore (5.1/9,030'). Both food lockers and a downright luxurious restroom are provided. Glacial polish and striations on the rock are evidence of the glacier that once carved this cirque. The summit visible southeast across the lake is Alta Peak (11,204').

Striking north, the trail winds among granite slabs and vibrant patches of seasonal wildflowers such as mountain pride, paintbrush, and meadow penstemon. Look here for Coville's columbine, a large cream-colored flower with five petals extending into backward-projecting spurs up to 1 inch long. Found only at rocky, high elevations in the southern Sierra Nevada,

it is closely related to, and can hybridize with, the crimson columbine, according to Richard Spellenberg in the *National Audubon Society Field Guide*. Magnificent examples of the rosy palette created by this cross-pollination can be found here soon after snowmelt—usually in late June and the first half of July. Do not pick the wildflowers.

Wrapping east, the trail passes a spur to seasonally staffed Pear Lake Ranger Station before turning southeast to reach the appropriately shaped Pear Lake (6.2/9,550'). A few lodgepole pines are sprinkled about the sloping granite shoreline; soaring ramparts of the basin heighten your sense of grandeur. The trail ends among the designated campsites near the lake's north shore (the "stem"), where food lockers and another plush outhouse can be found. Return the way you came.

Nearest Visitor Center Lodgepole Visitor Center, 559-565-4436, on the road to Wolverton 1.6 miles east of Generals Hwy., is generally open daily 8 a.m.–6 p.m. mid-June–mid-September, with reduced hours in early June and late September.

Backpacking Information The hike to Pear Lake makes for an ideal (and popular) 2-day trip. Wilderness permits are required and can be obtained from an office next to the visitor-center entrance, 559-565-4408. There is a fee of $15 per permit, and the office is open daily 7 a.m.–3:30 p.m. June–September. There is a trail quota of 25 people per day, but space is usually available except for the busiest weekends and holidays. Unlike other trailheads in the park, wilderness permits for this hike are first come, first served only. Due to heavy use, no fires are allowed, and camping is permitted at designated sites only.

Nearest Campground Lodgepole Campground (214 sites, $20) is adjacent to the visitor center. Reservations are essential for summer weekends, though space is often available during the week; for reservations, visit **recreation.gov** or call 877-444-6777.

Additional Information nps.gov/seki

HIKE 100 Moro Rock ↗

Highlights	Surmounting a precipitous granite fin and enjoying views of the Great Western Divide
Distance	0.6 mile round-trip
Total Elevation Gain/Loss	250'/250'
Hiking Time	1 hour
Recommended Map	USGS 7.5-min. *Giant Forest*
Best Times	June–September
Agency	Sequoia National Park
Difficulty	★★

A SHARP granite nubbin extending from the lip of the Giant Forest plateau, Moro Rock protrudes thousands of feet above the Kaweah River gorge. A narrow runway atop its prow offers superlative views of the jagged Great Western Divide.

The Hike climbs to the top of Moro Rock along precipitous ledges and up steps dynamited out of the rock. Among all the trails of Giant Forest with their ubiquitous crowds, this short climb to a unique viewpoint should not be missed. Giant sequoias grow elsewhere in greater seclusion (Hike 98), but there is only one Moro Rock. Crowds are always heavy.

To Reach the Trailhead Take Generals Hwy. to Giant Forest Village and turn east on Crescent Meadow Rd.; the turnoff is at the southern end of the complex. In 1.3 miles turn right onto the posted one-way loop for Moro Rock; park in the often crowded parking lot 0.4 mile farther along. A $20-per-vehicle entrance fee is charged for Sequoia National Park, valid for seven days.

Description Because Jeffrey pines, incense cedars, white firs, and sugar pines are thick at the outset, bare granite views through the trees provide little hint of the grandeur that awaits you. At step 21, a sign cries out WARNING— AREA OF EXTREME DANGER! Respect the warning about lightning strikes, and postpone your ascent if thunderstorms threaten. Past this sign, the magic begins.

Overhanging sections, narrow cracks, and concrete stairs allow almost everybody—be they sprinters and climbers, walkers and talkers, or huffers and puffers—to surmount the rock. Two of the many informative placards en route identify the peaks of the Great Western Divide (including Sawtooth Peak; see next hike) and detail the history of Generals Hwy., seen twisting tortuously below, where it climbs 4,000 feet in 19 miles. The pink flowers of mountain pride penstemon can be spotted in season sprouting from cracks in the rock. Climbers might also be seen clambering up the rock's steeper faces. At the summit, a 4-foot-wide level walkway with the trail's only bench distinguishes the edge of this precipitous granite blade.

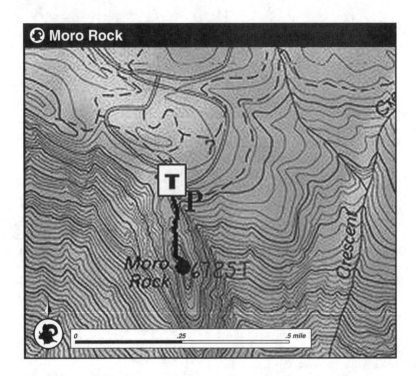

Nearest Visitor Centers The Giant Forest Museum in Giant Forest Village is open year-round, though hours vary by season. It's generally open daily 9 a.m.–5 p.m. May–June, and 9 a.m.–6 p.m. July–Labor Day, with reduced hours the rest of the year.

Other park visitor centers include the following: Kings Canyon Visitor Center at Grant Grove, 559-565-4307, 2 miles past the park entrance station along Hwy. 180, is open 365 days a year. Hours vary depending on the season, but it's generally open 9 a.m.–5 p.m. May–June and 8 a.m.–5 p.m. July–Labor Day, with reduced hours the rest of the year. Lodgepole Visitor Center, 559-565-4436, on the road to Wolverton 1.6 miles east of Generals Hwy., is generally open daily 8 a.m.–6 p.m. mid-June–mid-September, with reduced hours in early June and late September.

Nearest Campgrounds There are more than 2 dozen campgrounds in Kings Canyon and Sequoia National Parks and adjacent Sequoia National Forest. Check at one of the above visitor centers for current information and availability.

Additional Information nps.gov/seki

HIKE 101 Sawtooth Peak ⬈ 🚶

Highlight	A towering summit of the Great Western Divide
Distance	13.0 miles round-trip
Total Elevation Gain/Loss	4,500'/4,500'
Hiking Time	12–16 hours
Recommended Map	USGS 7.5-min. *Mineral King*
Best Times	July–September
Agency	Sequoia National Park
Difficulty	★★★★★

THE GREAT WESTERN DIVIDE towers more than 4,000 feet above the small hamlet of Mineral King in southern Sequoia National Park. The trail climbs up, straight up the divide's flanks, providing sweeping views of the soaring mountains and precipitous valleys. Beautiful Monarch Lake awaits at the base of 12,343-foot Sawtooth Peak, a jagged, trailless summit that offers magnificent and far-reaching views of the Sierra Crest, the Kern River Canyon, and the Great Western Divide.

The Hike ascends Sawtooth Peak from Mineral King. Epic but brutal, it gains 4,500 feet in less than 6 miles. Exceptional fitness and an early start are required for a one-day ascent. Lower Monarch Lake nestles at the mountain's base and provides a rest stop, or overnight campsite, 4.4 miles and 2,500 feet up from the trailhead. Some degree of acclimatization is important for the rarefied air above 10,000 feet; gaiters are useful for keeping grit out of your boots on the mountain's loose slopes. The last 1,500 feet of elevation gain is off-trail and involves considerable boulder-hopping and scrambling—wear the stiffest boots you own. No water is available at the trailhead; there is a faucet in front of the ranger station (see below). The first convenient trailside source is 1.3 miles distant and nearly 1,000 feet up.

To Reach the Trailhead From Hwy. 198 at Hammond, take the road to Mineral King—the turnoff is 4 miles northeast of the town of Three Rivers and 2 miles southwest of the

Ash Mountain Entrance Station to Sequoia National Park. While only 23 miles long, the narrow, winding Mineral King Rd. can take upward of 90 minutes to drive. You reach the park entrance station 12 miles past the turnoff, where a $20-per-vehicle entrance fee is collected. After another 6 miles, the road's surface alternates between dirt and pavement. The road soon passes through the tiny settlement of Silver City; a small general store here provides last-minute supplies. You pass Mineral King Ranger Station, where two large parking lots, an outhouse, and a pay phone are located, a short 0.9 mile before the desired trailhead.

Beware of lactating marmots! Throughout June and most of July, these critters develop a peculiar craving for antifreeze and brake fluid. Marmots will chew through coolant hoses, brake lines, and even spark plug wires seeking salts from this odd cocktail. Some people fence off the underside of their vehicles with chicken wire to avoid disaster. Some park in a less risky lot, while others just risk it. A safe parking alternative is the Tar Gap lot, 0.1 mile east of the ranger station, but it means a 0.7-mile road walk to the trailhead. Most active in June, marmots become more lethargic as July progresses. Ask at the ranger station for the most current marmot report.

Description The trail begins at the end of the north parking lot (0.0/7,820'), where current trail conditions are posted. The East Fork Kaweah River turns sharply west here, and

🌐 Sawtooth Peak

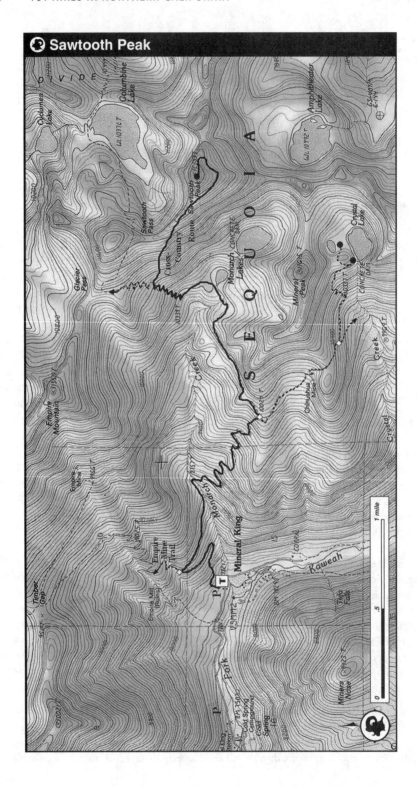

views south toward its headwaters are highlighted by the striking parabola made by Farewell Gap (10,586'), bordered west by the red metamorphic pyramid of Vandever Mountain (11,947').

Immediately climbing, the trail's first mile is the steepest, passing through open sage grassland with a few Sierra juniper. The distant pinnacle of Sawtooth Peak dominates the skyline east above Monarch Creek. Bouldery staircases help you ascend to a waterfall overlook. Now the trail traverses west and then—at the junction for Empire Mine Trail (0.6/8,320')—east back toward the creek. Ponderosa pines appear here and corn lilies, yarrow, Indian paintbrush, and lupine can be spotted underfoot. Climbing along the stream again, you pass a mossy spring gushing from the opposite hillside before the trail reaches creek level (1.3/8,760'). Imposing cliffs north, which tower 1,500 feet, actually represent only the lower southwest face of Empire Mountain, whose hidden slopes rise another 1,300 feet to the summit. Refill your water bottles here as this is your last opportunity before Monarch Lake.

Cross the stream and commence switchbacking up the slopes. At the 4th switchback western white pines appear, and by the 13th you've already ascended 700 feet above the creek. Traversing south, you cross a small ridgetop and then climb east below the ridgeline to reach the posted junction for Crystal Lake (2.6/9,860'). (The idyllic basin offers some exceptionally nice campsites near the south end of Crystal Lake, a 1.8-mile one-way journey from here.)

Continuing toward Sawtooth Peak, proceed straight on the main trail to begin a dramatic traverse beneath the lower flanks of Mineral Peak. Lower Monarch Lake remains hidden until you're almost upon it, when the red, jutting molar of Mineral Peak (11,615') also becomes visible for the first time south of the lake.

Lower Monarch Lake (4.4/10,380') straddles a geologic divide. The distinctive rock interface across the lake marks where overlying volcanic

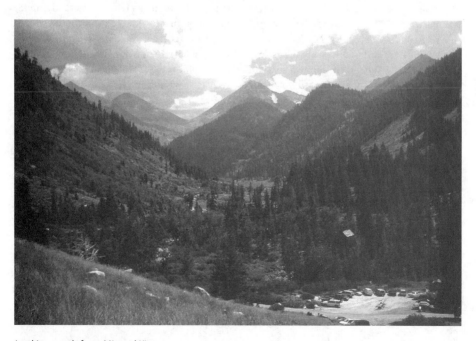

Looking south from Mineral King

rocks have been intruded by Sierra Nevada granite. Rarely is this geologic divide so pronounced. North, the granite mass of Sawtooth Peak rises dramatically above the lake, its summit just visible as the highest point on the ridge more than 2,000 feet above you. Several good campsites are scattered around the western shore, with food-storage lockers for bear and marmot protection. The lake, which can be circumnavigated with some scrambling, boils with small brook trout. Upper Monarch Lake is easily accessed by a use trail at the lake's far shore, north of the small inlet creek.

Briefly winding northwest away from the lake at the base of Sawtooth's slope, the posted trail to Sawtooth Pass begins climbing in an obvious spot. It completes five switchbacks before reaching a long swath of grit and dust extending upslope. The trail ascends this via numerous steep switchbacks, gaining 500 feet above the lake before—near the top of the loose sandy slope—spinning off various paths. While the actual trail over Sawtooth Pass heads upward and to the left from here, you should begin slowly bearing right as you ascend toward the summit. The last stand of foxtail pine, above you to the right, provides a good landmark for climbing and for the return descent.

Continue upward until you are nearly level with these trees, and then climb above and slightly to the right of them until you reach the ridge—a gain of around 1,000 feet from the top of the sandy slope. Incredible views east open up here, but they're better from the top. The peak is now clearly visible southeast, jutting from the ridge. To climb it, traverse below and then approach it from the south; the final scramble to the top is considerably easier from this direction. The last 100 feet require the most scrambling.

The view is epic. East lies the Kern River Canyon and its serrated eastern rampart, the Sierra Divide. Mount Whitney (14,494') can be spotted east-northeast. Looking north, barren and oft-frozen Columbine Lake (10,970') lies below you. The Great Western Divide strikes northeast beyond. On the divide's western slopes, Black Rock Pass Trail zigzags insanely up to its namesake. The large plateau that is home to Sequoia's Giant Forest is visible farther north-northwest, with the seemingly small knob of Moro Rock (see Hike 100) on its western edge. On a good day the Minarets and Ritter Range are visible on the northern horizon, a distance of more than 75 miles.

You should find the summit register in an ammo can among the giant slabs of granite. On your return, don't be tempted by sandy routes that drop directly down Sawtooth toward Upper Monarch Lake, because the unseen slope steepens precipitously below. Look for that foxtail pine stand (pointed out earlier) to guide your descent as you retrace your steps to the trailhead.

Nearest Visitor Center Mineral King Ranger Station, 559-565-3768, is open daily 8 a.m.–3:45 p.m. Memorial Day–late September.

Backpacking Information Wilderness permits are required and may be obtained from the park visitor centers and the Mineral King Ranger Station only during open hours. A quota of 20 people per day is enforced for this trailhead, although capacity is typically only exceeded in late August and on the busiest summer holidays. There is a fee of $15 per permit, regardless of trip length or group size. Three-quarters of permits can be reserved; the remainder are first come, first served. Reservations can be made for the entire season by mail or fax only beginning March 1 and no later than 2 weeks prior to the start of your trip; visit **nps.gov/seki** for more information and to download the application form.

Nearest Campgrounds Cold Springs Campground (40 sites, $12) is 0.1 mile west of the ranger station. If it's full, try Atwell Mills Campground (21 sites, $12), 4.1 miles farther west.

Additional Information **nps.gov/seki**

Appendix 1: Hikes by Theme

BACKPACKABLE

1 Upper Salmon Creek Falls, **Silver Peak Wilderness**
2 Vicente Flat, **Ventana Wilderness**
6 Pine Valley, **Ventana Wilderness**
9 Coit Lake, **Henry W. Coe State Park**
10 Coyote Creek, **Henry W. Coe State Park**
11 Sunol Regional Wilderness
18 Butano State Park
19 Castle Rock State Park
20 Big Basin Redwoods State Park
29 Marin Headlands
33 Alamere Falls, **Point Reyes National Seashore**
34 Sky and Coast Trails, **Point Reyes National Seashore**
37 Austin Creek State Recreation Area
38 Cache Creek Wilderness
42 Van Damme State Park
44 Yolla Bolly Wilderness
45 Lost Coast Trail, **Sinkyone Wilderness State Park**
46 Big Flat, **King Range Wilderness and National Conservation Area**
47 King Peak, **King Range Wilderness and National Conservation Area**
48 Punta Gorda Lighthouse, **King Range Wilderness and National Conservation Area**
53 Hogan Lake, **Russian Wilderness**
54 Canyon Creek Lakes, **Trinity Alps Wilderness**
55 Marble Rim, **Marble Mountain Wilderness**
56 Castle Dome, **Castle Crags State Park**
58 Mount Eddy, **Shasta-Trinity National Forest**
59 Hidden Valley, **Mount Shasta Wilderness**
64 Patterson Lake, **South Warner Wilderness**
66 Thousand Lakes Volcano, **Thousand Lakes Wilderness**
71 Feather Falls, **Plumas National Forest**
72 Sierra Buttes, **Tahoe National Forest**
73 South Yuba River, **South Yuba River Wild and Scenic Recreation Area**
74 Rubicon River, **Eldorado National Forest**
76 Mount Tallac, **Desolation Wilderness**
79 Grouse Lake, **Mokelumne Wilderness**
80 Mokelumne River, **Mokelumne Wilderness**
81 Hiram Peak, **Carson-Iceberg Wilderness**
82 Deadman Lake, **Emigrant Wilderness**
83 Green Creek, **Hoover Wilderness**
86 Half Dome, **Yosemite National Park**
88 Clouds Rest, **Yosemite National Park**
89 Ireland Lake, **Yosemite National Park**
91 Ediza Lake, **Ansel Adams Wilderness**
92 Balloon Dome, **Ansel Adams Wilderness**
93 Kaiser Wilderness
94 Little Lakes Valley, **John Muir Wilderness**
96 Palisade Glacier, **John Muir Wilderness**
98 Redwood Canyon, **Kings Canyon National Park**
99 Pear Lake, **Sequoia National Park**
101 Sawtooth Peak, **Sequoia National Park**

BEACHES

5 Molera Beach, **Andrew Molera State Park**
24 Phillip Burton Memorial Beach, **Golden Gate National Recreation Area**
26 San Francisco's Pacific Shore
33 Wildcat Beach, **Point Reyes National Seashore**
34 Kelham Beach, **Point Reyes National Seashore**
39 Bodega Dunes, **Sonoma Coast State Beach**
40 Sandy Cove, **Fort Ross State Historic Park**
41 Manchester State Park
45 Lost Coast Trail, **Sinkyone Wilderness State Park**
46 Big Flat, **King Range Wilderness and National Conservation Area**
48 Punta Gorda Lighthouse, **King Range Wilderness and National Conservation Area**
50 Klamath River Mouth, **Redwood National Park**

OTHER COASTSIDE HIKES

1 Silver Peak Wilderness
2 Vicente Flat, **Ventana Wilderness**
3 Cone Peak, **Ventana Wilderness**
4 Ewoldsen Trail, **Julia Pfeiffer Burns State Park**
22 Devil's Slide, **San Mateo County Parks**
27 Golden Gate Bridge
28 Point Bonita Lighthouse
29 Marin Headlands
35 Tomales Point, **Point Reyes National Seashore**
45 Lost Coast Trail, **Sinkyone Wilderness State Park**
47 King Peak, **King Range Wilderness and National Conservation Area**
51 Damnation Creek, **Del Norte Coast Redwoods State Park**

EPIC ADVENTURES

40 Sonoma's Lost Coast
44 North Yolla Bolly Mountain, **Yolla Bolly Wilderness**
80 Mokelumne River, **Mokelumne Wilderness**
86 Half Dome, **Yosemite National Park**
96 Palisade Glacier, **John Muir Wilderness**
101 Sawtooth Peak, **Sequoia National Park**

FISHING

9 Coit Lake, **Henry W. Coe State Park**
38 Cache Creek, **Cache Creek Wilderness**
53 Hogan Lake, **Russian Wilderness**

FISHING *(continued)*

54 The Trinity Alps
55 Marble Mountain Wilderness
57 Castle Lake, **Shasta-Trinity National Forest**
58 Mount Eddy, **Shasta-Trinity National Forest**
64 Patterson Lake, **South Warner Wilderness**
65 Burney Creek, **McArthur–Burney Falls Memorial State Park**
66 Thousand Lakes Wilderness
73 South Yuba River, **South Yuba River Wild and Scenic Recreation Area**
74 Rubicon River, **Eldorado National Forest**
77 Lake Tahoe, **D. L. Bliss and Emerald Bay State Parks**
79 Grouse Lake, **Mokelumne Wilderness**
80 Mokelumne River, **Mokelumne Wilderness**
89 Ireland Lake, **Yosemite National Park**
91 Ediza Lake, **Ansel Adams Wilderness**
92 San Joaquin River, **Ansel Adams Wilderness**
96 John Muir Wilderness
97 Kings River, **Sequoia National Forest**
99 Pear Lake, **Sequoia National Park**
101 Sawtooth Peak, **Sequoia National Park**

GEOLOGY

7 The Pinnacles, **Pinnacles National Park**
8 Fremont Peak, **Fremont Peak State Park**
14 Mount Diablo, **Mount Diablo State Park**
24 San Andreas Fault, **Golden Gate National Recreation Area**
33 Alamere Falls, **Point Reyes National Seashore**
35 Tomales Point, **Point Reyes National Seashore**
38 Cache Creek, **Cache Creek Wilderness**
39 Bodega Dunes, **Sonoma Coast State Beach**
54 The Trinity Alps
55 Marble Mountain Wilderness
56 Castle Dome, **Castle Crags State Park**
58 Mount Eddy, **Shasta-Trinity National Forest**
59 Hidden Valley, **Mount Shasta Wilderness**
61 Schonchin Butte, **Lava Beds National Monument**
62 Valentine Cave, **Lava Beds National Monument**
63 Glass Mountain, **Modoc National Forest**
66 Thousand Lakes Volcano, **Thousand Lakes Wilderness**
67 Chaos Crags, **Lassen Volcanic National Park**
68 Brokeoff Mountain, **Lassen Volcanic National Park**
69 Devils Kitchen, **Lassen Volcanic National Park**
70 Bidwell Park
72 Sierra Buttes, **Tahoe National Forest**
80 Mokelumne River, **Mokelumne Wilderness**
81 Carson-Iceberg Wilderness
82 Emigrant Wilderness
84 Mono Lake Tufas, **Mono Lake Tufa State Reserve**
86 Half Dome, **Yosemite National Park**
87 Sentinel Dome and Taft Point, **Yosemite National Park**
91 Ediza Lake, **Ansel Adams Wilderness**
94 Little Lakes Valley, **John Muir Wilderness**
96 Palisade Glacier, **John Muir Wilderness**
101 Sawtooth Peak, **Sequoia National Park**

GOOD FOR DOGS

1 Silver Peak Wilderness
2 Vicente Flat, **Ventana Wilderness**
3 Cone Peak, **Ventana Wilderness**
6 Pine Valley, **Ventana Wilderness**
11 Sunol Regional Wilderness
12 Coyote Hills, **Coyote Hills Regional Park**
13 Morgan Territory Regional Preserve
17 Wildcat Peak, **Tilden Regional Park**
22 Devil's Slide, **San Mateo County Parks**
30 Ring Mountain, **Ring Mountain Open Space Preserve**
38 Cache Creek, **Cache Creek Wilderness**
44 Yolla Bolly Wilderness
46 Big Flat, **King Range Wilderness and National Conservation Area**
47 King Peak, **King Range Wilderness and National Conservation Area**
48 Punta Gorda Lighthouse, **King Range Wilderness and National Conservation Area**
53 Russian Wilderness
54 Trinity Alps Wilderness
55 Marble Mountain Wilderness
57 Heart Lake, **Shasta-Trinity National Forest**
58 Mount Eddy, **Shasta-Trinity National Forest**
64 Patterson Lake, **South Warner Wilderness**
66 Thousand Lakes Wilderness
70 Bidwell Park
71 Feather Falls, **Plumas National Forest**
72 Sierra Buttes, **Tahoe National Forest**
73 South Yuba River, **South Yuba River Wild and Scenic Recreation Area**
74 Rubicon River, **Eldorado National Forest**
76 Mount Tallac, **Desolation Wilderness**
80 Mokelumne Wilderness
81 Carson-Iceberg Wilderness
82 Emigrant Wilderness
92 Balloon Dome, **Ansel Adams Wilderness**
93 Kaiser Wilderness
94 John Muir Wilderness

GOOD FOR KIDS

5 Molera Beach, **Andrew Molera State Park**
12 Coyote Hills, **Coyote Hills Regional Park**
14 Mount Diablo, **Mount Diablo State Park**
16 Cosumnes River Preserve
22 Devil's Slide, **San Mateo County Parks**
27 Golden Gate Bridge
28 Point Bonita Lighthouse
30 Ring Mountain, **Ring Mountain Open Space Preserve**
32 Martin Griffin Preserve, **Audubon Canyon Ranch**
39 Bodega Dunes, **Sonoma Coast State Beach**
40 Fort Ross State Historic Park
60 Tule Lake, **Tule Lake National Wildlife Refuge**
62 Valentine Cave, **Lava Beds National Monument**
65 Burney Falls, **McArthur–Burney Falls Memorial State Park**
84 Mono Lake, **Mono Lake Tufa State Reserve**

SWEEPING 360-DEGREE VISTAS

(continued)

91 Ediza Lake, **Ansel Adams Wilderness**
93 Mount Kaiser, **Kaiser Wilderness**
94 Little Lakes Valley, **John Muir Wilderness**
100 Moro Rock, **Sequoia National Park**
101 Sawtooth Peak, **Sequoia National Park**

TAKE IT EASY (THE 1-STAR HIKES)

8 Fremont Peak, **Fremont Peak State Park**
12 Coyote Hills, **Coyote Hills Regional Park**
14 Mount Diablo Summit, **Mount Diablo State Park**
16 Cosumnes River Preserve
27 Golden Gate Bridge
28 Point Bonita Lighthouse
39 Bodega Dunes
60 Tule Lake, **Tule Lake National Wildlife Refuge**
62 Valentine Cave, **Lava Beds National Monument**
63 Glass Mountain, **Modoc National Forest**
65 Burney Falls, **McArthur–Burney Falls Memorial State Park**
84 Mono Lake, **Mono Lake Tufa State Reserve**

WATERFALLS

1 Salmon Creek Falls, **Silver Peak Wilderness**
6 Pine Falls, **Ventana Wilderness**
20 Berry Creek Falls, **Big Basin Redwoods State Park**
54 Canyon Creek Falls, **Trinity Alps Wilderness**
65 Burney Falls, **McArthur–Burney Falls Memorial State Park**
85 Vernal and Nevada Falls, **Yosemite National Park**
99 Pear Lake, **Sequoia National Park**

WILDFLOWERS

1 Silver Peak Wilderness
2 Vicente Flat, **Ventana Wilderness**
5 Andrew Molera State Park
7 The Pinnacles, **Pinnacles National Park**
9 Coit Lake, **Henry W. Coe State Park**
10 Coyote Creek, **Henry W. Coe State Park**
11 Sunol Regional Wilderness
13 Morgan Territory Regional Preserve
15 Eagle Peak, **Mount Diablo State Park**
23 Montara Mountain, **San Pedro Valley County Park**
29 Marin Headlands
35 Tomales Point, **Point Reyes National Seashore**
37 Austin Creek State Recreation Area

46 Big Flat, **King Range Wilderness and National }Conservation Area**
54 The Trinity Alps
58 Mount Eddy, **Shasta-Trinity National Forest**
69 Devils Kitchen, **Lassen Volcanic National Park**
93 Kaiser Wilderness
96 John Muir Wilderness
97 Yucca Point, **Sequoia National Forest**
99 Pear Lake, **Sequoia National Park**
101 Sawtooth Peak, **Sequoia National Park**

WILDLIFE

16 Cosumnes River Preserve
32 Martin Griffin Preserve, **Audubon Canyon Ranch**
35 Tomales Point, **Point Reyes National Seashore**
38 Cache Creek, **Cache Creek Wilderness**
60 Tule Lake National Wildlife Refuge
84 Mono Lake Tufa State Reserve

AUTHOR'S FAVORITES

2 Vicente Flat, **Ventana Wilderness**
9 Coit Lake, **Henry W. Coe State Park**
11 Sunol Regional Wilderness
14 Mount Diablo, **Mount Diablo State Park**
26 San Francisco's Pacific Shore
28 Point Bonita Lighthouse
36 Table Rock, **Robert Louis Stevenson State Park**
37 Austin Creek State Recreation Area
44 Yolla Bolly Wilderness
54 The Trinity Alps
55 Marble Mountain Wilderness
56 Castle Crags, **Castle Crags State Park**
64 South Warner Wilderness
72 Sierra Buttes, **Tahoe National Forest**
80 Mokelumne River, **Mokelumne Wilderness**
85 Vernal and Nevada Falls, **Yosemite National Park**
86 Half Dome, **Yosemite National Park**
92 Balloon Dome, **Ansel Adams Wilderness**
93 Kaiser Wilderness
94 Little Lakes Valley, **John Muir Wilderness**
95 Ancient Bristlecone Pine Forest
96 Palisade Glacier, **John Muir Wilderness**
98 Redwood Canyon, **Kings Canyon National Park**
100 Moro Rock, **Sequoia National Park**
101 Sawtooth Peak, **Sequoia National Park**

Appendix 2: Selected Sources and Recommended Reading

Atlases

Benchmark California Road & Recreation Atlas. 8th ed. Benchmark Maps, 2013.

California Atlas & Gazetteer. 3rd ed., Yarmouth, ME: DeLorme, 2011.

Plant and Animal Identification

Johnson, Sharon G., Pamela C. Muick, Bruce M. Pavlik, and Marjorie Popper. *Oaks of California.* Los Olivos, CA: Cachuma Press, 1991.

Johnston, Verna R. *California Forests and Woodlands.* Berkeley, CA: University of California Press, 1994.

Keator, Glenn, Ruth M. Heady, and Valerie R. Winemiller. *Pacific Coast Fern Finder.* Rochester, NY: Nature Study Guild, 1981.

Lanner, Ronald M. *Conifers of California.* Los Olivos, CA: Cachuma Press, 1999.

Little, Elbert L. *National Audubon Society Field Guide to North American Trees, Western Region.* New York, NY: Alfred A. Knopf, 1998.

Lyons, Kathleen, and Mary Beth Cooney-Lazaneo. *Plants of the Coast Redwood Region.* Boulder Creek, CA: Looking Press, 1988.

Peterson, Roger Tory. *Field Guide to Birds of Western North America.* 4th ed. New York, NY: Houghton Mifflin, 2010.

Spellenberg, Richard. *National Audubon Society Field Guide to North American Wildflowers, Western Region.* New York, NY: Alfred A. Knopf, 2001.

Watts, Tom. *Pacific Coast Tree Finder.* 2nd ed. Rochester, NY: Nature Study Guild, 2004.

Geology

General California Geology

Alt, David D., and Donald W. Hyndman. *Roadside Geology of Northern and Central California.* 2nd ed. Missoula, MT: Mountain Press Publishing Company, 2000.

Harden, Deborah R. *California Geology.* 2nd ed. Upper Saddle River, NJ: Prentice-Hall, 2003.

McPhee, John. *Assembling California.* New York, NY: Farrar, Straus, and Giroux, 1993.

USGS. *Geologic Map of California.* 1:750,000. 1977.

Regional Geology

Durrell, Cordell. *Geologic History of the Feather River Country, California.* Berkeley, CA: University of California Press, 1987.

Galloway, Alan J. *Geology of the Point Reyes Peninsula.* Bulletin 202. California Division of Mines and Geology, 1977.

Konigsmark, Ted. *Geologic Trips: San Francisco and the Bay Area.* GeoPress, 1998.

Moore, James G., Warren J. Nokleburg, and Thomas W. Sisson. *Geologic Road Guide to Kings Canyon and Sequoia National Parks,* 1994.

Wahrhaftig, Clyde. *A Streetcar to Subduction and Other Plate Tectonic Trips by Public Transport in San Francisco.* Rev. ed. Washington, D.C.: American Geophysical Union, 1984.

Regional Information

The Central Coast, Bay Area, and Coast Ranges

California Coastal Commission. *California Coastal Resource Guide.* Berkeley, CA: University of California Press, 1987.

Cassady, Stephen. *Spanning the Gate.* Santa Rosa, CA: Squarebooks, 1993.

Elliot, Analise. *Hiking and Backpacking Big Sur: A Complete Guide to the Trails of Big Sur, Ventana Wilderness, and Silver Peak Wilderness.* 2nd ed. Birmingham, AL: Wilderness Press, 2013.

Golden Gate National Recreation Area Guide to the Parks. San Francisco, CA: Golden Gate Conservancy, 2000.

Lage, Jessica. *Point Reyes: The Complete Guide to the National Seashore and Surrounding Area.* Birmingham, AL: Wilderness Press, 2004.

Manning, Kathleen. *San Francisco's Ocean Beach.* Mount Pleasant, SC: Arcadia Publishing, 2003.

Paddison, Joshua. *A World Transformed: Firsthand Accounts of California Before the Gold Rush.* Berkeley, CA: Heyday Books, 1999.

Vanderwerf, Barbara. *The Coastside Trail Guidebook.* El Granada, CA: Gum Tree Lane Books, 1995.

Weintraub, David. *East Bay Trails: Hiking Trails in Alameda and Contra Costa Counties.* Birmingham, AL: Wilderness Press, 2005.

White, Peter. *The Farallon Islands: Sentinels of the Golden Gate.* San Francisco, CA: Scottwall Associates, 1995.

The North Coast and Klamath Mountains

National Park Service. *Official Redwood National and State Park Handbook.* 1996.

White, Mike. *Trinity Alps & Vicinity: A Hiking and Backpacking Guide.* 5th ed. Birmingham, AL: Wilderness Press, 2010.

Shasta and the Modoc Plateau

Boze, M. Jeanne. *The Nature of Bidwell Park.* 2nd ed. B. C. Publications, 1998.

Selters, Andy, and Michael Zanger. *The Mount Shasta Book: A Guide to Hiking, Climbing, Skiing, and Exploring the Mountain and Surrounding Area.* 3rd ed. Birmingham, AL: Wilderness Press, 2006.

White, Mike. *Lassen Volcanic National Park and Vicinity: A Complete Hiker's Guide.* 4th ed. Birmingham, AL: Wilderness Press, 2008.

The Sierra Nevada

Dinkey Creek: A Bridge from Past to Present. Kings River Ranger District, 1997.

Browning, Peter. *Sierra Nevada Place Names*. 3rd ed. Lafayette, CA: Great West Books, 2011.

Jenkins, J. C., and Ruby Johnson Jenkins. *Exploring the Southern Sierra: West Side*. Birmingham, AL: Wilderness Press, 1995.

Lamela, Susan, and Hank Meals. *Yuba Trails*. 1993.

Lekisch, Barbara. *Tahoe Place Names*. 2nd ed. Lafayette, CA: Great West Books, 1996.

Moore, James G., Warren J. Nokleburg, and Thomas W. Sisson. *Geologic Road Guide to Kings Canyon and Sequoia National Parks,* 1994.

Morey, Kathy. *Hot Showers, Soft Beds, and Dayhikes in the Sierra*. 3rd ed. Birmingham, AL: Wilderness Press, 2008.

———, Mike White, et al. *Sierra North: Backcountry Trips in California's Sierra Nevada*. 9th ed. Birmingham, AL: Wilderness Press, 2005.

———, Mike White, et al. *Sierra South: Backcountry Trips in California's Sierra Nevada*. 8th ed. Birmingham, AL: Wilderness Press, 2006.

Schaffer, Jeffrey P. *Desolation Wilderness and the South Lake Tahoe Basin: A Guide to Lake Tahoe's Finest Hiking Area*. 3rd ed. Birmingham, AL: Wilderness Press, 2003.

———. *The Tahoe Sierra: A Natural History Guide to 112 Hikes in the Northern Sierra*. 4th ed. Birmingham, AL: Wilderness Press, 1998.

———. *Yosemite National Park: A Complete Hiker's Guide*. 5th ed. Birmingham, AL: Wilderness Press, 2006.

Schifrin, Ben. *Emigrant Wilderness and Northwestern Yosemite*. Birmingham, AL: Wilderness Press, 1990.

Secor, R. J. *The High Sierra, Peaks, Passes, and Trails*. 3rd ed. Seattle, WA: The Mountaineers, 2009. Whitney, Stephen. *The Sierra Nevada*. San Francisco, CA: Sierra Club Books, 1979.

Index

About the Author

MATT HEID is the author of *One Night Wilderness: San Francisco Bay Area* and *AMC's Best Backpacking Trips in New England,* and is a contributor to *Backpacking California.* He holds a degree in earth and planetary science from Harvard University and stays busy pursuing a passion for outdoor writing and wilderness adventure in Northern California and New England. He currently lives in Bedford, Massachusetts.

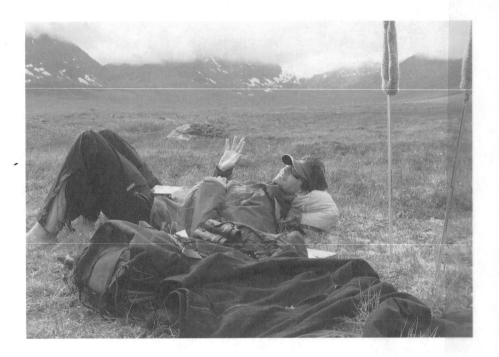